Conceptual Bases of
Professional Nursing

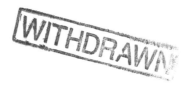

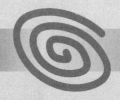

Conceptual Bases of
Professional Nursing

FOURTH EDITION

Susan Kun Leddy, R.N., Ph.D.

Professor
School of Nursing
Widener University
Chester, Pennsylvania

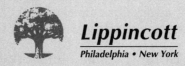

Lippincott
Philadelphia • New York

Acquisitions Editor: Lisa Marshall
Sponsoring Editor: Sandra Kasko
Project Editor: Jahmae Harris
Production Manager: Helen Ewan
Production Coordinator: Patricia McCloskey
Assistant Art Director: Kathy Kelley-Luedtke
Indexer: Lynne Mahan

Fourth Edition

Library of Congress Cataloging-in-Publications Data

Leddy, Susan.
    Conceptual bases of professional nursing / Susan Leddy. — 4th ed.
        p.   cm.
    Includes bibliographical references and index.
    ISBN 0-397-55277-7
    1. Nursing.   I. Title.
    [DNLM: 1. Nursing.   2. Nursing Theory.   WY   16   L472c   1998]
    RT41.L53   1998
    610.73—dc21
    DNLM/DLC
    for Library of Congress   97-42746
                                                                          CIP

Care has been taken to confirm the accuracy of the information presented and to describe generally accepted practices. However, the authors, editors, and publisher are not responsible for errors or omissions or for any consequences from application of the information in this book and make no warranty, express or implied, with respect to the contents of the publication.

The authors, editors and publisher have exerted every effort to ensure that drug selection and dosage set forth in this text are in accordance with current recommendations and practice at the time of publication. However, in view of ongoing research, changes in government regulations, and the constant flow of information relating to drug therapy and drug reactions, the reader is urged to check the package insert for each drug for any change in indications and dosage and for added warnings and precautions. This is particularly important when the recommended agent is a new or infrequently employed drug.

Some drugs and medical devices presented in this publication have Food and Drug Administration (FDA) clearance for limited use in restricted research settings. It is the responsibility of the health care provider to ascertain the FDA status of each drug or device planned for use in their clinical practice.

9   8   7   6   5   4   3   2   1

To the memories of three people whose beliefs and values helped to shape my professional identity: my father, Dr. Bert B. Kun; my baccalaureate program chairperson at Skidmore College, Miss Agnes Gelinas; and Mae Pepper, my colleague, coauthor, mentor, and friend.

To the late Janis H. David, a mentor who taught Mae the essence of professional nursing, helped her develop as a nurse educator, demonstrated what it means to be an advocate for patients, and served as a guide throughout Mae's professional growth.

In Memory
J. Mae Pepper
January 18, 1936–March 19, 1997

For twenty years, Mae was my colleague, co-author, mentor, and friend. We met in 1977, when Mae joined the faculty at Mercy College in Dobbs Perry, New York. Mae's previous teaching experience at the University of North Carolina-Chapel Hill, New York University, and Bronx Community College, as well as her vision, wisdom, and dedication were crucial to the development and accreditation of our new baccalaureate program for registered nurses, and to the subsequent development of the first master's program at the College.

Mae held the position of Chairperson of the Nursing Program from 1981 until her sudden death in March 1997 from a ruptured aortic aneurysm. Although she talked for years about leaving administration in order to do more scholarly work, she continued to serve as Chair out of a sense of duty and responsibility. She was devoted to the students and faculty, and very conscientious in her service to the College and many civic and professional organizations.

Mae also found time to read voraciously, listen to music, care for animals, and to enjoy outdoor white-water rafting, camping, and bird-watching. She loved her garden, was a careful craftsperson in furniture refinishing, and liked to go to garage sales and flea markets looking for collectibles. Mae had a good sense of humor and loved a good time. I remember a trip we took to a convention in Las Vegas. Mae "knew" which slot machines were ready to pay off, and she won over $900. Devoted to her friends and family, she willingly gave time and attention to anyone who asked.

Mae was an irreplaceable intellectual mentor as well as a friend. She was a great listener, and her counsel was always wise and kind. Mae lived her belief in mutuality, genuineness, and respect for others. She is missed greatly.

Contributors

Susan E. Gordon, R.N., Ed.D.
Professor
Lienhard School of Nursing
Pace University
Pleasantville, New York

Lucy J. Hood, R.N., D.NSc
Assistant Professor
St. Luke's College
Kansas City, Missouri

Carol R. Sando, R.N., D.NSc
Coordinator, Learning Resource Center
School of Nursing
Widener University
Chester, Pennsylvania

Preface

Mae Pepper died suddenly on March 19, 1997, before she was able to write her contributions to this fourth edition. I have tried to keep as much of her voice as possible, while updating all chapters, making major revisions of four chapters, and adding two new chapters. In addition, efforts have been made to make this edition more "user friendly" by way of brief clinical vignettes to introduce many chapters, a second type color, and extensive use of concise bulleted or numbered lists.

Section 1, *The Dynamics of Professional Development,* focuses on the professional nurse; contextual and philosophical influences on professional nursing practice; historical perspectives on the profession; the nurse's socialization for practice; and the nurse's professional self-development. Section 2, *The Knowledge Bases of Professional Practice,* presents theoretical bases such as patterns of knowing and nursing science; the research process in nursing (revised to emphasize research utilization); nursing models and theories; processes of professional nursing (revised to include cognitive, interpersonal, and patterning processes); and the health process (revised to include worldviews of health, and health promotion, protection, and patterning). Section 3, *The Changing Healthcare Context,* includes the health care delivery system (thoroughly updated and revised, with contributions from Carol Sando), and a new chapter on health care policy, contributed by Lucy Hood. Section 4, *Professional Practice Strategies,* addresses the professional nursing role with family and community clients; accountability (contributed by Susan Gordon); communication in helping relationships; processes of teaching–learning and leadership; a new chapter on management of client care, emphasizing intrapersonal and interpersonal processes; and visions for the 21st century.

As Mae and I noted in the preface to the third edition, "During these changing times, we have been pleased with the utilization of our book in many educational settings, particularly in baccalaureate and graduate programs. Although the first edition of the book was targeted for upper division RN baccalaureate programs, we have become aware of its utilization in generic baccalaureate programs, masters programs, and practice settings . . . . It is our hope that this [fourth] edition of *Conceptual Bases of Professional Nursing* will continue to make a contribution to the profession."

S.K.L.

Preface to the First Edition

In the last quarter century, nursing has moved decisively toward becoming a scientific discipline. It has begun to develop and test its own theoretical bases, to promote scholarly development of its professional practitioners, and to apply its own theory to its practice. Although progress in attaining control of its own practice has been slow and is still not completely accomplished, a clearer picture of the special service offered to society by the profession is emerging. As the autonomous body of knowledge that is called nursing is developed and disseminated, and as the profession assumes accountability to the public it services by requiring excellence in the education of its practitioners and the delivery of its services, control of its practice is more likely to be completely accomplished. Acknowledging the absolute necessity for the profession to practice from its own body of knowledge, we have recognized the need to emphasize the conceptual bases from which professional nursing is practiced.

Conceptual Bases of Professional Nursing represents our efforts to present an overview and synthesis of professional concepts that we believe to be basic to the development of professional practitioners. This book was originally conceived to assist the registered nurse engaged in baccalaureate nursing education to become resocialized into the full professional role. In the process of writing, however, it seemed to us that the contents of this book could serve as a useful resource to all professional nursing education programs; to facilitate resocialization in "second step" programs, to serve as a resource at multiple points in the educational development of students in first professional degree programs, and to provide a professional review with a consistent framework in the early part of the education of graduate students from diverse baccalaureate nursing programs.

The book is organized into four sections. Section 1 addresses the nature of the profession through exploration of historical influences, philosophical perspectives, factors that influence socialization into the profession, and the development of a professional self concept by the practitioner. Section 2 focuses on theoretical bases of professional nursing, with separate chapters related to scientific thought and theory development, the research process, theories applicable to nursing, and models of nursing. Section 3 addresses concepts relevant to the delivery of professional nursing, the health process, the health care delivery system, and accountability. Finally, in Section 4 the components and roles of professional nursing are considered. These include nursing process; communication and helping relationships; leadership; and the roles of change agent, client advocate, and contributor to the profession. Future perspectives are then projected briefly.

The book has been written as an integrated text with a common framework and liberal use of cross references; however, each chapter can "stand alone," and thus the content can be read in any order. If the contents are assigned in a different sequence from that presented, however, we would encourage an early review of our conceptual framework for nursing, which is found at the end of Chapter 2.

We have been fortunate to have received feedback from a number of our professional colleagues. Special appreciation is expressed to Sharron Humenick, Donea Shane, Roanne Dahlen, Carolyn Lansberry, Hanna Jacobson, and Carol Lofstedt, who all critiqued parts of the manuscript; however, we take full responsibility for the philosophical and conceptual views expressed.

We could not have completed this book without the support and tangible assistance provided by Ed and Carol, to whom we express our heartfelt appreciation and love.

The contents of this book reflect the current synthesis of ideas, knowledge, and values that we began to articulate seven years ago, as we struggled with the development of a new curriculum. Our conceptions are continuing to evolve. We eagerly anticipate the debate and dialogue we hope this book will engender, in order to further the development and refinement of nursing science.

Susan Leddy, R.N., Ph.D.
J. Mae Pepper, R.N., Ph.D.

Contents

The Dynamics of Professional Development

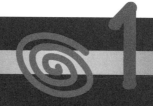

The Professional Nurse

LEARNING OUTCOMES

By the end of this chapter, the student will be able to:

1 Identify the characteristics of professional practice.

2 Appreciate how the Code for Nurses affects a nurse's practice.

3 Know what ethical principles form the basis for the moral dimension of professional nursing practice.

4 Know what determines the legal parameters of professional nursing practice.

VIGNETTE

Sue graduated from an associate degree program 3 years ago and has been working on a medical–surgical unit at the community hospital. She is concerned about losing her job and thinks that a baccalaureate degree might be a good "insurance policy." However, Sue says, "I am a good nurse, even if I don't have a BSN. I don't see how more school will make me more professional!"'

Nurse, nourish, and nurture—all are derived from the same Latin source. These words have been so closely associated through the years that some people label any caregiver a "nurse." Thus, some historians have identified the roots of modern nursing in the care given to the sick by military camp followers or religious sisters, or even in the nurturance of children by their mothers. The assumption that nursing is an art possessed inherently by any female has hindered development of a concept of nursing as a profession with an organized body of knowledge and specialized skills.

In contrast, the Social Policy Statement (American Nurses Association [ANA], 1995) stresses that nurses provide care that promotes well-being in both healthy and ill people, individually or in groups and communities. Four "essential features of contemporary nursing practice" are cited (ANA, 1995, p. 6):

> Attention to the full range of human experiences and responses to health and illness without restriction to a problem-focused orientation
>
> Integration of objective data with knowledge gained from an understanding of the patient's or group's subjective experience
>
> Application of scientific knowledge to the processes of diagnosis and treatment
>
> Provision of a caring relationship that facilitates health and healing

◎ Characteristics of a Profession

Although nursing has been called a profession for many years, an assessment of the characteristics of a profession indicates that it should more accurately be considered an "emerging profession." Characteristics of a profession have been described (Freidson, 1994; Miller, Adams, & Beck, 1993) as:

- Authority to control its own work
- Exclusive body of specialized knowledge
- Extensive period of formal training
- Specialized competence
- Control over work performance
- Service to society
- Self-regulation
- Credentialing system to certify competence
- Legal reinforcement of professional standards
- Ethical practice
- Creation of a collegial subculture
- Intrinsic rewards
- Public acceptance

These characteristics of a profession can be categorized as intellectual; personal and interpersonal; characteristics reflecting commitment to serve society; characteristics emphasizing autonomy; and characteristics that reflect shared personal values. Personal values that characterize professional practice will be discussed later in this chapter.

INTELLECTUAL CHARACTERISTICS

This category really has three components: (1) a body of knowledge on which professional practice is based; (2) specialized education to transmit the body of knowledge; and (3) use of knowledge in critical and creative thinking.

Body of Knowledge

Professional practice is based on a body of knowledge derived from experience (leading to expertise) and research (leading to theoretical foundations for knowledge). This knowledge base contributes to judgment and a rationale for modifying actions according to a specific situation. However, nursing education has often emphasized proven methods for responding to particular kinds of situations. This approach to education may explain why many nurses seem unwilling or unable to apply knowledge to clinical problem-solving, contributing to dependence in practice. They seek the "right" answer and do things the way they always have been done. Thus, for example, clients may be discharged without self-care teaching because "the doctor didn't write an order," and pain medication is withheld because "it isn't 4 hours yet."

An important component of professional education is liberal studies in the arts, sciences, and humanities. Liberal education "leads to a greater personal and professional contribution to nursing and society" (Bottoms, 1988, p. 124) and to the continued development of personal values and coherence of knowledge. Desired outcomes of baccalaureate education in any major toward which liberal components contribute include the development of thinking and communication skills, historical consciousness, understanding of what science is, exploration of personal values, appreciation of fine art, and appreciation of ethnic diversity (Association of American Colleges, 1985, pp. 18–26).

In the past, it has been debated whether nursing's body of knowledge was unique to nursing or was an application of knowledge borrowed from behavioral and physical sciences and medicine. Previously, nursing derived its knowledge base through intuition and experience and by borrowing from other disciplines. In recent years, however, nursing theorists have developed frameworks, or models, that are uniquely relevant for nursing (see Chap. 8). Because nursing now has theory-building research that provides a basis for practice and knowledge, this debate is no longer relevant.

Specialized Education

Nursing transmits knowledge through specialized education. However, there are five levels of basic education for registered nursing, all of which prepare for one licensing examination—the National Council Licensure Examination for Registered Nursing (NCLEX). Three of the five levels (diploma, associate degree, and baccalaureate degree) accept high school graduates, whereas the other two (master's degree and doctoral degree) accept college graduates with liberal arts majors.

In the mid-1980s, a project to differentiate practice for the associate degree–prepared nurse (ADN) and the bachelor's of science degree–prepared nurse (BSN) agreed on the role competencies described on page 7. (Primm, 1987, p. 222).

Recently, the PEW Health Professions Commission (1995) recommended focusing "associate preparation on the entry-level hospital setting and nursing home practice, baccalaureate on the hospital-based care management and community-based practice, and master's degree for specialty practice in the hospital and independent practice as a primary care provider" (p. 34).

Power, authority, and professional status usually are associated with a postgraduate educational base, yet in 1992* only 38% of actively licensed nurses had baccalaureate or higher education in nursing (Division of Nursing, 1994). How can nursing be considered a true profession when (1) a high school diploma gains entry into three different kinds of educational programs, all of which permit the candidates to take the licensing examination for registered nursing, and (2) the majority of graduates possess an associate degree or less? Much controversy has focused on presumed quality of the various education patterns rather than on their differences of purpose.

According to Newman (1990, p. 167), "the time is long overdue for the profession to move from having nurses with various levels of preparation doing the same thing, or nurses with one level of preparation doing everything, to practitioners with different levels of preparation doing different, interrelated things."

Newman proposes a trilevel model with three different practice roles, each with different educational preparation:

1. Professional nursing clinician, who has "direct responsibility to clients over time for the determination of both short- and long-term nursing care across multiple practice settings . . . . Educational preparation needed for this role is a postbaccalaureate professional degree based on a curriculum that is person-centered and focused on health" (Newman, 1990, p. 170).
2. Team leader, who "provides clinical leadership within institutional settings . . . and is responsible around the clock for the quality of

(text continues on page 8)

In 1992, of practicing nurses, 34% had a diploma, 28% had an associate degree, and 38% a baccalaureate or higher degree in nursing.

ADN

The ADN will become a licensed registered nurse (RN) who provides direct care based on the nursing process and focused on individual clients who have common, well-defined nursing diagnoses. Consideration is given to the client's relationship within the family.

The ADN functions in a structured health care setting that is a geographic or a situational environment where the policies, procedures, and protocols for provision of health care are established. In the structured setting there is recourse to assistance and support from the full scope of nursing expertise.

The ADN uses basic communication skills with focal clients and coordinates with other health team members to meet focal clients' needs.

The ADN recognizes the focal client's need for information and modifies a standard teaching plan.

The ADN recognizes that nursing research influences nursing practice and assists in standardized data collection.

The ADN organizes for focal clients those aspects of care for which the nurse is responsible.

The ADN maintains accountability for her own practice and for aspects of nursing care delegated to peers, licensed practical nurses, and ancillary nursing personnel.

Within a specified work period, the ADN plans and implements nursing care that is consistent with the overall admission to postdischarge plan.

The ADN practices within accepted ethical and legal parameters of nursing.

BSN

The BSN will become a licensed RN who provides direct care based on the nursing process and focused on clients with complex interactions of nursing diagnoses.

Clients include individuals, families, groups, aggregates, and communities in structured and unstructured health settings. The unstructured setting is a geographic or a situational environment that may not have established policies, procedures, and protocols and has the potential for variations requiring independent nursing decisions.

The BSN uses complex communication skills with focal clients, collaborates with other health team members, and assumes an accountable role in change.

The BSN assesses the need for information and designs comprehensive teaching plans individualized for the focal client.

The BSN collaborates with nurse researchers and incorporates research findings into nursing practice.

The BSN manages comprehensive nursing care for focal clients.

The BSN maintains accountability for her own practice and for aspects of nursing care delegated to other nursing personnel consistent with their levels of education and expertise.

The BSN plans for nursing care based on identified needs of the focal client from admission to postdischarge.

The BSN practices within accepted ethical and legal parameters of nursing.

nursing care administered by a team of staff nurses and auxiliary personnel . . . . Preparation needed for this role is a baccalaureate in nursing" (Newman, 1990, pp. 170–171).

3. Staff nurse, who is "responsible for the implementation of delegated medical and nursing care for designated clients within a specified setting and who function as members of a nursing team . . . . Preparation needed for this role is the associate degree in nursing" (Newman, 1990, p. 171).

In this model there is no competition between the practice roles because all three roles are essential. Because the practice roles are different, the educational preparation for each role must be different, as must the credentialing and titling process.

Newman's model is one way that nurses can refute the persistent assumption that "a nurse is a nurse" and move toward unambiguous acceptance of the differentiation between professional practice and supporting practice in nursing roles.

Critical and Creative Thinking

A logical and critical thinking process is one essential component of professional practice. The nursing process is a problem-solving approach, a system to:

1. Collect and organize information derived from multiple sources
2. Decide what is needed, based on that information
3. Select and implement one approach from among many possible approaches
4. Evaluate the results of the process

Most nurses solve problems every working day. However, there may be a tendency to act hastily on the basis of both inadequate information and insufficient brainstorming for alternative approaches. For example, given the following problem, the nurse could take either of two actions:

Problem: What would you (the nurse) do with a hospital patient who keeps his television on after "lights out"?

■ Possible action 1: Tell him that he must adhere to hospital policy and turn off the television.

■ Possible action 2: Allow him to watch as long as no one else is inconvenienced.

Discussion: Both actions would have been taken before enough information has been collected to know why the client keeps the television on. If it turns out that he is anxious, nursing intervention should be directed toward relieving his anxiety, or at least helping him relax and sleep despite it, instead of toward the symptom (the television). If he is not tired because his sleep–wake pattern is different than hospital policy, the television might be allowed, along with an effort to let him sleep later in the morning. The point is that the appropriate action depends on the reason for the problem and the generation of reasonable alternatives derived by logical thinking. (See Chap. 9 for a more detailed discussion.)

PRACTICE COMPONENTS

Health care delivery systems are being "redesigned" and "reenginee~ increase cost effectiveness, productivity, and efficiency. Greenberg (1994, p 28A) identified several rules for reengineering including organizing around outcomes and not tasks and cross-training staff, shifting from specialized care providers to generalist providers. Expecting to reduce operational cost, many acute care institutions have hired large numbers of unlicensed assistive personnel (UAP) who are used not only for nonnursing tasks such as transportation and answering phones, but also for skilled interventions such as inserting a urinary catheter or administering oxygen. Ironically, UAP substitution for RNs is not cost effective when training, supervision, and unoccupied time are considered. In addition, "patient morbidity and mortality is significantly adversely affected by lowering the registered nurse staffing level or skill mix ratio" (Zimmermann, 1995, p. 210). However, the trend toward use of UAPs in hospitals seems to be accelerating.

Nurses who continue to practice in hospital settings must be aware of the delegation issues of potential for harm, complexity, and required problem-solving in working with UAPs. It must be remembered that "final accountability for the appropriateness of the delegation decision, adequacy of nursing care, and UAP actions and outcomes cannot be delegated" (Zimmermann, 1995, p. 209). (Delegation to UAPs is discussed further in Chap. 18.)

As a result of reengineering and managed care changes, in 1996, only 60% of American nurses were employed in hospitals. According to the Division of Nursing, almost 45,000 jobs were eliminated in U.S. hospitals between 1993 and 1995. It has been suggested that "the hospital of the future will concentrate on four areas—trauma, sophisticated diagnostics, critical care, and operative procedures that are unsuitable for ambulatory care" (*Nursing Spectrum*, 1996, p. 9). In 1996, 16% of nurses were working in community settings, 8.5% were employed in ambulatory care, and 8% were working in long-term care facilities (Division of Nursing, 1997). The new jobs will be in outpatient centers, home health care, hospice, occupational settings, long-term care facilities, and ambulatory clinics, with new opportunities for nurse entrepreneurs.

The downsizing of acute care positions makes it essential that RNs develop new skills for ambulatory care settings. Core dimensions of the current clinical practice role in ambulatory care have been identified (Haas & Hackbarth, 1995, p. 232):

1. Enabling operations (eg, maintain safe work environment)
2. Technical procedures (eg, assist with procedures)
3. Nursing process (eg, develop nursing care plan)
4. Telephone communications (eg, telephone triage)
5. Advocacy (eg, act as client advocate)
6. Teaching (eg, instruct client on self-care)
7. Expert practice (eg, serve as preceptor for students)

ـnical role dimensions were identified, they were similar ـ ـion of the client teaching dimension with greater empha- ـ learning needs and following through with teaching, and the expert practice dimension into outreach to the commu- ـ ـ as skill in primary care and advanced nursing practice. High- ـedures are emerging as an entirely new dimension of future practice in ambulatory care.

ـ SOCIETY

Since the days of Florence Nightingale, nursing has been associated with service to others. Many students still enter nursing "to help people," an image of the nurse shared by the public.

But the intrinsic motivation "to care" is only one conceptualization of caring currently receiving much attention in the nursing literature. Morse and colleagues (1991, p. 122) have identified five conceptualizations of caring: (1) caring as a human trait, (2) caring as a moral imperative, (3) caring as an affect, (4) caring as an interpersonal interaction, and (5) caring as a therapeutic intervention. Obviously, caring is much more complex than just intuitive concern for others. Several nurse theorists have even developed conceptual models for nursing that include caring as a major concept. (See Chap. 8 for a more detailed discussion.)

Professional service to society requires integrity and responsibility for ethical practice and a lifelong commitment. Nursing has been viewed by many of its practitioners as a job rather than a career. In 1992, 83% of licensed RNs were actively employed in nursing, 69% of them full-time (Division of Nursing, 1994). Many nurses either leave the profession (at least temporarily) to raise a family or work primarily to supplement family income. Because professional commitments may be secondary to other concerns, these nurses may tend to seek job security and avoid "rocking the boat." This attitude is easily exploited by the employing agency. Regardless of such difficulties as high client–nurse ratio, rotating shifts, reassignment to provide adequate coverage of other units (floating), and constant change in client assignments, some nurses will make do and maintain the status quo. For those nurses, the service orientation has shifted from the responsibility to an individual client and the welfare of all clients to the welfare of the employing institution.

Service to people involves ethical responsibility. The nurse must have the integrity to do what is right, often in situations that cause real moral dilemmas. Codes for nurses have been developed by the International Council of Nurses and the ANA. Intrinsic to these codes is the belief that the recipient of nursing care has basic rights and that a nurse's primary responsibility is to the client. (The ANA code is discussed later in this chapter.)

Service to society also requires legal assurances that practitioners are competent. A credentialing system, such as licensure, provides a system for certifying minimal safe practice by a person legally permitted to be

called a "registered nurse." Nurse
forcement against incompetence by
ical or negligent practice.

AUTONOMY

Autonomy means that practitioners hav
in the work setting. Autonomy involves iı
risks, and responsibility and accountabil.
as self-determination and self-regulation.
also obligated to collaborate with others fo.

For the past 50 years, most nurses have ı
where authority is vested in administrative
ganization. This is in contrast to medicine, w   ̨olitical
power and professional credibility through te̩   ̩petence and specialized knowledge. Nurses have sought statu̩ ̩.ɾough increased rank in
the hierarchy rather than through expert practice. Now, the changes in
health care delivery toward managed care in community health settings
provide new threats to autonomous practice for nurses. As Aroskar (1995,
p. 67) states, "Nurses' autonomy is at stake in managed care arrangements
in which nurses may be used merely as means to the ends of cost control—
a negation of nurses as moral agents who are responsible and accountable
for nursing care delivered." Nurses need to advocate for clients to ensure
that health care access, equity, and quality are not co-opted by the system
emphasis on controlling costs.

However, nursing lacks a collective professional identity. Although
united action by over two million potential practitioners represents enormous potential power, nursing has been fragmented by internal dissension
and rivalry. Instead of presenting a united front, each subgroup maintains
its own turf. The result is political impotence and professional powerlessness. A major goal for nursing must be the development of strength that
can be translated into legislative power to increase legal autonomy and
provide for third-party reimbursement for nursing services.

This section has focused on the composite character of the nursing
profession. The following section examines characteristics of the nurse as
a member of the profession, what Styles (1982, p. 8) terms "profession-
hood."

The Professional Nurse

CHARACTERISTICS OF PROFESSIONAL NURSING PRACTICE

For some nurses, work is a job that provides financial return and some degree of satisfaction. Professional practice, on the other hand, requires a
"deep and abiding awareness of purpose and direction in place of a spe-

objectives or standards" (Styles, 1982, p. 57). For a profes-
work is a component of a career plan and an integral part of the
on's being.

Styles has explored the idea that involvement, motivation, and commitment are separate components of a person's sense of vocation. Involvement is viewed as a quantitative measure; for example, how much time or
energy does the person devote to nursing? Motivation is the driving force
suggested by the question "what's in it for me?" Motives might include
prestige, financial gain, or even just keeping busy, or they might include
the opportunity for self-expression and achievement of excellence. Commitment is defined as the "intimacy of the perceptions about nursing to
the very core of the self" (Styles, 1982, p. 107). It is unlikely that a person
could achieve a professional self-identity without great involvement and a
sense that nursing is a major component of her or his life.

Styles suggests that it is time to "reinstate the service ideal in its proper
primary relationship to our science and practice on the one hand, and to
our legitimate claims to self-determination and reward on the other"
(Styles, 1982, p. 60). Components of this service ideal include a sense of
purpose, a sense of capability, and a concern for others demonstrated as
caring. According to Koldjeski (1990, p. 49), caring includes interpersonal
valuing and involvement; experiencing with the other; instillment of faith,
concern, and love for another; and actualization. This concern for others,
although by itself not sufficient to form a professional purpose, is basic to
a service ideal. Whether a person could be a professional nurse without
possessing genuine warmth and caring for others is questionable.

The concept of a professional includes accountability and autonomy
for personal actions. Accountability means that the nurse is answerable
for her own behavior.

Autonomy means the freedom and the authority to act independently
and to control one's own life and not the lives of others. For example, an
autonomous nurse might make a judgment about a client's possible health
"problem(s)" but would work with the client to identify the client's perceptions and priorities.

Unfortunately, nurses collectively have been characterized by feelings
of inadequacy, powerlessness, and frustration and avoidance of accountability for autonomous practice. Competition for status has interfered
with a spirit of collegiality and shared respect. As a result, nursing has
been largely a labor force rather than a significant influence on the health
care delivery system.

Collaboration with members of the health professions, especially
physicians, has been promoted as an appropriate approach to teamwork.
True collaboration involves the potential for equally valued contributions
by the parties. Yet the typical medical curriculum provides physicians
with little experience with or knowledge of the potential contributions of
colleagues in other disciplines. Most nurses have much less education
than do physicians and thus usually are not viewed as physicians' equal

colleagues. By emphasizing cooperation and collaboration, nurses have used their potential power to "maintain the very system which has oppressed . . . rather than change the system" (Ashley, 1973, p. 638).

The health care delivery system has embraced the concept of managed care, in an effort to constrain the escalation of health care delivery costs. In principle, managed care provides for planned organization and coordination of client care across delivery settings. Unfortunately, in practice, managed care largely has been directed to management of medical care to provide "a controlled balance between quality and cost" (Giuliano & Poirier 1991, p. 52). The managed care role is the role envisioned by Newman for the professional nursing clinician. If implemented widely, this role could increase autonomous nursing practice, enhance professional collaboration among nurses in various settings, and facilitate achievement of desired health outcomes and client satisfaction.

Large numbers of nurses have not been ready risk takers. Seeking to cooperate with other health professionals may represent less risk than autonomous practice, but professionals need the ability to manage ambiguity and diversity to make sound judgments and decisions in practice. They also need knowledge and skills to use the political process for power. The unwillingness to take risks (based on sound knowledge) and use political power are the greatest barriers to autonomous and assertive nursing practice.

Professional nursing practice is subject to legal prescriptions and moral dilemmas. These areas will be discussed in the following section.

MORAL DIMENSIONS OF PROFESSIONAL PRACTICE

Ethical Systems

Ethics is the philosophical study of morality. *Morals* are the "standards of right and wrong that one learns through socialization" (Catalano, 1995, p. 2). Ethics is a system of valued behaviors and beliefs for determining right or wrong and for making judgments about what should be done to or for other human beings. Because there is no arbitrary standard of right and wrong, the study of ethics helps nurses identify their own moral positions and biases and assists decision-making in ethical dilemmas.

There are often ambiguities in the setting and conflicts of values and between rights and obligations. As a result, there usually is no clear-cut single answer for a given moral dilemma. Because people may disagree as to the best decision, many moral decisions require an agonizing personal choice among imperfect and conflicting alternatives.

Dominant definitions of managed care stress the administrative and financial aspects of health care delivery, with emphases on efficiency and effectiveness. They do not include the humane caring values of respect for persons, protection of healing relationships, providing benefits for the sick and vulnerable, and general concerns of justice and fairness that have traditionally been assumed in nursing and medical care. Within the managed care context there is a critical need for nurses to advocate for the needs of individuals and to participate in professional efforts to establish work environments that support high-quality nursing care (Aroskar, 1995).

"Effective nurses function as moral agents . . . concerned with doing good and avoiding harm" (Bandman & Bandman, 1995, p. 46). To protect the rights of clients and provide ethical guidelines for the nursing profession, the Ethical Code for Nurses was first developed by the ANA in 1950 and periodically revised since then. Catalano (1995, p. 18) lists the key ideas of this code as:

- Respect for human dignity
- Patient's right to privacy and confidentiality
- Patient and public safety
- Responsibility and accountability of nurses
- Nursing competency
- Participation in research
- Quality of patient care
- Nursing's integrity
- Collaboration with members of the health care team

ETHICAL CODE FOR NURSES
The ANA Code for Nurses (ANA, 1985, pp. 1–16) is as follows:

1. The nurse provides services with respect for human dignity and the uniqueness of the client unrestricted by considerations of social or economic status, personal attributes, or the nature of the health problems
2. The nurse safeguards the client's right to privacy by judiciously protecting information of a confidential nature
3. The nurse acts to safeguard the client and the public when health care and safety are affected by the incompetent, unethical, or illegal practice of any person
4. The nurse assumes responsibility and accountability for individual nursing judgments and actions
5. The nurse maintains competence in nursing
6. The nurse exercises informed judgment and uses individual competence and qualifications as criteria in seeking consultation, accepting responsibilities, and delegating nursing activities to others
7. The nurse participates in activities that contribute to the ongoing development of the profession's body of knowledge
8. The nurse participates in the profession's efforts to implement and improve standards of nursing
9. The nurse participates in the profession's efforts to establish and maintain conditions of employment conducive to high-quality nursing care
10. The nurse participates in the profession's effort to protect the public from misinformation and misrepresentation and to maintain the integrity of nursing

11. The nurse collaborates with members of the health professions and other citizens in promoting community and national efforts to meet the health needs of the public

The "Interpretive Statements" distributed with the code emphasize clients' rights and nurses' responsibilities. Clients' rights include:

1. Respect for human dignity, and adequately informed consent
2. Full involvement in the planning and implementation of health care
3. Nursing care based on need, irrespective of social and economic status, personal attributes, or the nature of the health problem
4. Privacy and confidentiality of information
5. Protection from unsafe or unethical health care practices

Nurses' responsibilities include:

1. Assuming accountability and responsibility for giving safe and competent care, delegating activities to others, and maintaining the integrity of nursing
2. Participating in research while protecting the rights of human subjects
3. Establishing and maintaining employment conditions conducive to high-quality nursing care
4. Promoting collaborative planning for availability and accessibility to quality health services for all citizens

REEXAMINATION OF ETHICAL STANDARDS

Together, the ANA Code and the Interpretive Statements "provide a framework within which nurses can make ethical decisions and discharge their responsibilities to the public, to other members of the health team, and to the profession" (ANA, 1985, p. iii). An ethical code defines a professional standard, but it does not provide specific guidelines for how the nurse should act in a given situation, nor is it legally binding. Individual decisions, if moral, are based on ethical principles and can be enforced only by the nurse's conscience.

Ethical Principles
AUTONOMY

Autonomy is a basic ethical principle. An autonomous person is capable of making rational and unconstrained decisions and acting on those decisions. Belief in autonomy means that the nurse respects the client and the choices that the client may make. However, as with most rights, autonomy is not an absolute right. "Under certain conditions, limitations can be imposed upon it, such as when one individual's autonomy interferes with another's rights, health, or well-being" (Aiken & Catalano, 1994, p. 23). Interference with a person's autonomy, whatever the reason, is *paternalism.*

A person can be constrained from acting autonomously through lack of knowledge just as well as by coercive force. Thus, the nurse is obligated to share all relevant information and alternatives for action with the client so that informed choices can be made. The nurse also is obligated to respect the client's decisions, even when disagreeing with them. This may mean that nurses are forced to choose between doing something they believe to be in the client's best interests and respecting the client's decision to do otherwise.

BENEFICENCE AND JUSTICE

Another ethical principle, *beneficence*, relates to the nurse's duty to do good and not harm. However, it is difficult sometimes to determine what exactly is good for another person and who can best make the decision about this good (Aiken & Catalano, 1994). This principle is closely related to the principle of *justice*, which is the obligation to be fair to all people. The concept of distributive justice states that "individuals have the right to be treated equally regardless of race, sex, marital status, medical diagnosis, social standing, economic level, or religious belief" (Aiken & Catalano, 1994, p. 23).

The preceding principles are based on the assumption that all persons have certain ethical "rights," which are really privileges, concessions, or freedoms. There are three types of rights (Aiken & Catalano, 1994, p. 26):

1. *Welfare rights* (also called legal rights) are rights based on a legal entitlement to some good or benefit. These rights are guaranteed by law. For example, U.S. citizens have a right to equal access to housing regardless of race, sex, or religion.
2. *Ethical rights* (also called moral rights) are rights that are based on a moral or ethical principle. Ethical rights usually do not have the power of law to enforce the claim, although, over time, popular acceptance of an ethical right can give it the force of a legal right. For example, health care is really a long-standing privilege for Americans that is sometimes viewed as a right.
3. *Option rights* are based on a belief in the dignity and freedom of human beings. Option rights give individuals in free and democratic societies the freedom of choice and the right to live their lives as they choose, as long as they stay within a set of prescribed boundaries. For example, people may wear whatever clothes they choose, as long as they wear some type of clothing.

Individual rights are associated with a number of concerns. For example, what kinds of entities have rights and what kinds do not? Does a fetus have rights? When a conflict of rights arises, how should the conflict be resolved? Obligations to clients may seem to conflict with obligations to the physician or to the institution. This is not really a moral dilemma although the decision may be an agonizing one. An important distinction is made between doing what is morally right and what is least difficult practically. As a professional, the nurse's primary ethical obligation is to the client. However, the nurse may have legal obligations to both the client and the institution. These legal obligations are discussed in the next section.

LEGAL DIMENSIONS OF PROFESSIONAL PRACTICE

Licensure

Licensure refers to "a legal process by which a designated authority grants permission to a qualified individual to perform designated skills and services in a given jurisdiction" (Catalano, 1995, p. 82). Thus, a license is a legal document that certifies that minimal standards for qualified practitioners have been met. Licensure is a function of the state, based on the state's obligation to protect its citizens from incompetent or unsafe health care practitioners.

Requirements for licensure as an RN are included in each state's nurse practice act. Most nursing practice acts have basically the same major components: "legislative mandate (why have this law?), definition of nursing, requirements for licensure, exemption from licensure, grounds for revocation, suspension or conditioning of the license, provision for endorsement for persons licensed in other states, creation of a board of examiners, responsibilities of the board, and penalties for practicing in violation of the act or without a license" (Kelly & Joel, 1995, pp. 468–469).

All states use the National Council Licensure Examination for Registered Nurses (NCLEX-RN) for licensure purposes. The test includes two components: nursing process and client needs. To be eligible, a student must be a graduate of a state-approved school of nursing and be approved by the State Board of Nursing. Since 1993, a computerized examination has been administered to permit individuals to take the examination at any time at an approved testing site. Thus, passing the examination not only permits licensure and registration in the state in which the examination is written, but also permits later registration (listing on the official roster) in other states if desired. Although licensure is permanent (unless the license is revoked for illegal or immoral behavior), registration must be renewed periodically (usually every 1–2 years) by payment of a fee to each state in which current registration is desired. All that is needed is to fill out forms and pay the required fee to become licensed "by endorsement."

All 50 states have mandatory licensure. This means that anyone who practices nursing according to the legal definition of practice must be licensed, except for students in their course of study, employees of the federal government, and persons performing in an emergency situation. Only in North Dakota is a baccalaureate degree in nursing a requirement for licensure as an RN. All other states license and register graduates of all educational programs.

In the 1980s, momentum appeared to be developing toward mandatory continuing education in every state. However, according to a 1995 survey, only 25 state boards of nursing had continuing education requirements for renewal of license registration, and 33 state boards of nursing had continuing education requirements for reentry into active practice (Annual CE Survey, 1996). In addition, concern has been expressed with the lack of data linking continuing education to patient care outcomes (Hewlett & Eichelberger, 1996). At least one state (Colorado) has repealed mandatory continuing education for licensure, and only one state has instituted mandatory continuing education for licensure since 1991 (Hewlett & Eichelberger, 1996).

Most states have revised their nurse practice act several times since the first acts were written in the early 20th century. In 1990, the ANA published a revised model nursing practice act, which defined the practice of nursing as "the performance of services for compensation in the provision of diagnosis and treatment of human responses to health or illness. This practice includes, but is not limited to:

1. Assessment, diagnosis, planning, intervention, and evaluation of human responses to health or illness
2. The provision of direct nursing care to individuals to restore optimum function or achieve a dignified death
3. The procurement, coordination, and management of essential client resources
4. The provision of health counseling and education
5. The establishment of standards of practice for nursing care in all settings, including the development of nursing policies, procedures, and protocols for a specific setting
6. The direction of nursing practice, including delegation to those practicing technical nursing
7. The supervision of those who assist in the practice of nursing
8. Collaboration with those who assist in the practice of nursing
9. The administration of medication and treatments as prescribed by those professionals qualified to prescribe under the provision of (cite state statute[s]; American Nurses Association, 1990)."

Legal Responsibility

Licensure as an RN carries with it the responsibility for safe and competent practice. If injury, unnecessary suffering, or death should occur as a result of care given by a nurse, the nurse legally may be held responsible for malpractice or negligence. Negligence is "the omission of an act that a reasonable and prudent person would perform in a similar situation" (Catalano, 1995, p. 73). Malpractice, a form of negligence, is "the failure of a professional to act as a reasonable and prudent professional with the same education and experience would have acted in a similar situation" (Catalano, 1995, p. 75). Some of the most common acts of negligence by nurses involve burns; falls; wrong dosage, concentration, or kind of medication; mistaken identity; blood administration; failure to communicate effectively with the client, the client's family, or health team members; failure to observe and take appropriate action; failure to observe defects in equipment; and failure in reasonable judgment.

Nurses are legally responsible for their own actions. But because in most cases nurses also are employees of an institution, the question may arise as to whether the institution and the client's physician also are legally responsible. This is due to the legal *respondeat superior* (master–servant) rule, which states that the master is responsible for the acts of the servants. Based on this rule, the nurse's employer also is held responsible for the nurse's acts.

Negligence is based on four doctrines of liability, master–servant, borrowed servant and captain of the ship, ostensible agency, and *res ipsa loquitur* ("let the thing speak for itself") (Catalano, 1995). According to the master–servant doctrine (*respondeat superior* or "let the master answer"), an employer is also liable, along with an employee, for the employee's negligence on the job. RNs who also are students are considered employees if they usually work for pay in that institution. On the other hand, the contract between the nursing school and the clinical agency usually specifies that basic students are not employees of the agency and must carry their own liability insurance. (Often, a blanket school policy covers all students and faculty.) However, precedent cases have held institutions (as well as the students and possibly the faculty) responsible for the actions of nursing students acting as agents of the institution in the provision of care.

Nursing students are accountable and personally liable for their actions. In cases involving alleged negligence, the court will try to establish the standard of care against which the student's actions will be evaluated. The actions of nursing students will be judged by their experience and the amount of their education. This is based on the standard of reasonable care, which is concerned with the degree of skill and knowledge customarily used by a competent practitioner of similar education and experience in the community. However, "the student is held to the standards of care (standards of reasonableness) of an RN if performing RN functions" (Kelly & Joel, 1995, p. 499). Thus, individual limits of experience and education must be known by the student, who must be adequately prepared for clinical assignments. If questions arise about how to proceed with an activity, the faculty must be contacted.

Ethical and legal considerations may at times overlap. The Tuma case, widely reported in the literature in the early 1980s, is an example. Tuma was a registered nurse employed as an instructor in an associate degree nursing program. A student was assigned to care for a woman who had been told the day before by her physician that she was dying of leukemia and that the only hope for prolonging life was chemotherapy. The client had consented, and Tuma and the student were to begin the treatment.

The client was very upset about receiving chemotherapy, as she had lived with her disease for 12 years with the help of prayer and natural foods. While the treatment was being started, Tuma discussed alternative treatments with the client, who asked her to return that evening to continue the discussion with her children. Tuma did return, but she did not discuss her intervention with the physician and asked the student to "forget" that she had heard the discussion. The client's children told the physician, who complained that the nurse had interfered with the client–physician relationship. As a result of the complaint, Tuma was suspended from her job and her license to practice was suspended for 6 months. Tuma appealed her case to the state supreme court, which upheld her appeal on the grounds that the state's practice act did not define unprofessional conduct.

This case raised concerns because it seemed to indicate that the nurse does not have a legal right to give information about medical treatment to a client even though the client had requested that information; but that was not the issue in this case. Tuma not only gave the requested information but also deliberately withheld information from the physician. She was aware that the consent the physician had received was not informed consent, but she did not alert the physician to the client's concerns, nor did she refuse to start the treatment.

Nurses must know and function within the legal parameters of practice in their state. If nurses have moral or legal concerns about medical treatment, they must share those concerns and the reasons for them with the physician and, if necessary, with nursing, medical, or hospital authorities. Nurses may refuse to carry out a treatment, but must not attempt to circumvent the physician by interfering with treatment without the physician's knowledge. The goal should be collaboration, not competition.

◎ Conclusion

The process of becoming a professional nurse involves change and growth at various stages throughout a career. Through educational and occupational experiences, the nurse gains attitudes, beliefs, knowledge, and skills that, when integrated with moral and legal standards, characterize competent and committed professional service.

THOUGHT QUESTIONS

1 Should nursing be considered a profession? Why?

2 Is differentiated practice a good idea? Can it work given today's managed care environment?

3 Do you have what Styles calls a "professional self-identity?" How can this be cultivated?

4 Nursing practice is heavily regulated legally. What are the strengths and weaknesses of this system?

5 How would you respond to Sue's comments in the vignette that opens this chapter?

REFERENCES

Aiken, T. D., & Catalano, J. T. (1994). *Legal, ethical, and political issues in nursing.* Philadelphia: Davis.

American Nurses Association. (1985). *Code for nurses with interpretive statements.* Kansas City, MO: Author.

American Nurses Association. (1990). *Suggested state legislation: Nursing practice act, nursing disciplinary diversion act, prescriptive authority act.* Washington, DC: Author.

American Nurses Association. (1995). *Social policy statement.* Washington, DC: Author.

Annual CE Survey. (1996). *The Journal of Continuing Education in Nursing, 27,* 4–7.

Aroskar, M. A. (1995). Managed care and nursing values: A reflection. *Journal of Nursing Law, 2,* 63–70.

Ashley, J. (1973, October). This I believe about power in nursing. *Nursing Outlook, 21,* 637–637.

Association of American Colleges. (1985, February 13,). Integrity in the curriculum. *Chronicles of Higher Education,* pp. 12–30.

Bandman, E. L., & Bandman, B. (1995). *Nursing ethics through the life span* (3rd ed). Norwalk, CT: Appleton & Lange.

Bottoms, M. S. (1988). Competencies of a liberal education and registered nurses' behavior. *Journal of Nursing Education, 27,* 124–129.

Catalano, J. T. (1995). *Ethical and legal aspects of nursing* (2nd ed.) Springhouse, PA: Springhouse.

Freidson, E. (1994). *Professionalism reborn: Theory, prophecy, and policy.* Chicago: University of Chicago.

Division of Nursing. (1992, 1994). *National sample survey of registered nurses.* Washington, DC: Department of Health and Human Services.

Division of Nursing. (1996, 1997). *Advance notes from the national sample survey of registered nurses.* Washington, DC: Department of Health and Human Services

Giuliano, K. K., & Poirier, C. E. (1991). Nursing case management: Critical pathways to desirable outcomes. *Nursing Management, 22,* 52–55.

Greenberg, L. (1994). Work redesign: An overview. *Journal of Emergency Nursing, 20,* 28A–32A.

Haas, S. A., & Hackbarth, D. P. (1995). Dimensions of the staff nurse role in ambulatory care: Part III—Using research data to design new models of nursing care delivery. *Nursing Economics, 13,* 231–241.

Hewlett, P. O., & Eichelberger, L. W. (1996). The case against mandatory continuing education. *Journal of Continuing Education in Nursing, 27,* 176–181.

Kelly, L. Y., & Joel, L. A. (1995). *Dimensions of professional nursing* (7th ed.). New York: McGraw-Hill.

Koldjeski, D. (1990). Toward a theory of professional nursing caring: A unifying perspective. In M. Leininger & J. Watson (Eds.). *The caring imperative in education* (pp. 45–57). New York: National League for Nursing.

Miller, B. K., Adams, D., & Beck, L. (1993). A behavioral inventory for professionalism in nursing. *Journal of Professional Nursing, 9,* 290–295.

Morse, J. M., Bottorff, J., Neander, W., & Solberg, S. (1991, Summer). Comparative analysis of conceptualizations and theories of caring. *Image, 23,* 119–126.

Newman, M. A. (1990). Toward an integrative model of professional practice. *Journal of Professional Nursing, 6,* 167–173.

Nursing Spectrum. (1996). Career/fitness guide, pp. 8–10.

PEW Health Professions Commission. (1995). *Critical challenges: Revitalizing the health professions for the twenty-first century.* San Francisco CA: UCSF Center for the Health Professions.

Primm, P. L. (1987). Differentiated practice for ADN- and BSN-prepared nurses. *Journal of Professional Nursing, 3,* 218–224.

Styles, M. M. (1982). *On nursing: Toward a new endowment.* St. Louis: Mosby.

Zimmermann, P. G. (1995). Replacement of nurses with unlicensed assistive personnel: The erosion of professional nursing and what we can do. *Journal of Emergency Nursing, 21,* 208–212.

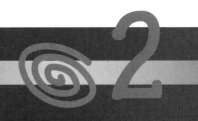

Contextual and Philosophic Elements of Nursing

LEARNING OUTCOMES

By the end of this chapter, the student will be able to:

1 Identify factors in the environment that constitute the context within which nursing is practiced.

2 Appreciate why a personal philosophy of nursing is significant to the individual nurse.

3 Know the essential elements of a philosophy of nursing.

4 Know the essential steps in analyzing ethical dilemmas.

5 Understand how demographic, cultural, and economic factors in the environment create ethical dilemmas for nurses.

6 List some of the fallacies that occur in the ethical decision-making process.

7 Appreciate how knowledge, freedom, and choice operate in the nursing process.

Nursing is a science focused directly on humanity in a highly complex and technologic world. This focus means that values and beliefs are important. Professional nurses are feeling and thinking providers of health care, and clients are feeling and thinking participants in nursing care. Each has values and beliefs that strongly influence their lives.

A person's values and beliefs interact directly with conditions in the environment. These environmental conditions are called the *context* of nursing. One definition of context is the circumstances or setting in which an event occurs (Soukhanov, 1992)—in other words, the environment. Each nurse brings to the professional practice arena a set of beliefs about people, the world, health, and nursing. This set of beliefs is called the philosophy of nursing. While giving nursing care, nurses continuously interact with the environment, which is characterized by contextual conditions or factors. The pragmatist or operationalist part of the professional self pays serious attention to the context of practice. The idealist part of the professional self pays serious attention to the ideal conceptions of practice. Some degree of congruence between the pragmatist and visionary selves is desirable for genuine and humane practice.

This chapter includes a discussion of both the context and philosophy of nursing; a description of selected contextual elements of practice; indications of the ethical nature of nursing and the dilemmas confronting the nurse in practice in a contextual world; elaboration of a process for ethical decision-making in nursing; and finally, a set of guidelines for developing a personal philosophy of nursing.

◎ The Contextual Basis of Nursing Practice

What is the world of nursing like today? That question can only be answered if we first look at what the world in general is like, because this world is the environment or the larger context for nursing.

Naisbitt and Aburdene (1990) believe that several dramatic changes have occurred in the past 20 years. Society moved from being industrial to becoming an information society. As high technology developed, the need for maintaining personal contact with people was intensified. The United States moved from a national to a world economy, characterized by more focus on long-term than short-term concerns. Organizational structures became more decentralized. People began to accept responsibility for self-help rather than depending on institutions to provide help. They began to value participatory democracy more than representative democracy. Networking became more valued than climbing hierarchical ladders. The mentality of decision-making changed from seeing only "either–or" options to envisioning multiple options in efforts to solve problems.

These trends indicate that changes have been many, that they have occurred rapidly, and that changes can be predicted to be even more intense and occur even more rapidly in the future.

WORLD TRENDS IN THE LATE 1990S

According to Naisbitt and Aburdene (1990, p. 13), "events do not happen in a vacuum, but in a social, political, cultural and economic context." Having been mostly on target in predicting the trends of the 1980s, Naisbitt and Aburdene projected what they believe will be the next changes in social, political, cultural and economic contexts. Some of the trends they predicted have been selected because of their special potential significance for nursing.

Communications

Noting, for example, that one fiberoptic cable across the Pacific Ocean could carry some 8,000 conversations (in 1989) simultaneously, while the old copper wire could carry only 48 conversations, Naisbitt and Aburdene (1990, p. 23) state that "telecommunications—and computers—will continue to drive change, just as manufacturing did during the industrial period." This development makes it possible for people to "communicate anything to anyone, anywhere, by any form—voice, data, text, or image— at the speed of light" (Naisbitt & Aburdene 1990, p. 23). Because of these communication developments, people have the ability to readily participate in the global economy.

It is predicted that the ability to communicate easily and to travel rapidly will lead to more similar, global, lifestyles. However, a strong countertrend has been recognized, in the form of cultural nationalism, marked by "a desire to assert the uniqueness of one's culture and language" (Naisbitt & Aburdene, 1990, p. 119).

In the delivery of health care, nurses will need to respect the cultural nationalism of clients.

Women as Leaders

Another trend predicted by Naisbitt and Aburdene was that the 1990s would be a decade of women in leadership. Women would no longer be a minority in the work force. Perhaps more importantly, women have a slight advantage over men because they do not have to unlearn authoritarian behaviors: "To be a leader . . . it is no longer an advantage to have been socialized as a male" (Naisbitt & Aburdene, 1990, p. 217).

Leadership today does not involve using authority to tell people what to do. Rather, leaders must coach, inspire, and gain people's commitment. "The dominant principle of organization has shifted, from mangement in order to control an enterprise to leadership in order to bring out the best in people and to respond quickly to change" (Naisbitt & Aburdene, 1990, p. 218). This suggests that the moral development of women as caring, responsible persons may prove to be an asset.

Caring in the nursing environment should be supported by the changing view of leadership in the world. (This changing view is discussed in Chap. 17.)

The Biology Metaphor

Naisbitt and Aburdene believe that the entire world, not only nursing, is shifting from the models and metaphors of physics to those of biology to help understand the dilemmas and opportunities inherent in living. The metaphor of physics suggests "energy-intensive, linear, macro, mechanistic, deterministic, outer-directed"; in contrast, the metaphor of biology suggests "information-intensive, micro, inner-directed, adaptive, holistic" (Naisbitt & Aburdene, 1990, p. 241).

This biology metaphor is congruent with nursing's move from the military model to an advocacy model.

The Ethical Individual

The final trend Naisbitt and Aburdene cite is the triumph of the ethical individual. Living in a global world, individuals will be responsible for "preserving the environment, preventing nuclear warfare, and eliminating poverty" (Naisbitt & Aburdene, 1990, p. 299). In this kind of world, people not only are responsible but also are empowered to accomplish their goals.

Nurses' movement from oppressed persons to caring, empowered persons is supported by this trend.

DEFINITIONS OF CONTEXTUAL ELEMENTS OF NURSING

Five factors that shape the context within which nursing occurs have been chosen for discussion in this chapter. These elements are identified as demographic, economic, cultural, environmental, and ethical factors in health and the health care environment.

Demographics is defined as "the characteristics of human populations and population segments, especially when used to identify consumer markets" (Soukhanov, 1992, p. 497). These characteristics reflect social and economic conditions. The demographics of a population influence the opportunities an individual has to form or maintain cooperative and interdependent relationships with fellow human beings. In this chapter, the human groups considered to be at high risk will be identified, and the demographic factors associated with increasing risks to health will be discussed.

Economic contexts are the social processes involved in the production, distribution, and consumption of goods and services (Soukhanov, 1992, p. 583). In nursing's case, the service is health care. Economics is primarily focused on the considerations of costs and return for the services provided. Health services are viewed as commodities; therefore, providers must be reimbursed for their services. This chapter will include a brief overview of costs, distribution, and quality of health care.

Cultural contexts are defined as "the totality of socially transmitted behavior patterns, arts, beliefs, institutions, and all other products of human work and thought" (Soukhanov, 1992, p. 454). Sometimes these traditions are described as standardized social characteristics of a specific group of people. Cultural aspects of nursing will be discussed in this chapter. The nurse needs to be able to control the conflicts of behavioral patterns and values that result when cultural beliefs clash.

Environmental contexts are the global influences on health when the focus is on the health of the human species, rather than on an individual, small group, or single community. Given that information has become global, threats to health cannot be confined or dealt with solely behind local or national boundaries. In an ecocentric view, "the environment is considered to be whole, living, and interconnected" (Kleffel, 1996, p. 1). This chapter will consider selected threats to health from the perspective of the global environment.

Ethical contexts are the moral duties and obligations emerging from a person's dealing with good and bad, and right and wrong. To be ethical, the nurse must act in accord with approved standards of behavior or a professionally accepted code of behavior. Morality in nursing practice will be discussed in this chapter. An ethical decision-making process will be reviewed, and ethical dilemmas that nurses confront every day will be discussed. A dilemma is said to exist if the nurse is confronted with a situation involving choosing between equally unsatisfactory alternatives.

Nurses' abilities to reason logically, and their morality and sense of ethics, shape their values. These values are constantly either reinforced or challenged in nursing practice. One primary source of reinforcement or challenge is the environmental context within which nurses practice. The contextual factors identified above, and the nurse's values and belief system, are continuously interacting forces in the nursing process.

Below is an introductory discussion of the philosophical basis of nursing practice, followed by further description of contextual variables affecting nursing practice.

◎ The Philosophic Basis of Nursing Practice

The nurse's philosophy of nursing is critical to the practice of professional nursing. Philosophy encompasses the belief system of the professional nurse as well as a quest for knowledge. A person's belief system and understanding are strong determinants of the way he or she thinks about a phenomenon or a situation. The way someone thinks is a strong determinant of his or her actions.

Because professional nursing can be defined as a process of purposeful actions between the nurse and the client, the nurse needs to understand the definition, purposes, significance, and elements of philosophy in order to thoughtfully develop a personal philosophy of nursing. Thus, this section will present a definition of philosophy and discuss the significance of philosophy to human systems and nursing.

It is generally accepted that philosophy encompasses three areas: concern with knowledge, values, and being, or one's beliefs about existence. In all three areas, intellectual processes underlie the methods of philosophy. Concern with knowledge is important to nursing because nursing is a science, and the nursing process is based on logic and the scientific method. Emphasis on values is important to nursing because nurses continuously make attitudinal, preferential, or value choices as they commit themselves to nurse–client relationships. Focus on being or existence is significant to nurses, clients, and the profession because being is the manifestation of life.

PHILOSOPHY DEFINED

The meaning of philosophy, derived from the Greek, is "lover of wisdom" (Soukhanov, 1992, p. 1360). *Philosophy* is defined as "love and pursuit of wisdom by intellectual means and moral self-discipline" (Soukhanov, 1992, p. 1360). Philosophy is a science that comprises logic, ethics, aesthetics, metaphysics, and the theory of knowledge (epistemology).

For clarity, *philosophy of nursing* is defined as the intellectual and affective outcomes of the professional nurse's efforts to:

1. Understand the ultimate relationships between humans, their environment, and health
2. Approach nursing as a scientific discipline
3. Integrate a sense of values; and
4. Articulate a personal belief system about human beings, environment, health, and nursing as a process

THE SIGNIFICANCE OF PHILOSOPHY FOR NURSING

To achieve intellectual enlightenment is considered better protection against calamitous mistakes than ignorance. Thus, over time, the study of philosophy has accrued great benefits for individuals, societies, and, particularly, the specific sciences. Pursuing the objectives of philosophy, the individual is afforded an opportunity to exercise both understanding and value judgments. Understanding is developed by the quest for reasons. Value judgments are developed by the quest for ethical and aesthetic decisions. Society is improved when members grow in knowledge. Sciences benefit from philosophy essentially because philosophy governs their methods through logic and ethics.

The nursing profession needs leaders who are philosophers of nursing. Nursing must prepare nurse practitioners who have:

Visions for nursing as a scientific discipline
Concern for the ultimate good of humankind
Belief systems reflecting sound ethics
Developed and reflect on their own philosophies of nursing

These practitioners need personal philosophies of nursing that reflect a belief in leaders who are more concerned about recasting health care institutions for the benefit of humankind than about ruling the institutions. These practitioners are more concerned with creating new systems of thought than with developing dogmas to direct nursing practice, research, and education. They also are concerned with the morality of nursing and health care, and promote practice based on a professional code of ethics.

Rafael (1996) has coined the term "empowered caring" for leadership as a unity of power and caring that values the characteristics and experiences of women, and, as a system of ethics, "stems from a heightened awareness of interrelatedness and emerges as a sense of responsibility toward others" (p. 15). These ideas are discussed further in Chap. 17.

Nursing leaders have defined values as "beliefs or ideals to which an individual is committed and which guide behavior" and state that they are "reflected in attitudes, personal qualities, and consistent patterns of behavior" (American Association of Colleges of Nursing, 1986, p. 5). A national panel for determining the essentials of college and university education for professional nursing recommended that seven values are essential (American Association of Colleges of Nursing, 1986, pp. 5–7):

Altruism
Equality
Aesthetics
Freedom
Human dignity
Justice
Truth

◎ Major Contextual Elements Affecting Nursing Practice

To understand the moral or ethical dimensions of nursing more fully, the nurse needs to understand the contextual elements of nursing that either reinforce or challenge belief and value systems. This section discusses selected demographic, economic, cultural, environmental, and ethical factors that characterize the context of nursing practice. Public policy, another significant contextual element, is discussed in Chapter 12.

Although the following discussion is not comprehensive and is presented only as an overview, the factors chosen are those believed to be the most influential in the achievement of professional practice goals.

DEMOGRAPHIC ELEMENTS

The demographic profile of the U.S. population is changing significantly. In a major document for nursing, *Healthy People 2000* (U.S. Department of Health and Human Services, 1990a, pp. 2–3), the Bureau of the Census projected several demographic changes by the year 2000:

1. A 7% growth in the total population, to nearly 270 million people
2. A median age of 36, as compared to 29 in 1975
3. Declining household size to 2.48, with husband–wife households continuing to decrease to 53% of all households
4. A 30% increase in persons over age 85, to a total of 4.6 million
5. An increase in those over age 65 to 13% of the population—35 million people
6. Declining number of children under age 5, from 18 million in 1990 to fewer than 17 million
7. Racial and ethnic changes:
   a. Declining proportion of whites, from 76% to 72%
   b. Increasing proportion of Hispanics, from 8% to 11.3%
   c. Increasing proportion of African Americans, from 12.4% to 13.1%
   d. Increasing proportion of Native Americans, Alaska Natives, Asians, and Pacific Islanders, from 3.5% to 4.3%
8. Women as the major source of new entrants into the work force
9. A 6 million-person increase in new immigrants, with the east and west coasts of the United States expected to receive most of them

These demographic changes essentially change the context for strategic planning for health programs and services that will maximize the health of all people in this country. Chapter 11 presents further discussion of these demographic factors in relation to the health care delivery system.

Implications for Nursing
What are the implications for nursing that emerge from these demographic changes?

POPULATION INCREASES
The increased size of the population mandates increased health care services. The larger population will need more health care. We suggest, however, that the increased quantity of health care is not nearly as significant as is the change in quality of care that is mandated.

As people all over the world assume more responsibility for their health and become more informed about caring for themselves, the nature of their nursing care needs changes dramatically. Despite the fact that people live in a high-technologic environment and need technical experts as caregivers, they need professional nurses more. All clients need a special primary health care provider who focuses on their whole life experience and clearly understands how they experience their own well-being or threats to that well-being. Who can serve this function better than the professional nurse?

THE AGING POPULATION
The increasing age of the population poses special demands on nursing. The older people are, the more at risk they are to suffer chronic health impairments. Clearly, those aged 65 and over have higher rates of hospital-

ization and use the entire spectrum of health care services more than any other population group. Those aged 85 and over will have, in addition, greater needs for assistance in negotiating the activities of daily living.

Preziosi (1991) verifies that the increasing population of older adults, and the parallel increase in persons with chronic diseases, require nurses to research and provide new methods of health care delivery. He notes, for example, how "32 percent of Americans aged 75 and older cannot climb ten stairs, 40 percent are unable to walk two blocks," and "42 percent of nursing home residents cannot get out of a chair without help" (Preziosi, 1991, p. 1).

Perhaps the most important need is for health promotion and illness prevention services. That means that the primary goal for nurses should be to improve the quality of life for every older adult client with whom they interact. Professional knowledge will be called on not only to help these clients learn to use their strengths more effectively, but also to engage the collaborative efforts of those clients and their social support systems.

Some believe that the increasing population of older adult clients will mandate that professional nurses use the managed care approach. These nurse managers will need to coordinate the care of clients "with physicians, social workers, physical therapists, and other professionals" (U.S. Department of Health and Human Services, 1990b, p. III-B-4).

CHANGING HOUSEHOLD AND FAMILY STRUCTURES

Declining household sizes translate into increased nursing care needs. Because more adult members of a household are engaged in work outside the home, and because some family members outlive others, often fewer family members are available to serve as caregivers in the event that one family member needs such assistance. Even if the needs can be met by nonprofessional personnel, the care will need to be mutually planned with the client and monitored by professional personnel. Thus, primary care responsibilities and "managed care" responsibilities lie with professional nurses.

Consider, for example, the needs of Ms. M, an 88-year-old, independent, woman who managed to remain in her home, conduct her own business affairs, and live the kind of life she desired to live, with the help of neighbors who became surrogate family members as she grew older.

Ms. M lived alone on the first two floors of a large, three-story home and had a tenant renting the third floor. In the final 6 months of her life, however, she needed help with her personal care and activities of daily living, and required special care as a result of a malignant neoplasm. Her surrogate family (four neighbors) all had professional work responsibilities and could not provide the direct care she needed.

The Visiting Nurse Service was asked to evaluate Ms. M's needs and became her most significant health care delivery system, with a primary professional nurse becoming her most significant provider. Along with daily visits, during which she provided the professional care Ms. M needed, the professional nurse:

1. Collaborated with the family doctor, the oncologist, the radiologist, and the four neighbors serving as surrogate family
2. Supervised the care provided by home health care aides
3. Mutually planned with Ms. M to engage hospice care
4. Finally collaborated with the hospice nurse who shared the primary care responsibilities with her

In this case, the client had sufficient financial resources to cover all expenses involved in carrying out the preferred plan of care. Ms. M was able to stay in her own home, stay in control of many decisions despite the fact that she was highly dependent on the care providers for personal care, and enjoy her friends, until she peacefully died during sleep.

There were two critical factors in this example of high-quality nursing care: (1) The professional nurses were highly knowledgeable, sensitive to Ms. M's human needs, and committed to fully implementing the role of client advocate; and (2) Ms. M could afford to pay for all services required.

This real-life example points out two important challenges to the nursing profession:

Can we prepare enough professional nurses to handle these responsibilities?

What happens to clients who do not have the financial resources, and what is our responsibility for those without resources?

The role of the professional nurse as care manager is discussed further in Chapter 18.

DECLINING POPULATION OF CHILDREN

As other population groups increase and the proportion of children decreases, a serious challenge occurs: to maintain and to increase the human and financial resources needed to provide critically needed health care services for children. There is concern that the care of older adults could reduce the care available for children.

Atkinson (1991, p. 16) declares that

proof of a crisis in children's health isn't hard to find. The U.S. infant mortality rate continues to be an embarrassment. A crisis in the country's childhood immunization program has led to epidemics of measles and other preventable diseases.

Preziosi (1991) notes that low birth weight is responsible for the deaths of 45,000 infants annually in the United States.

Beyond these crises is a major social problem in the United States today: homelessness, which affects some 3 million persons, of whom 30% are families with children (Berne et al., 1990). Nurses are in the forefront trying to find solutions to the health problems associated with homelessness. They have developed models for addressing the health needs of the homeless (Berne et al., 1990), have begun to plan educational experiences for student nurses in homeless shelters (Witt, 1991), and have identified admission criteria and policies of shelters to determine access options for all persons needing shelter services (Barge & Norr, 1991).

Barge and Norr found that the most difficult of all shelter policies are those admission policies regarding children. They found that "women with male children more than 7 years old, pregnant women, and substance abusers were less likely to be admitted" (Barge & Norr, 1991, p. 145). Nurses are challenged to imagine the plight of homeless persons and to continue initiatives not only to deliver primary health care to this population, but also to shape social policy to prevent the crisis of homelessness.

The implications of racial, ethnic, and immigration trends for nursing are covered in the discussion of the context of culture.

SELECTED WORLD DEMOGRAPHIC FACTORS

It is important that nurses know that, despite the fact that women live longer than men, there are fewer women than men in the world. According to a United Nations report, "women now outlive men almost everywhere, but they are still in the minority in many developing regions because of higher female mortality in the past" (United Nations, 1991, p. 12). It is significant that the median age of women is rising rapidly in every part of the world except Africa (United Nations, 1991, p. 13). Perhaps the fact that Africa has the world's highest reported fertility rate accounts for the lower longevity of women there.

The lowest fertility rates occur in the developed countries. According to the United Nations (1991, p. 12), everywhere in the world except Africa

> the proportion of women aged 60 and over is rising because of longer life expectancy and lower childbearing rates . . . . For every 100 elderly men, there are 152 elderly women in the developed regions, 116 in Africa and in Latin American and the Caribbean, and 107 in Asia and the Pacific.

It is equally important to know that more than half of the world's population lives in developing countries.

One statistic that indicates the health of a nation is the maternal death rate. Despite the fact that the United States is one of the world's most developed countries, it does not have the lowest maternal death rate. According to the United Nations (1991), the U.S. rate is 8 maternal deaths per 100,000 births; the lowest rate (3 per 100,000 births) is in Sweden. Eleven developed nations have lower maternal death rates than the United States. Bangladesh has the highest reported maternal death rate in the world (600 per 100,000 births), according to the United Nations data.

These worldwide demographic data suggest that nurses must differentiate health care planning strategies among different countries on the basis of their level of development. Nurses in the United States are further challenged to answer the question of why one of most developed nations in the world does not demonstrate the best rates on all major health indices.

ECONOMIC ELEMENTS

Tracking the cost of health care, the Robert Wood Johnson Foundation (1991) identified costs to the nation and to U.S. business, government, and consumers; it also compared the costs to other nations. In the last 20 years, the proportion of the gross national product (GNP) devoted to health care has increased 50% "even after adjusting for economywide inflation and even though many Americans still receive inadequate care" (Robert Wood Johnson Foundation, 1991). During that same period, costs to the federal government more than tripled; costs to state and local governments more than doubled; and

> employers now pay not only for the health insurance premiums . . . but also the employer share of public payroll taxes for Medicare, the medical portion of workers' compensation, temporary disability insurance and, in some cases, the costs of on-site health services. Finally, from a global perspective, the U.S. spent more per capita than any other country, paying $2,140 per capita on health care. That rate was $546 higher than Canada, which has the second highest per capita expenditure for health (Robert Wood Johnson Foundation, 1991, p. 9).

Further information on the economic context of health care is provided in Chap. 11.

Implications for Nursing

The economic context of health care has two major implications for nursing:

1. Professional nurses must become more aware of the impact of costs on the public and determine if the health care delivery system operates efficiently or if it wastes money
2. Professional nurses must seize the opportunity to provide primary health care to many who really need nursing care more than medical care

According to the Public Citizens Foundation (1991, p. 5), an organization founded by Ralph Nader, "the U.S. health care system will waste an estimated $136 billion on administrative red tape" in 1991. This group further suggests that $459 to $540 per person could have been saved on paperwork alone in one year if national health insurance had been enacted.

The Public Citizens Foundation (1991, p. 5) also reported a rather startling finding: "Blue Cross/Blue Shield of Massachusetts insures 2.7 million subscribers and employs 6,682 people—more than are employed by the entire Canadian nation health program to administer coverage for more than 26 million residents." If these data are valid, nurses must act as citizens to stop the waste and as professionals to provide health care in efficient and cost-effective ways.

One of the nation's best known health care economists, Uwe E. Reinhardt (1991, p. 3B), suggests that the Canadian system may be more effective because Canada has a parliamentary system and that the U.S. public is focused on the wrong issue. He believes that the debate in the United States should be about the cost–benefit ratio, stating that "we have a cost–benefit crisis in health care, not necessarily a spending crisis . . . . The debate should be about this" (Reinhardt, 1991, p. 3B).

Better efficiency in care delivery is needed, but the current practice of downsizing the number of staff RNs, and replacing them with unlicensed assistive personnel (UAP), is a short-sighted bureaucratic strategy that diminishes quality of care. The best return for the dollars paid for nursing care will occur if the number of well-prepared professional nurses is increased. Knowledge pays dividends. This belief is congruent with the trend that the provision of information now far outweighs technical production in all fields of human endeavor. Nurses prepared to provide preventive services through sharing information with clients could significantly reduce the need for acute and long-term care. This in return would reduce costs and improve the economic context in which nursing practice occurs.

CULTURAL ELEMENTS

By the year 2000, the minority-group population in the United States will include approximately 80 million racially and ethnically diverse people. People's habits of promoting health, their ways of behaving when sick, their ways of recognizing and responding to illness, and their ways of defining health are strongly determined by their sociocultural background. Because nursing today exists within a pluralistic cultural context, professional nurses must understand specific cultural factors to "provide culturally appropriate nursing care for each patient" (Giger & Davidhizar, 1995, p. 5). Thus, it has become important for nurses to develop and use assessment measures that recognize the diversity among cultures.

With the changes occurring in the U.S. population, all nurses have the opportunity to interact with people of many cultures—some of whom follow values, beliefs, norms, and practices very different from the nurse's own. Because professional nurses always hope to promote change directed toward maximum well-being, they must interact with clients in ways that fully support the client's integrity. Supporting clients' integrity means allowing clients to maintain their own values, norms, beliefs, and traditions. Changes in health behaviors should not force clients to give up their unique cultural assets. Differences need to be viewed as assets, not liabilities.

If a cultural phenomenon is viewed as a liability, to be effective with a client of another culture the nurse must immediately attempt to reframe the perceived liability into an asset. Consider a client who screams loudly throughout much of labor. A nurse may perceive the screaming as negative and disruptive behavior in the labor room environment.

Before acting on her belief as truth, this nurse needs to assess the client's cultural attributes. If the nurse determines that, in the client's culture, screaming is believed to ward off evil happenings, the nurse can start to reframe her original perceptions into perceptions that the client is taking charge of the situation and doing everything she knows to achieve her goal of bearing a healthy baby. The reframing process can be enhanced by using a valid assessment tool for evaluating cultural variables and their influence on the client's health.

The synthesis of borrowed concepts from anthropology, sociology, and biology with the nursing concepts of caring, nursing process, and interpersonal communications is the basis for the theory of transcultural nursing (Boyle & Andrews, 1989). Transcultural nursing concepts derived from this synthesis, according to Boyle and Andrews (1989), include cultural beliefs and values, health and illness systems, nurse–client interactions, and culture-specific nursing care. The quality of the nurse–client relationship depends on how closely the nursing care matches the client's expectations. The degree to which expectations are shared and met is related to how much agreement there is between the nurse and the client on cultural symbols of health, healing, illness, disease, and caring.

Giger and Davidhizar (1995) propose six cultural phenomena that the nurse must understand to be effective with clients of another culture:

1. Communication: meanings of both verbal and nonverbal behavior
2. Space, particularly the comfort level related to personal space
3. Social organizations: patterns of cultural behavior learned through enculturation
4. Time: concept of the passage of time, duration of time, and points in time
5. Environmental control: abilities of persons to control nature
6. Biologic variation: racially related body structure, skin color, and other physical characteristics; enzymatic and genetic variations; electrocardiographic patterns; susceptibility to disease; nutritional preferences and deficiencies; and psychological characteristics

Consistent with cultural phenomena, Boyle and Andrews (1989, pp. 24–25) propose that nurses need to assess eight areas reflecting cultural variation. They have proposed an assessment model encouraging the nurse to gather the following data:

1. History of the origins of the client's culture
2. Value orientations, including view of the world, ethics, and norms and standards of behavior, as well as attitudes about time, work, money, education, beauty, strength, and change
3. Interpersonal relationships, including family patterns, demeanor, and roles and relationships
4. Communication patterns and forms
5. Religion and magic

6. Social systems, including economic values, political systems, and educational patterns
7. Diet and food habits
8. Health and illness belief systems, including behaviors, decision-making, and use of health care providers

Most American nurses "are immersed in a value system of rational analytic, biomedical principles, which is reflected in their attitudes and behaviors" (Boyle & Andrews, 1989, p. 50). Cultural encounters occur when nurses of one culture care for clients from other cultures. These encounters can result in learning by both the nurse and the client. On the other hand, "ineffective interethnic relations can lead to prejudice, discrimination, and racism" (Boyle & Andrews, 1989, p. 51).

Using Dibble's framework, Boyle and Andrews (1989, p. 52) define prejudice as "a hostile attitude toward individuals simply because they belong to a particular group presumed to have objectionable qualities." They define discrimination as "the differential treatment of individuals because they belong to a minority group," and racism as "a mixed form of prejudice (attitude) and discrimination (behavior) directed at ethnic groups other than one's own."

Other ineffective outcomes of interethnic nurse–client relationships occur when nurses exhibit cultural blindness. In cultural blindness, the nurse "ignores differences and proceeds as if these did not exist" (Boyle & Andrews, 1989, p. 53). The entire U.S. health care delivery system can be accused of expecting all clients to manage equally well with methods and materials originally designed for white, Anglo-Saxon Protestant Americans.

Implications for Nursing

Clearly, the assessment step of the nursing process is extremely important in interethnic relationships between clients and nurses. To gather data about a client of a culture different from the nurse's, the nurse needs to view clients as experts on their own life and the contexts within which they exist. If the nurse views each client as an expert and communicates with empathy, genuineness, and respect, then both participants in the interethnic relationship will grow. Prejudice, discrimination, racism, and cultural blindness will be controlled, and learning will be the outcome.

Communication is the interpersonal process that actualizes the nursing process. In this process, the nurse's and client's ability to be accurately and fully understood assumes critical significance. If the nurse and the client come from different ethnocultural backgrounds, the validation that must occur to ensure understanding is more difficult.

As Geissler (1991, p. 191) states, "certainly, [the] inability to use the dominant language of the health care system providers and/or cultural differences in verbal and nonverbal expressions between the patient and provider must be taken into account" to implement all steps of the nursing process. Nurses must understand that a language difference does not mean that the client has a problem communicating verbally, but rather that both the nurse and the client have a barrier to mutual understanding. The nurse must ensure that appropriate translators or interpreters are used as needed to facilitate good communication.

ENVIRONMENTAL ELEMENTS

A number of environmental factors affect global health. In addition to overpopulation (discussed above), these factors include socioeconomic considerations, pollution and global warming, deforestation of the rain forests and species extinction, and availability of primary health care.

Socioeconomic Considerations

Some of the problems of poverty include (Helman, 1994):

Unemployment
Limited education and literacy
Inadequate diet (including lack of breast-feeding)
Poor housing (inadequate sanitation and water)
Overcrowding
Lack of waste disposal
Stress-related psychosocial problems (marital breakdown, domestic violence, depression, alcoholism, and drug addiction)
Lack of confidence due to repeated defeat

Socioeconomic conditions also affect the infrastructure of the setting, including physical structures such as roads, electrical power, and hospitals. In addition, personnel such as nurses and doctors tend to be concentrated in more affluent areas. Violence is a major concern, with war causing 15 to 50 million refugees worldwide, landmines threatening life and limb, and children killed in drive-by shootings. Accidents may be associated with burns from open fires or a kerosene stove (Lane & Rubinstein, 1996). Motor vehicle accidents are prevalent in congested cities. People are exposed to environmental toxins such as lead, pesticides, and chemicals on a daily basis.

Pollution and Global Warming

Major contributors to global warming, a problem of international concern, are culturally derived "needs" rather than necessities of life. Chlorofluorocarbon aerosols are used to prevent body odor (deodorants), present a youthful appearance (hair lacquer), and portray order, affluence, and social respectability through shiny furniture (furniture polish). Automobiles represent prestige, power, autonomy, individualism and mobility, and not just transportation. The environment has a limited capacity to deal with waste, and currently critical resources such as the ozone layer, carbon cycle, and Amazon rain forests are being depleted, with catastrophic implications for future generations.

Deforestation and Species Extinction

Indigenous peoples are causing major destruction of rain forests to obtain land to farm for food for the rapidly increasing population. However, much of the former forest areas are poorly suited for farming, and soil erosion from the lack of trees reduces productivity. The loss of trees increases air carbon pollution and contributes to global warming. The destruction of habitat for animals, birds, plants, and microbes, and the killing of animals for trophies and animal parts, is inadvertently leading to species extinction at the rate of 74 per day, so that within 50 years, one-fourth of all species are expected to become extinct (Helman, 1994). However, two-thirds of the world's population relies almost exclusively on traditional medicines derived from plants in the rain forests (Helman, 1994). What is our ethical obligation to future generations and other organisms on the planet?

Availability of Primary Health Care

There are difficulties with the two major approaches to primary health care used worldwide. The World Health Organization has advocated a comprehensive, community-based strategy that targets improved health education, nutrition, sanitation, immunizations, family planning, maternal and child health, and supply of essential drugs (Lane & Rubinstein, 1996). However, this approach is expensive, there is a shortage of personnel to provide the needed services, and it is difficult to get community participation.

The United Nations International Children's Emergency Fund (UNICEF) has approached preventive health care selectively, with child survival considered paramount (Helman, 1994). Targeted interventions include:

Growth monitoring
Oral rehydration
Promotion of breast-feeding
Immunization against infectious and parasitic diseases
Family planning
Food supplements

However, this approach has encountered problems with cultural beliefs. For example, growth monitoring (height and weight) is a western, culture-bound way of defining "health." A mother may be concerned that if her child is more "normal" than others, there will be envy. If the child is less "normal" than others, this may be perceived as due to the "evil eye" of witchcraft (Helman, 1994).

IMPLICATIONS FOR NURSING

Unfortunately, many health promotion programs designed by middle-class individuals assume that people will "invest" in themselves through education, savings, diet, avoiding smoking, or using condoms, and defer gratification, to reap a future benefit such as better physical health, better quality of life, or increased life expectancy. People who live in poor socio-economic conditions lead precarious lives. Because the struggle for survival is the main concern, the focus is on a short time span and short-term benefits. Nurses need to consider the client's motivation when intervening to promote health.

The availability of health care is a significant factor when considering utilization of the delivery system. Compliance with weekly clinic visits is unlikely if the clinic is 10 miles away from the client's home and the client does not have the money for bus fare.

Cultural beliefs must be considered when intervening for health. Many times, an intervention is rejected by the community because of lack of trust in "outsiders." The value of children as proof of male virility, a visible sign of adult status, and a way to ensure future economic and social standing (Helman, 1994) must be considered as part of family planning. In addition, nurses must be aware that some religions disapprove of artificial birth control and must incorporate cultural beliefs about the body in their care.

All the issues discussed in this section involve ethical issues, and nurses are intimately involved in all of the ethical dilemmas surrounding health care today. The following section presents a brief overview of the ethical context of nursing.

VIGNETTE

Stephen is often the only RN on duty during evenings in the nursing home in which he works. Lately he has become increasingly concerned about one of his patients, Miss Moore, a 77-year-old woman with advanced emphysema, who has been restrained because she wants to pull out her feeding tube and be allowed to die. He agonizes about what he should do.

ETHICAL ELEMENTS

In conducting the process of nursing, professional nurses act on the basis of their own moral beliefs and their cognitive and interpersonal abilities. These abilities are continuously shaped by the development of knowledge, relationships, and values. Given the dynamic nature of the interactions among knowledge, relationships, and values, nurses often experience ethical dilemmas in the caring process.

Major ethical issues in nursing have been identified by Bandman and Bandman (1995) as:

- Quantity vs. quality of life
- Pro-choice vs. pro-life
- Freedom vs. control
- Truth-telling vs. deception
- Allocation of limited resources
- Empirical knowledge vs. personal belief (pp. 7–10)

Each of these issues generates a dilemma for nurses who care. The following section discusses caring as an ethical issue that creates a dilemma for professional nurses; it identifies selected issues that pose further dilemmas for the nurse who cares. This section is presented to stimulate readers to consider the moral foundations of nursing and to further develop their own values as guides to their own practice.

The Ethical Dilemma of Caring

Referring to pride as a component of one's healthy self-image, former U.S. congresswoman, professor, and orator Barbara Jordan (1988), addressing the American Nurses Association (ANA) convention, stated: "You have reason to be proud of your profession, proud of the service you provide to men and women all over the country, all over the world, and you have every reason in the world to be proud to care—because when you care, things happen." She also pointed out that the corollary of that statement is also true: "When you don't care, things happen." Articulating her belief that we have been socialized to care for people with whom we share the world, Jordan professed that people in our government gave life to the ethic of caring, noting that if the people of the world are to continue to survive, rules and order must be maintained to prevent the alternative—anarchy, disorder, and the breakdown of civilization.

Reverby (1987), explaining the dilemma of caring, focuses on the limitations society has imposed on nursing by creating conditions that do not value the desire to care. Reverby and Jordan agree that nurses care:

> Nurses, whatever else can be charged against them, continuously try to meet their obligations to care (Reverby, 1987, pp. 1–2).
> While many things have changed about society, one thing has not changed. One thing has remained constant—a nurse cares, and we who are your patients count on you to keep caring (Jordan, 1988).

The dilemma, then, emerges from the conflict between the imposed limitations of society and the expected socialization of the nurse. Reverby (1987, p. 2), noting the intertwined nature of the history of women and the history of nursing, has identified four major constraints on caring as a professional value: "limitations—of imagination, of cultural ideology, of economics, and ultimately of political power."

For caring to be a moral value, Fry (1987, p. 48) asserts that it must be viewed as good or right for four specific reasons:

1. It must be "viewed as an ultimate or overriding value to guide one's action"
2. It must be "considered as a universal value and, hence, applied to all persons in similar circumstances"
3. It must be "considered prescriptive in that certain behaviors (empathy, support, compassion, protection, etc.) are preferred"
4. It must "consider the human flourishing of others and not just one's own welfare"

As a possible explanation of the dynamics of the caring dilemma, Gilligan (1982) recognized the possible differences in the moral development of men and women in our society. She postulated that women have based their moral development on the capacity for responsibility and care, whereas men's basis for moral development is the advancement of rights. She further suggests that women, accepting conventional interpretations, have confused responsibility "with a responsiveness to others that impedes a recognition of self" (Gilligan, 1982, p. 127). Writing about nursing, Reverby (1987, p. 203) adds, "The tradition of obligation made it very difficult for nurses to speak about rights at all, or to articulate a vision of caring that acknowledged the need for the right to determine duty."

What women really want may be the opportunity to continue to value caring while gaining the right to be autonomous. If so, they will recognize and seek to implement the empowerment of others in a way that does not have to be at the expense of self. However, in order to achieve this, the broader social problems of gender and class must be solved. According to Reverby (1987, p. 207), nursing would not be alone in benefiting from such an effort: "If nursing can create the vision of autonomy and altruism as linked qualities, and achieve the power to forge this unity, all of us have much to gain." Gilligan (1982, p. 127) perhaps explains the advantages of the unification of autonomy and altruism:

> The truths of relationships return in the rediscovery of connection, in the realization that self and other are interdependent, and that life, however valuable in itself, can only be sustained by care in relationships.

Pointing out that the demands for health care continue to increase and that nurses are indispensable to the U.S. health care delivery system, Jordan (1988) professed that without nurses there is no health care system. At the conclusion of her address to nurses at the ANA convention, she acknowledged the interdependence of society and nurses and the need for the moral value of caring:

> You are nurses. I've said that you care and you do, but it is time for us, the people, to care about you. It is time for us to care about your future, your dignity, your opportunity, your autonomy—care about you, because, when you care, things happen (Jordan, 1988).

It is also time for professional nurses themselves to confront the dilemmas associated with caring as a central value for nursing.

◎ Morality in Nursing Practice

Morality is "the oughts of a given society" (O'Neil, 1995, p. 224). Because nursing decisions always involve choices to be made by the nurse and the client, morality, in which the decisions to be made are matters of conscience, is an important characteristic.

According to Packard and Ferrara (1988, p. 61), the key moral ideas that have been recognized for centuries are "goodness, justice, freedom, equality, and respect for human beings." They link nursing to these great moral ideas through the concept of health: "Since it seems obvious that nursing is related to human health and that both individual and collective health figure prominently in the ability to live well, then it is certain that nursing links with the great moral ideas" (Packard & Ferrara, 1988, p. 61). They further assert that nurses have indisputable obligations to act in some positive direction to affect health and thus must consider the morality of their actions and be able to work through moral problems.

Taylor (1985, p. 13) states that "the nature of the nurse–patient relationship is undergoing renewed examination as the paradigms in use change." She suggests that nursing ethicists need to consider particularly the tension between the arguments of rights and responsibilities:

> If nursing is to be the close personal relationship with the patient . . . our ethics should focus on responsibilities and obligations. If nursing is described as a trade relationship, on the other hand, the ethics of rights is most appropriate.

Taylor's directive to nursing ethicists is based on the work of Gilligan (1982), who distinguishes two ways of thinking about moral development. She associates these conceptions of morality with male and female modes of describing relationships between others and self (Gilligan, 1982, p. 19):

1. Fairness: connecting moral development to the understanding of rights and rules (male mode)
2. Concern with the activity of care: connecting moral development to the understanding of responsibilities and relationships (female mode)

Gilligan suggests that Kohlberg's view of moral development (1981) (ie, "rights") is a male mode of describing relationships between others and self. She suggests that women predominantly describe their relationships in terms of "responsibilities."

> Clearly, these differences arise in a social context where factors of social status and power combine with reproductive biology to shape the experience of males and females and the relations between the sexes (Gilligan, 1982, p. 2).

Rafael (1996, p. 4) associates patriarchy (a "perpetuation of male dominance through valuing men, their characteristics, and their activities while at the same time devaluing women and their characteristics and activities") with "denigration of women and that which is feminine" (p. 6), contributing to feelings of powerlessness and disenfranchisement. Gilligan's framework provides one possible guide for constructing a theory of ethical nursing practice within an ethic of care.

Among the several moral principles central to health care today are beneficence, fidelity, and veracity. According to Flynn (1987, p. 62), "the general principle of beneficence states that we must do good and, on the other hand, must act to prevent harm." Fidelity is viewed by Aroskar (1987, pp. 79–82) as primary loyalty and faithfulness to clients. Veracity is the important moral principle of truth-telling (Aroskar, 1987, p. 85). Each of these principles seem straightforward and clearly acceptable to professional nurses.

Every ethical principle poses serious issues for the nurse. Flynn (1987, p. 63), speculating about beneficence, states that disagreements commonly occur about "what is meant by the good, about how to go about doing good, and how to interpret the clinical situation." Aroskar (1987, p. 84) points out that competing loyalties create difficulties for nurses to demonstrate fidelity to clients: "These conflicting loyalties may include loyalties to oneself and one's personal principles and values, loyalty to physician and nurse colleagues, and loyalty to one's employers." Asserting that nurses commonly find themselves in the middle of situations in which clients or their families have not been told the truth about their conditions or treatments for those conditions, Aroskar (1987, pp. 85–86) alerts nurses to two problems encountered in their efforts to act out of the principle of veracity: (1) withholding of information and (2) deception.

Additionally, Keegan (1995) discusses the principle of double effect in which "nurses are involved in actions that have untoward consequences" (pp. 139–140) and suggests that four conditions must be met before an act can be justified (Keegan, 1995, p. 140):

1. The act itself must be morally good or at least indifferent
2. The good effect must not be achieved by means of the bad effect
3. Only the good effect must be intended, although the bad effect is foreseen and known
4. The good effect intended must be equal to or greater than the bad effect

To resolve the dilemmas resulting from an effort to care in morally principled ways, the nurse must know how to make ethical decisions. Following is a brief discussion of the theoretical basis for ethical decision-making and a suggested process for making ethical decisions.

THE BASIS FOR ETHICAL DECISION-MAKING

Ethics in nursing is concerned with doing good and avoiding harm (Bandman & Bandman, 1995). Choice is an essential element of ethical behavior and the nurse's responsibility for valuing a client's choices:

Nursing strategies for facilitating patients' choices enhance the values of personhood, especially at critical times in a person's life, when he or she is ill, incapacitated, dying, or vulnerable due to age, mental disability, or socioeconomic status (Bandman & Bandman, 1995, p. 114).

Nurses, like all other scientists and philosophers, base decisions on outcomes of inquiry. Munhall (1988, p. 151) says that nursing inquiry is linked to ethical reflection, the ethical question being "toward what goal and for what end?" She states that "many of our research endeavors focus on facilitating 'health.' The search for a means to produce a desired health outcome requires critical ethical reflection" (Munhall, 1988, p. 152).

Three Perspectives

Three perspectives that provide a background for and influence ethical thinking are:

Principlism
Care
Contextualism

The most prevalent organizing framework is *principlism,* "an orientation incorporating duties, rights, and principles" (O'Neil, 1995). The principlist perspective values rational thinking. However,

where the principlist perspective values impartiality and detachment when arriving at ethical decisions, the care perspective stresses that each situation is unique and requires sensitivity to others' needs and to the dynamics of particular relationships (O'Neil, 1995, p. 232).

The *care* perspective values dialogue to meet the needs of the particular person(s) involved. Finally, in *contextualism,* individual situations become paradigm cases that provide "rules of thumb" to follow. In the contextualist perspective, practical experience in patient care is valued (O'Neil, 1995).

A Process for Making Ethical Decisions

Nurses encounter moral problems frequently in practice, thus creating the need for a workable method with which to analyze and resolve ethical dilemmas. Fowler (1987, pp. 183–184) has proposed a method for ethical decision-making that incorporates all three perspectives to help nurses thoughtfully consider moral problems:

1. *Identify the problem.* Clearly identify the ethical problem; determine whether there is more than one ethical concern; examine any sense of conflict with duties and personal or professional values; and determine whether the ethical conflict rightfully belongs to you
2. *Identify the morally relevant facts.* Examine the context of the dilemma (how it occurred, likelihood of it arising again, who the key players are as well as their views and vested interests); and iden-

tify other considerations such as administrative, political, economical, legal, medical, or aesthetic concerns

3. *Evaluate the ethical problem.* Examine the ethical norms by reviewing the literature, codes of ethics for nursing, and moral traditions in the profession. From this review, identify the guides for moral action that are appropriate for the situation. Consider broader ethical principles, such as justice and autonomy, for giving direction to your action; consider the aspects of the dilemma that individualize it; examine the dilemma according to ethical principles; and assign priority to these principles, according to both the professional and the personal ethical demands of the situation

4. *Identify and analyze action alternatives.* Determine actions that are open to you; consider new or creative actions that could be taken; determine the harms and benefits likely to result from each alternative action (who will be harmed and who will be helped); identify which actions will likely produce subsequent dilemmas; ethically analyze each alternative; and consider institutional procedures that could help with the particular dilemma

5. *Choose and act.* From your ethical evaluation of the dilemma and alternative actions, choose a plan of action; modify the plan in accordance with legal or other values while remaining true to your moral norms; and act

6. *Evaluate and modify the plan.* Identify the results of your actions; clarify your moral feelings about your actions; consider modifications for future situations; consider how to prevent such dilemmas in the future; and modify your plan of action in the current situation if necessary

Bandman and Bandman (1995, pp. 110–114) warn nurses about pitfalls that can occur in the ethical decision-making process. They label these pitfalls "fallacies" or errors in reasoning. Such errors in reasoning include:

1. Arguing that because something (X) is the case, therefore, something (X) ought to be the case
2. Making someone accept the conclusion of another on the basis of force alone (appealing to force)
3. Abusing the person rather than the person's reasons for making a particular decision
4. Arguing that since everybody does something, that something must be good
5. Appealing to inappropriate authority to justify a decision
6. Assuming that if one exception is made to a rule, then uncontrolled events with unwanted circumstances will occur (called the "slippery slope fallacy")
7. Refusing to allow evidence to be shared if it contradicts one's personal position

Bandman and Bandman (1995) suggest that fallacies can be avoided if certain principles are consistently used as the basis for ethical decision-making:

1. Valuing and respecting the client's self-determination
2. Serving the client's well-being in practice in a manner that prevents harm and does good (beneficence)
3. Treating clients fairly and with equity by respecting their rights and treatment options, making them equal participants in shared health care decisions

Nursing practice, education, and research provide many opportunities for the professional nurse to make ethical decisions and to experience the satisfactions of resolving ethical dilemmas. Situations that generate ethical dilemmas arise from the nurse's efforts to determine what is right. In dealing with each of these ethical issues, the primary responsibility of the professional nurse in caring for the client is always to respect the human as a unified being. Despite variations in the definition of responsibility in nursing, all nursing leaders would probably agree that the structure of the professional nurse's responsibility is to self, to clients, and to the profession, always for the purpose of the improvement of health.

Developing a Personal Philosophy of Nursing

To develop a personal philosophy of nursing, the professional nurse must focus on concern about the nature of human beings and the life process. From the perspective of nursing, the nurse must attempt to answer the following questions, which reflect the fundamental elements of nursing:

1. What is society—of whom is it composed, and what is the nature of the relationships among its constituents?
2. What is your central belief about the individual person, and that individual's potential? The family? The community?
3. What constitutes the environment?
4. How do human beings and the environment interact?
5. What is your view of health? Is it a continuum? A unidirectional phenomenon? A state? A process?
6. How do illness and wellness relate to health?
7. What is the central reason for the existence of nursing?
8. Who is the recipient of nursing care?

From the perspective of a philosopher's concern with knowledge, the nurse must attempt to answer the following questions that reflect the essential elements of the scientific discipline:

1. What is the nursing process?
2. From what cognitive base does the professional nurse operate?

3. How is the nursing process implemented? What is necessary in the application of knowledge?
4. How is the theory base for nursing derived?
5. What is the theoretical framework for the profession?
6. What are the purposes and process of nursing research?

From the philosopher's concern with ethics and aesthetics, the professional nurse must attempt to answer the following questions reflecting the valuation elements of nursing:

1. What are the essential rights and responsibilities of the professional nurse?
2. What are the essential rights and responsibilities of the recipients of nursing care?
3. What are the governing ethical principles in the delivery of nursing care and the conduct of nursing research?
4. What are your beliefs about the educational requirements for the practice of the profession?
5. What are your beliefs about the teaching–learning process?

The greatest opportunity to begin to develop answers to the preceding questions is provided in the nurse's educational experience. Built on the nurse's entire life experience as well as on his or her professional education experience, the nurse's professional self-concept allows realization of a dynamic philosophy of nursing by caring for clients, peers in nursing, and other health care providers.

◎ Conclusion

In giving care to individuals, groups, and communities, the professional nurse is influenced by environmental contextual elements that affect people's lives and create difficult ethical decisions. Nurses who have considered their beliefs, and have developed a philosophy to guide their practice, have a basis for action related to ethical issues.

THOUGHT QUESTIONS

1 Why is a personal philosophy of nursing significant to the individual nurse?

2 How can it be argued that nursing is a moral art?

3 What are the principal ethical values that affect professional nursing practice?

4 What are the ethical implications in Stephen's vignette regarding Miss Moore?

REFERENCES

American Association of Colleges of Nursing. (1986). *Final report: Project on the essentials of college and university education for professional nursing.* Washington, DC: Author.

Aroskar, M. A. (1987). Fidelity and veracity: Questions of promise-keeping, truth-telling, and loyalty. In M. D. M. Fowler & J. Levine-Ariff (Eds.). *Ethics at the bedside—A sourcebook for the critical care nurse.* Philadelphia: Lippincott.

Atkinson, C. (1991, November/December). Kids in crisis: Can we stop the slide in children's health care? *Public Citizen, 11,* 16–19.

Bandman, E. L., & Bandman, B. (1995). *Nursing ethics through the life span* (3rd ed.). Norwalk, CT: Appleton & Lange.

Barge, F. C., & Norr, K. F. (1991, Fall). Homeless shelter policies for women in an urban environment. *Image, 23,* 145–149.

Berne, A. S., Dato, C., Mason, D. J., Rafferty, M. (1990, Spring). A nursing model for addressing the health needs of homeless families. *Image, 22,* 8–13.

Boyle, J. S., & Andrews, M. M. (1989). *Transcultural concepts in nursing care.* Glenview, IL: Scott, Foresman/Little, Brown College Division.

Flynn, P. A. R. (1987). Questions of risk, duty, and paternalism: Problems in beneficence. In M. D. M. Fowler & J. Levine-Ariff (Eds.). *Ethics at the bedside—A sourcebook for the critical care nurse.* Philadelphia: Lippincott.

Fowler, M. D. M., & Levine-Ariff, J. (Eds.). (1987). *Ethics at the bedside—A sourcebook for the critical care nurse.* Philadelphia: Lippincott.

Fry, S. T. (1987). Autonomy, advocacy, and accountability: Ethics at the bedside. In M. D. M. Fowler & J. Levine-Ariff (Eds.). *Ethics at the bedside—A sourcebook for the critical care nurse.* Philadelphia: Lippincott.

Geissler, E. M. (1991, April). Transcultural nursing and nursing diagnosis. *Nursing and Health Care, 12,* 190–192, 203.

Giger, J. N., & Davidhizar, R. E. (1995). *Transcultural nursing: Assessment and intervention* (2nd ed.). St. Louis: Mosby-Year Book.

Gilligan, C. (1982). *In a different voice—Psychological theory and women's development.* Cambridge, MA: Harvard University Press.

Helman, C. G. (1994). *Culture, health and illness* (3rd ed.). Oxford: Butterworth-Heinemann.

Jordan, B. Keynote speech at the 1988 ANA Convention, Louisville, KY: June 11, 1988.

Keegan, L. (1995). Holistic ethics. In B. M. Dossey, L. Keegan, C. E. Guzzetta, & L. G. Kolkmeier (Eds.). *Holistic nursing: A handbook for practice* (2nd ed.). Gaithersberg, MD: Aspen.

Kleffel, D. (1996). Environmental paradigms: Moving toward an ecocentric perspective. *Advances in Nursing Science, 18,* 1–10.

Kohlberg, L. (1981). The philosophy of moral development: Moral stages and the idea of justice. New York: Harper & Row.

Lane, S. D., & Rubinstein, R. A. (1996). International health: Problems and programs in anthropological perspective. In C. F. Sargent & T. M. Johnson (Eds.). *Medical anthropology. Contemporary theory and method* (Rev. ed.). Westport, CT: Praeger.

Munhall, P. L. (1988). Ethical considerations in qualitative research. *Western Journal of Nursing Research, 10,* 150–162.

Naisbitt, J., & Aburdene, P. (1990). *Ten new directions for the 1990s: Megatrends 2000.* New York: Morrow.

O'Neil, J. A. (1995). Ethical decision making and the role of nursing. In G. L. Deloughery (Ed.). *Issues and trends in nursing* (2nd ed.). St. Louis: Mosby-Year Book.

Packard, J. S., & Ferrara, M. (1988). In search of the moral foundation of nursing. *Advances in Nursing Science, 10,* 60–71.

Preziosi, P. (1991, May/June). *Public policy bulletin* (pp. 1–4). New York: National League for Nursing.

Public Citizen Foundation. (1991, July/August). Health care wasteland, Upfront news. *Public Citizen, 11*, 5.

Rafael, A. R. F. (1996). Power and caring: A dialectic in nursing. *Advances in Nursing Science, 19*, 3–17.

Reinhardt, U. E. (interview with K. Anderson). (1991, May 6). Pressures build with rising costs. *USA Today*, p. 3B.

Reverby, S. M. (1987). *Ordered to care—The dilemma of American nursing, 1850–1945.* New York: Cambridge University Press.

Robert Wood Johnson Foundation. (1991). Tracking the cost of health care. *Advances—Newsletter of the Robert Wood Johnson Foundation*, p. 9.

Soukhanov, A. H. (Ed.). (1992). *The American heritage dictionary of the English language* (3rd ed.). Boston: Houghton Mifflin.

Taylor, S. G. (1985). Rights and responsibilities: Nurse–patient relationships. *Image, 17*, 9–13.

United Nations. (1991). *The world's women—Trends and statistics 1970–1990.* New York: Author.

U.S. Department of Health and Human Services. (1990a). *Healthy people 2000: National health promotion and disease prevention objectives.* Washington, DC: U.S. Government Printing Office.

U.S. Department of Health and Human Services. (1990b). *Seventh report to the President and Congress on the status of health personnel in the United States.* (Executive Summary). Washington, DC: U.S. Government Printing Office.

Witt, B. S. (1991). The homeless shelter: An ideal clinical setting for RN/BSN students. *Nursing and Health Care, 12*, 304–307.

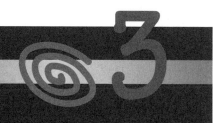

Dynamics in the Development of Professional Nursing

LEARNING OUTCOMES

By the end of this chapter, the student will be able to:

1 Discuss the factors that led to the establishment and perpetuation of nursing education within a service-dominated model.

2 Discuss the factors that led to the establishment of levels of nursing practice and education.

3 Identify the factors inherent in the formation of the American Nurses Association, the National League for Nursing, and their competition today.

4 Describe the factors that led to the dominant position of the hospital as an employer of nurses.

5 Discuss trends in the delivery of health care over the past 50 years.

VIGNETTE

Martha, Carol, and Joe are new RN–BSN students. In their "transition" course they sign up to do a presentation on nursing history. They hope this will help them to better understand current and evolving issues affecting the profession.

Nursing as an organized occupation began in America in 1873 with the formation of educational programs based on the British model inspired by Florence Nightingale. Because of enormous social and technologic changes occurring at that time, nursing was rapidly manipulated for the profit and advantage of other groups. Given both the dependent position of women in Victorian society and the lack of a conceptual base for practice, nursing education was vulnerable to control by hospital administrators and physicians. These same forces have continued to influence the development of nursing; it is only now, 125 years since its beginning, that nursing is finally emerging into professional status. This chapter presents a historical perspective on the forces currently influencing the growth and development of the nursing profession.

 ## The 1860s to 1960s

THE INFLUENCE OF THE HEALTH CARE DELIVERY SYSTEM

Home as a Setting for Care

Nurses were first trained in the United States in the 1870s. At that time, medical care was provided in the home for paying patients ("clients"), with nursing care provided primarily by female members of patients' families. As nurses began to graduate from training schools, they were hired to provide nursing care in the home, under the supervision of a physician.

The only alternative for those too poor to afford a physician and nurse in the home was to go to a hospital, where care was provided only by untrained medical students and slovenly attendants. It was not until 1886 that the first organized district nursing organizations were formed in Boston and Philadelphia to provide care to all who were sick, regardless of ability to pay. Nurses followed physicians' orders, gave treatments, recorded temperature and pulse, and taught hygiene to clients and their families (Moore, 1900, pp. 18–20).

Lillian Wald and Mary Brewster opened a Nurses' Settlement House in New York City in 1893 and used the term "public health nurse" for the first time to describe their trained nurses. The nurses responded to calls from clients as well as physicians, giving services in the home to all who needed them, with no distinction between those who could pay and those who could not. In 1895, they moved to larger accommodations that became known as the Henry Street Settlement House. By 1900, 20 district nursing organizations employed 200 nurses across the United States (Roberts, 1954, p. 14). In 1906, the first African American public health nurse, Elizabeth Tyler, was appointed to the staff of the Henry Street Visiting Nurse Service (Carnegie, 1986, p. 148).

Some of the basic principles of public health nursing were becoming apparent. It was increasingly evident that nursing should be available to all who were sick, regardless of ability to pay or religious affiliation; a definite distinction was being made between nursing and almsgiving; nurses were beginning to recognize the importance of keeping records; the importance of cooperation with other groups in the community was being stressed in order to avoid gaps and duplication of services; and the family began to emerge as the unit of service (Spradley, 1990). It was recognized that district nurses needed more preparation than they received in hospital programs.

Public health nursing continued to prosper from 1900 until the time of World War I. Social consciousness was widespread, and social and legislative reform were encouraged. In 1910, the Department of Nursing and Health was established at Teachers College in New York, the first nursing department in a college. Post-basic nursing courses to prepare teachers, administrators, and public health nurses were offered. Voluntary agencies developed rapidly in this climate. The National 0rganization for Public Health Nursing (NOPHN) was established in 1912, with membership open to public health nurses, public health agencies, and interested citizens.

Care by trained private-duty nurses and public health nurses continued to be provided primarily in patients' homes until the Great Depression of the 1930s. As hospitals and the medical profession developed during the 1930s and 1940s, hospitals became respected community institutions for all classes of patients. The home then decreased in importance as a care setting until the 1980s, when emphasis on reduction of costs for health care delivery stimulated earlier hospital discharge, ambulatory diagnostic laboratory testing, and long-term intravenous therapy in the home. In recent years, the expansion of in-home care has produced a critical need for professional nursing input and care.

The Hospital as an Employer

While nursing in the home setting was undergoing some modifications, dramatic change was affecting hospital nursing. By the beginning of the last quarter of the 19th century, hospitals were mainly charity institutions "that provided care for indigent patients who had nowhere else to go" (Kalisch & Kalisch, 1986, p. 157). Most hospitals were dirty, unventilated, and contaminated by infection. The causes for infectious diseases such as typhoid fever, cholera, and diphtheria were not discovered for another 10 years. Rubber gloves for use in surgical operations were not invented until 1891. Even the thermometer and the hypodermic syringe were not commonly used until the 1880s. The major treatment for most illnesses was bloodletting, which certainly killed more patients than it helped. Hospital conditions were so miserable that people began to demand reform.

The hygienic hospital practices demonstrated by Florence Nightingale and her small group of self-proclaimed nurses during the Crimean War (1854–1856) drew attention to the potential for nursing to bring about hospital reform. Nightingale and her apprentices reduced the mortality rate in British military hospitals from 42% to just over 2% (Kalisch & Kalisch, 1986, p. 51). Several years later, during the American Civil War (1861–1865), women volunteers demonstrated their ability to handle hard work and improve conditions in military hospitals. After the war, the movement to establish nurse training schools was seen as a way to improve hospital conditions while also providing a respectable occupation for women.

Hospital growth was also promoted by the tremendous scientific discoveries and social changes occurring in the last quarter of the 19th century. The discovery of radiography, anesthetics, and the value of aseptic procedure led to the development of aseptic surgery, requiring specialized equipment that seldom could be found outside of the hospital.

Furthermore, the Industrial Revolution caused an influx of people to the cities, increasing the demand for medical care. Previously, physicians had cared for paying patients at home, and only those too poor to pay for a private physician went to a hospital. But improving conditions in hospitals, combined with the need to centralize medical care, led to rapid growth of hospitals. From 1873 to 1923, the number of hospitals in the United States grew from 149 to 6,762 (Bullough & Bullough, 1978, p. 132), many under the proprietary ownership of physicians. That enormous growth could not have occurred without the cheap, efficient service provided by nursing students in hospital training schools.

The untrained attendants who had dominated hospital nursing care were rapidly replaced by nursing students. However, there were few opportunities for hospital work for the trained graduates. After graduation, a few nurses were retained to fill head nurse positions, but almost all graduates worked in homes as private-duty nurses. In addition, many hospitals sent their students into patients' homes, keeping the students' pay for hospital income. The nurse moved in with the family and was on duty 24 hours a day, for an average of 3 weeks. By 1920, the average pay was $120 a month. Although the nurse was overworked for some months, she often was idle while waiting for a new case. As they grew older, many nurses found themselves unable to cope with the all-night vigils and the hard work (Goldmark, 1923, pp. 168–169).

Over the next 50 years, most trained nurses were employed in private duty. However, by the end of the 1920s, many private-duty nurses were in desperate financial straits. Because of the development of specialized equipment and services, an increasing number of patients were being treated in hospitals rather than in physicians' offices or at home. The number of hospitals increased dramatically, with a concomitant increase in the number of nurse training programs. The number of student nurses to staff the hospitals increased steadily, despite the lack of jobs for nurses when they completed their training. "The typical hospital connected with a school of nursing during 1938 employed an average of ten graduate nurses for general duty or bedside nursing" (National League for Nursing Education, 1939, p. 898).

By the Great Depression, some trained nurses were willing to work for hospitals for just room and board. Despite resistance by some hospitals, graduate nurses were allowed to remain in the hospital, often with little more pay than they had received as students. The hospitals without training schools could pay graduate nurses less than they had been paying untrained attendants. The movement toward hospital employment for graduate nurses accelerated as the scientific discoveries after World War II increased medical care specialization.

The growth of third-party reimbursement, first through private insurance after World War II and then through Medicare and Medicaid insurance in the 1960s, led to enormous growth in the number and profitability of hospitals. Hospitals provided a centralized location for proliferating medical technology, with unlimited, retrospective cost reimbursement by insurers.

Growth of the Nursing Team

By the time the United States entered World War II, graduate RNs had become accepted as part of the hospital staff. Many hospitals had closed their schools of nursing when they discovered that they could hire graduate nurses more cheaply than the cost of staffing with students. Thus, when large numbers of graduate RNs joined the armed forces, a serious shortage of nurses developed in civilian hospitals. Nursing schools received federal monies to increase student nurse enrollment, and, at the request of the Office for Civilian Defense, trained volunteer nurses' aides were hired to assist nurses. In addition, certificate holders from Red Cross home nursing classes began volunteering for nonprofessional duties and later were paid as auxiliary workers.

Early federal concern for production of adequate numbers of nurses led to the Nurse Training Act of 1964 (P.L. 88-581).

> Adding Title VIII to the Public Health Service Act, it authorized (1) grants to assist in the construction of teaching facilities, (2) grants to defray the costs of special projects to strengthen nurse education programs, (3) formula payments to schools of nursing, and (4) extension of professional nurse traineeships. Subsequent enactments, in 1966, 1968, 1971, 1975, and 1981 reauthorized and revised provisions of the nurse training program. Between 1965 and 1982, almost $1.6 billion was appropriated under the Nurse Training Act (Institute of Medicine, 1983, p. 231).

After World War II, the nurse shortage intensified as demand for hospital beds increased. Many nurses retired from nursing because of marriage or better-paying employment outside the field; others retired from hospital nursing for nursing positions in industry or public health, which offered more autonomy.

In addition, hospitals had found that many duties could be performed by aides and auxiliary workers, at a perceived lower cost. Many hospital administrators and physicians also were angered by the aggressive push by the professional nursing association, the American Nurses Association (ANA), for an 8-hour day and 40-hour week, improved salaries, and a voice in the planning and administration of hospital nursing services.

One way to obtain relatively low-cost service and maintain control over the worker was to establish schools for practical nurses. In 1947, there were 36 training schools for practical nurses. Between 1948 and 1954, 260 more were established, mostly in hospitals. Local public schools also established programs affiliated with hospitals to take advantage of federal vocational education funds. By 1952, there were more than 144,000 practical nurses, comprising 52% of nursing service personnel. Aides trained in a 6-week course had replaced the wartime auxiliary workers. With graduate RNs, graduate licensed practical nurses (LPNs), students, and aides all giving nursing service in the same setting, hospitals began to use a team plan for efficient care of a group of patients. This approach is still used in many hospitals today.

The proliferation of workers giving nursing care made it possible for hospitals to increase their operating profits. Graduate RNs were increasingly assigned managerial roles that took them away from the bedside. The public, confronted with an array of caregivers, confused the nursing aide with the professional nurse. The image of nursing held by nurses and the public became increasingly blurred.

Models for Nursing Practice

Since the Depression, the vast majority of nurses have worked in the hospital setting. During this time the structure of the work environment has undergone numerous revisions related to changes in prevalent social values and management theories. For the first half of the 20th century, functional nursing delivery was used, based on the management beliefs of Weber (1964) in an environment of immigrants adapting to an emerging industrialized society. The functional pattern was based on a pyramidal management structure, heavy supervision, and a heavy reliance on rules, policies, and procedures. In the late 1940s and early 1950s, under the influence of the humanistic values of Maslow (1954) and in an environment of a nurse shortage, team nursing was introduced. Team nursing was meant to increase attention to the individual needs of clients, maximize the capabilities of each team member, and augment the role of the professional nurse team leader. This pattern took advantage of the increasing numbers of differentiated health workers such as practical nurses, nursing assistants, and aides (Stillwagon, 1989).

Development of the Medical Profession

The current venerated status of medical education and the medical profession seems incredible when compared with the situation in the United States just after the Civil War. At that time, as a rule, a medical school conferred a degree on completion of "annual courses of four months' duration over a two-year period. Both first- and second-year students attended the same lectures each year" (Kalisch & Kalisch, 1986, p. 35). It was hoped that in between the two courses of lectures, the students would spend some time observing patients with a physician preceptor, but there was no systematic hospital teaching.

Medical schools of that period were proprietary schools, not associated with universities or hospitals. The best medical schools finally began to strengthen their links with hospitals in the 1870s and 1880s, but regular class attendance was not required and examinations were cursory. Admissions standards varied from some high school to college education. A common saying of the time was that "a boy who is unfit for anything else must become a doctor" (Kalisch & Kalisch, 1986, p. 35).

By the beginning of the 20th century, medical education reform had focused on upgrading the standards of entry "to level the whole profession above a recognized base rather than create an educational elite" (Stevens, 1971, p. 38). (As is shown later in this chapter, that is exactly the emphasis in nursing education some 100 years later.) In the 1870s, reforms at Harvard led to a graded medical school curriculum, lengthening of the curriculum to 3 years, administration of regular examinations, and the requirement of a college degree for entry.

These reforms marked the beginning of a new movement toward a genuine university medical education (Stevens, 1971, p. 41). Between 1900 and 1926, the number of medical schools decreased from 160 to 79 and the number of yearly graduates fell from 5,214 to 3,962 (Burgess, 1928, p. 35). The rapid increase in the knowledge base for practice mandated both an increase in admission and graduation standards and an increased emphasis on quality.

Thus, through a coincidence of history, the late 1800s were a crossroads for both nursing and medicine. The establishment of hospital-based nurse training programs provided nursing students with constant access to patients. This was threatening to physicians, most of whom had little practical training. All efforts to increase the education in nurse training were resisted strenuously by physicians and organized medicine. Domination effectively prevented competition. At the same time, the exploding scientific and technologic revolution, as well as rapid urbanization and immigration, "sparked the development of hospitals and medicine" (Stevens, 1971, p. 34). Medical education moved into the postgraduate university, which led to true professional education. Yet nursing education remained apprenticeship training, which maintained the subservient relationship with hospitals and physicians.

Why didn't nurses break out of the apprenticeship mold? Why didn't nursing education move into the university, as had medical education? The simple answer is that nursing was composed almost solely of women, and in the 19th century women had limited opportunities. In the absence of nursing theory to provide a power base separate from medicine, nursing was easily controlled by hospitals and physicians.

THE DEVELOPMENT OF NURSING EDUCATION

The Influence of the Role of Women

In the mid–19th century, white, middle-class women led circumscribed lives. Legally, a woman was considered a ward of her father or her husband. She had no independent rights because common law stated that "the husband and wife are one, and that one is the husband" (Kalisch & Kalisch, 1986, pp. 84–85).

The Victorian era also produced exaggerated chivalry and etiquette. The "lady" was considered fragile and physically weak. The American woman was expected to be modest, humble, pious, and chaste. "Regarded as inferior to men, in mind as well as in body, women were declared unsuited for intellectual development" (Kalisch & Kalisch, 1986, p. 84).

The woman's role was in the home; her primary duty was fulfilled in motherhood. It was not considered proper for respectable women to have careers or even to be educated. In fact, there was some concern that education would interfere with childbearing by focusing energy on the brain instead of the reproductive organs. Even working as a governess in a socially acceptable home was suspect. Few women ever went beyond grammar school, although a few attended finishing school, where they learned social graces and the art of piano playing and singing.

Thus, in the 1870s, women who had to work were in a difficult position. The choices for untrained working-class women outside of the home were "virtually limited to retail clerking, factory labor, domestic service, or prostitution" (Bullough & Bullough, 1978, p. 118), because teaching or even office work required some education. For these reasons, nursing training seemed to be a reasonable alternative for women of modest means who wanted or needed a career.

Until that time, however, nursing had been considered an inferior, undesirable occupation. Much of the care of the sick in hospitals was provided by women paupers from workhouses, who had neither the experience nor the desire to be good nurses. In New York, female criminals who had been arrested for drunkenness or vagrancy were required to work in Bellevue Hospital for 10 days instead of serving a jail term. In 1910, Charles Dickens's Martin Chuzzlewit immortalized Sairey Gamp and Betsy Prig (two sloppy, careless, and slovenly old women) as a "fair representation of the hired attendant on the poor in sickness." Certainly, no respectable woman would have stooped to hospital nursing had it not been for the example of Florence Nightingale.

The example of Miss Nightingale's service in the Crimean War began the change in the public's image of nursing. "She made public opinion perceive, and act upon the perception, that nursing was an art, and must be raised to the status of a trained profession" (Kjervik & Martinson, 1979, p. 22). A product of an upper-class English Victorian upbringing, Florence Nightingale saw nursing as closely related to mothering because both used the "natural feminine characteristics of nurturance, compassion, and submissiveness" (Kjervik & Martinson, 1979, p. 38).

Although she developed a theoretical model for nursing (in which the environment influenced health outcomes), Nightingale believed that the nurse's role should be to follow protocol rather than to use independent decision-making. Thus, she believed that the emphasis of nurses' training should be on carrying out orders. This belief set a crucial precedent in defining nurses as subordinate to physicians—even in giving basic nursing care, an area in which physicians lacked expertise.

Nightingale's determination to improve the dismal reputation of nursing led her to propose stringent policies which were appropriate at that time, but which were perpetuated to the detriment of the professional development of nursing. Good character was emphasized in the selection of student applicants, but intellectual characteristics were ignored. The nursing residence was instituted to protect and monitor morality, but it also promoted the dependence and isolation of students and gave the hospital control over all aspects of their lives. The strict nursing service hierarchy, which was established to maintain discipline in nursing, emphasized a deference to authority rather than the development of individual leadership qualities. Despite these drawbacks, however, Florence Nightingale's example led to the popular image of the nurse as the "lady with the lamp," with saintlike qualities of selfless compassion and endless toiling to ease suffering. Nightingale (with the help of untrained volunteers, including at least one black woman, Mary Grant Seacole) had made nursing respectable, and women were attracted in droves.

In the United States, the nurse training system was instituted at the very time that college education was becoming available for upper-class women. By the end of the 1870s, most state universities were admitting women, and colleges for women began to be established. Vassar opened in 1865, followed by Smith in 1871 and Wellesley in 1875. Because these colleges were in the process of establishing themselves, they did not want to be associated with an occupation of questionable reputation. They were also financially out of reach for the working-class women who were attracted to nursing as a way to improve their status. Ironically, at the same time that medical education moved into the postgraduate university, nursing education became established as apprenticeship training under the control of physicians and hospitals.

Hospital Training Programs

The first nursing training programs were established in America in 1872 and 1873 in Boston, in New Haven, and in New York City. In 1880 there were 15 programs, and by 1900 there were 432 programs with 3,456 graduates (Burgess, 1928, p. 35).

The early training programs were semiautonomous in relation to their affiliated hospitals. However, they lacked financial endowments and independent budgets, and rapidly became dependent on the hospitals for support. What had begun as separate and relatively autonomous programs became nursing service departments in hospitals. Because the hospital controlled service and so-called education, the students worked 7 days a week, 50 weeks a year for 1 to 2 years in exchange for on-the-job training, a few lectures, and a small allowance. It is not surprising that offering a training school became essential to the financial success of a hospital.

The number of training schools increased dramatically from 15 schools in 1880 to 2,155 schools in 1926 (Burgess, 1928, p. 35). The quality of the schools varied considerably, as documented by a survey of nursing education published in 1923 (Goldmark, 1923) and a 1925 study done by the Committee on the Grading of Nurses (Burgess, 1928). Of the schools responding, 42% had no regular nurse instructor and an additional 42% had only one. Of the instructors, 42% had less than a high school diploma, only 16% had some college education, and 85% had not had any continuing education after beginning to teach.

The varied and generally poor quality of training programs caused widespread concern about the care of the public and the future of nursing. From the time the Flexner report on medical education revolutionized that profession in 1910 (Flexner, 1910), nursing leaders have encouraged studies that they hoped would lead to improved quality of nursing education. After the Goldmark report of 1923, numerous studies and surveys indicated that the root of most difficulties was nursing schools' dual purpose of service and education. However, the studies resulted in limited reform. Diploma schools remained the dominant educational pattern for registered nursing until the early 1970s.

Associate Degree Programs

In 1951, Montag published her doctoral dissertation "The Education of Nursing Technicians," which proposed education for the technician RN in community colleges. The program was to completely prepare the nurse for immediate employment. The concept was researched for 10 years, after which community college nursing flourished in the growing societal emphasis on educational accessibility and mobility. The Brown (1948) and Ginsberg (1949) reports had stressed movement of professional registered nursing education into the college, with the eventual end of technical practical nursing education. Instead, Montag simply replaced the technical hospital RN with a technical college-prepared nurse. Registered nursing was splintered into three modes of educational preparation, while practical nursing continued to flourish in vocational and hospital settings.

Baccalaureate Education

In 1893, the first diploma program within a university setting was established by the School of Medicine at Howard University. The program, designed for African American students, only lasted 1 year within the university setting before being assumed by Freedmen's Hospital. In 1909, the University of Minnesota established a 3-year diploma program in nursing within the College of Medicine. In the years that followed, a common pattern in colleges was a combined academic and professional course of 4 or 5 years leading to a nursing diploma and a bachelor of science degree. The college of liberal arts and hospital-based nursing studies were completely separate, a pattern that has again recently surfaced and is being promoted as "innovative."

"The first university school to be established on an independent basis with its own dean, a substantial endowment, and all students entered in the degree program, was opened in Yale University in 1923" (Dock & Stewart, 1938, p. 179). By 1929, a bachelor's degree was required for admission. Although truly collegiate schools were established at Western Reserve University (1923), Vanderbilt University (1930), and the University of Chicago (1925), there was opposition from physicians who argued that "intelligence and sound knowledge of theory were unnecessary and might handicap the prospective nurse" (Kalisch & Kalisch, 1986, p. 381). Nursing education remained associated with the hospital diploma school in the minds of the public, and the number of nurses graduated from baccalaureate programs remained a small percentage of total graduations.

ORGANIZATIONAL INFLUENCES

There were no national women's organizations of any kind in the United States before the Civil War. The nursing associations were the first professional groups to be organized and controlled by women (Bullough & Bullough, 1978, p. 135).

In 1894, the Society of Superintendents of Training Schools for Nurses of the United States and Canada (which became the National League of Nursing Education [NLNE] in 1912) was established. Two years later, this organization sponsored a conference of representatives of nursing school alumnae associations. They organized the Nurses' Associated Alumnae of the United States and Canada, which was to become the ANA in 1912 (Bullough & Bullough, 1978, p. 136). Thus, from the very start of organized nursing, nurses were separated into two national nursing organizations: one for graduate nurses, and the other for the leadership group. The following section briefly describes the development of the National League for Nursing (NLN), the ANA, and the international honor society in nursing, Sigma Theta Tau.

National League for Nursing
The Superintendents Society concentrated on the improvement of nursing education. Through their efforts, a course in hospital economics was offered by Teachers College, Columbia University, "to prepare potential teachers and administrators." The course was later (1905) lengthened to a 2-year program, which for many years was the only source of advanced education available to nurses.

Improvement of the hospital training programs focused on requirements for admission (high school graduation), limitation of work hours of students (first to 12 and then to 8 hours a day), and efforts to close the wide gap between good schools and poor ones. However, as late as 1949, only about 25% of state-approved schools met or approached standards set 12 years earlier, 50% were nearer to standards set 22 years earlier, and 25% were still struggling to meet these earlier standards (School Improvement Program, 1963, pp. 3–4).

In 1949, the National Nursing Accrediting Service, established by the NLNE in association with the Association of Collegiate Schools of Nursing (ACSN) and the NOPHN, ranked schools based on 1937 and 1942 criteria. No programs were accredited until 1952, when an accrediting service became part of the new NLN, which was formed by combining NLNE, ACSN, NOPHN, Joint Committee on Practical Nurses and Auxiliary Workers in Nursing Service, Joint Committee on Careers in Nursing, National Committee for the Improvement of Nursing Services, and National Nursing Accrediting Service. The accreditation process was influential in improving educational quality. It is still a major function of the NLN.

American Nurses Association

The Associated Alumnae concentrated their early efforts on obtaining state registration of nurses in an effort to differentiate trained nurses from those with no formal training. Separate drives for registration were mounted in each state, and the first registration acts were passed in 1903 in North Carolina, New Jersey, New York, and Virginia. An RN was defined as someone who had attended an approved or registered nursing program (although most states placed absolutely no restrictions on the scope or quality, and some nurses were "grandfathered" in with no formal training) and, in some states, had passed a board examination. None of the original registration acts defined the scope of professional nursing practice (Am J Nurs, 1903, pp. 562–564).

In 1938, New York began a new phase by mandating the licensure of all who sought to give nursing care. This act, which made it illegal for any others to practice nursing, was the first nursing practice act to define the practice of nursing (Hicks, 1938, p. 563). Unfortunately, the new practice acts specified rigid hour and subject requirements that had to be completed. The apprenticeship system of education was legally mandated, and the rigidity made curriculum experimentation almost impossible.

Later, many states incorporated into their nursing practice acts the language of a 1955 ANA "model definition of nursing," which included the disclaimer: "The foregoing shall not be deemed to include acts of diagnosis or prescription of therapeutic or corrective measures" (ANA Board, 1955, p. 1474). This created many problems as nursing responsibilities began to expand.

The state association as the basic unit of membership for ANA was established in 1916, at a time when many states, particularly but not exclusively in the South, barred membership to African American nurses. A separate national organization, the National Association of Colored Graduate Nurses (NACGN), was established in 1908 under the leadership of

Martha M. Franklin. This organization established a central registry for African American nurses, supported civil rights activities, promoted educational opportunities for African Americans, and played a pivotal role supporting the establishment of the Cadet Nurse Corps (1943), making it possible for African American nurses to serve in the armed services. The NACGN dissolved in 1951. "By that time, provisions had been made for black nurses to bypass those southern states that denied them membership and join the ANA directly as individual members" (Carnegie, 1986, p. 99).

Sigma Theta Tau

As a specialty discipline, nursing was recognized as equal to other disciplines with a scholarship base when Sigma Theta Tau was founded in 1922 by six students at the Indiana University Training School for Nurses to encourage and recognize superior scholarship and leadership achievement at the undergraduate and graduate levels in nursing. The name comprises the initials of the Greek words storga, (love), tharos (courage), and tima (honor).

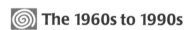 ## The 1960s to 1990s

CHANGES IN THE HEALTH CARE DELIVERY SYSTEM

The 1960s

At the start of the 1960s, the health care delivery system was comprised primarily of independent, not-for-profit hospitals, small private practices of office-based physicians, and neighborhood drug and medical supply stores. Bywords of physician practice were authority, prerogative, autonomy, free choice, solo practice, and fee for service. Biomedical breakthroughs proliferated, leading to high- technology intensive care units and specialty surgery, but consumers paid little. Hospitals and physicians billed private insurers like Blue Cross (associated with the American Hospital Association) and Blue Shield (associated with the American Medical Association), and received retrospective, cost-based reimbursement. Competition was minimal. However, in 1965, the federal government became a major payer, through the Medicare and Medicaid programs, for coverage of the poor and elderly. By 1969, concern was being expressed about the rapidly mounting costs of health care.

The 1970s

The 1970s were characterized by inflation and unemployment, and consumers revolted against tax increases. Mechanisms such as utilization review to reduce the length of hospital stay, regulation of hospital construction, and peer review of physician services under Medicare were tried in efforts to restrain rising health care costs but were not very effective.

Insurers carried increased risk because they were under pressure not to increase premiums. Blue Cross, which had been criticized as simply passing on increased hospital costs to a helpless public, legally separated from the American Hospital Association in 1972. In 1974, the Employee Retirement Income Security Act added incentives to businesses to self-insure. A few investor-owned hospitals were established, but medicine and hospital care, although under pressure, went on as usual.

The 1980s

Costs continued to skyrocket during the 1980s, although the economy was weak. In 1983, Medicare prospective payments (diagnosis-related groups [DRGs]) were instituted to reduce the rate of increase of Medicare hospital costs, and in 1989, tighter control of Medicare physician payments was instituted. The emphasis of reimbursement policies shifted from promoting access to care toward containing costs by reducing the length of hospital stay. By the end of the decade, hospitals were experiencing decreased profits and shortened hospital stays, which led first to empty hospital beds and then to hospital consolidation. Many acutely ill patients were shunted to ambulatory and home care.

Increasingly, the insurance industry was influenced by commercial (for-profit) companies and businesses trying to reduce the costs for coverage of their employees. Selective contracting reduced consumer choice, but allowed insurers to choose which providers they would pay on the basis of low-cost bidding. As a result, fierce competition for contracts developed. In addition, managed care became a burgeoning movement. However, the costs of health care also grew enormously, especially in hospital expenses, stimulating the federal government to try to decrease hospitalization and hospital care as a way to limit costs.

The 1990s

By 1990, "95% of insured employees were enrolled in some form of managed care, including fee-for-service plans with utilization management, preferred provider organizations, and HMOs" (Bodenheimer & Grumbach, 1995, p. 87). Providers created integrated health networks, in which hospitals, insurance companies, and physicians join forces by merging or affiliating with one another. Large surpluses of specialist physicians and a shortage of generalists were forecast. Physicians increasingly practiced in large groups, while major commercial companies dominated insurance coverage through managed care plans. A majority of nursing homes, home health care companies, and multihospital systems were for-profit companies, but 85 million Americans were uninsured, underinsured, or enrolled in Medicaid (Ginsberg, 1995). Risk management tactics were increasingly used to avoid enrolling potentially high users of services.

Despite high patient acuity, and ample documentation that RNs improve quality of patient care (Brooten & Naylor, 1995), by the mid-1990s,

RNs were being replaced by unlicensed assistive personnel (UAP), resulting in changed skill mix, reduced nurse staffing levels (with many nurses out of work), and economic devaluation of RNs (Buerhaus, 1995).

CHANGES IN NURSING PRACTICE

The thrust in the 1960s and 1970s was toward primary nursing, based on the principles of Herzberg (1966). This pattern was set up for a primary nurse who was responsible for planning client care throughout the hospitalization. However, because the hospital organization was still pyramidal and bureaucratic, nurses were still bound by the constraints of lack of control over time, and the system was modified in many settings into total patient care during an 8- or 12-hour shift.

In the late 1980s, under the impetus of DRGs and cost constraints, the case manager concept became popular. Case management combined managed care with an emphasis on outcomes with consultation among various providers to enhance the quality of patient care. The intent of case management was to promote coordination and continuity of nursing care (reminiscent of primary nursing), but as the emphasis shifted to controlling short-term costs of care, "work redesign" models for "patient-focused care" were being developed.

The key elements of patient-focused care (Greenberg, 1994) are:

■ Patients with similar diagnoses are grouped on the same units
■ Ancillary and support services are decentralized to the nursing unit
■ Staff are cross-trained, shifting from specialized care providers to generalist providers
■ Patient care teams of cross-trained providers give the majority of care for a group of patients

As a result of work redesign efforts, the skill mix has been reduced, with RNs and licensed vocational nurses (LVNs) being replaced by UAP who have received minimal on-the-job training in such areas as patient hygiene, patient mobility, and determining and recording vital signs and intake/output. In addition, nonnursing personnel such as respiratory therapists, social workers, housekeeping, dietary, and clinical laboratory workers have been reassigned to the nursing department under the supervision of the nurse manager.

As a result, profound changes in responsibility, authority, and accountability are occurring. RNs are now expected to assume significant responsibility for allocation of personnel and resources, delegation of patient care responsibilities, supervision of the direct patient care provided by others, and evaluation of patient outcomes. Competence in supervising UAP and personnel from other health care disciplines, using leadership, communication, care management, and health teaching skills is crucial to these new roles (McLaughlin, Thomas, & Barter, 1995).

Although the majority of nurses have been employed in acute care institutional settings in the past, the ongoing downsizing of hospitals and professional staff requires that nurses consider the developing opportunities in community-centered care. Some of the evolving opportunities for employment include:

Home care via visiting nurse associations, public health agencies, or for-profit organizations

Nurse-managed centers

Physician office practices or health maintenance organizations (HMOs)

Community health centers; migrant worker health centers

Specialty clinics—women's health, family planning, renal dialysis, birthing center

Hospice

Schools

Occupational settings

Ambulatory care clinics, surgical centers

Regardless of setting, the issue for the nursing profession has been to promote a work environment and organizational model that promotes "accountability with control, authority, and autonomy over factors related to the professional's work" (Porter-O'Grady, 1987, p. 281). Participation in decision-making through access to information, task identity, links between performance and reward, and challenge also is needed to enhance professional job satisfaction and growth. The challenge is to foster professional care regardless of the structural model for nursing practice.

Specialty Certification

Specialization indicates continued development in a particular special interest area of practice and may be recognized through job descriptions, educational programs, specialty organizations, state certification, or national certification through the American Nurses Credentialing Center (ANCC). The American Association of Nurse Anesthetists began its certification program in 1945. By 1990, there were at least 56 certification opportunities available (Fickeissen, 1990), and by 1994, more than 300,000 nurses were certified in a specialty area (Nicholas, 1995).

The rapid growth of certification has led to a number of questions and concerns:

■ Labels for specialty areas are overlapping and duplicative (eg, certifications exist for a practitioner, nurse practitioner, advanced practitioner, family practitioner, pediatric practitioner, adult practitioner, and medical–surgical practitioner). It is also difficult to differentiate between specialties and subspecialties (eg, for pediatric oncology certification, which is the specialty and which is the subspecialty?)

- Should certification continue as a voluntary process or be replaced with licensure for advanced practice?
- Educational, practice, and experience requirements vary widely, leading to confusion among nurses and consumers. The establishment of the American Board of Nursing Specialties (ABNS) in 1991 as a national peer review program for specialty nursing certification bodies provides a mechanism to address these issues (Parker, 1994)

Although certification is supposed to attest to knowledge and skills in a specialty field, the rewards are largely intrinsic. Few positions require or reward financially for certification. However, many individuals consider certification to be prestigious, and it has been viewed by some as a way to improve the image of the profession.

THE CHANGING EDUCATIONAL SYSTEM

Undergraduate Education

Since 1965, when nursing began to develop as a scientific discipline, baccalaureate nursing education has grown and developed to approximately one-third of nursing admissions, where it has stabilized. Three factors contributed to this growth:

The Brown report and the Bridgman study
Accreditation standards formulated by the NLN
Federal monies to increase the pool of nurses eligible for graduate study

Concurrently, the ANA report published in 1965, "Educational Preparation for Nurse Practitioners and Assistants to Nurses: A Position Paper," concluded the following:

> The education for all of those who are licensed to practice nursing should take place in institutions of higher education; minimum preparation for beginning *professional* nursing practice should be a baccalaureate degree; minimum preparation for beginning *technical* nursing practice should be an associate degree in nursing; education for assistants in health service occupations should be short, intensive preservice programs in vocational education rather than on-the-job training.

This report intensified the conflict over the future role of hospital diploma programs and the "professional/technical" language widened the schism in nursing education. However, it fostered the growth of associate degree programs.

"In 1962, students from associate degree programs constituted 3.7 percent of the graduating registered nurses. By 1972 they were 37 percent of the graduating class" (Facts About Nursing, 1982–83, p. 78). By 1993, they constituted almost 64% of graduations (Nursing Data Review 1996, p. 43) (Table 3-1).

TABLE 3-1

Graduations from Baccalaureate, Associate Degree, and Diploma Programs of Nursing*

Years	Baccalaureate		Associate Degree		Diploma		Total Number
	Number	Percent of Total	Number	Percent of Total	Number	Percent of Total	
1960-61	4,031	13%	917	3%	25,071	84%	30,019
1965-66	5,488	16%	3,349	10%	26,072	74%	34,909
1970-71	9,856	21%	14,534	31%	22,065	48%	46,455
1975-76	22,579	29%	34,625	45%	19,861	26%	77,065
1980-81	24,370	33%	36,712	50%	12,903	17%	73,985
1985-86	25,170	33%	41,333	54%	10,524	14%	77,027
1990-91	19,264	27%	46,794	65%	6,172	8%	72,230
1993-94	28,912	30%	58,839	62%	7,118	8%	94,870

*Data modified from Nursing Data Book, 1982, pp. 39 and 56; and Nursing Data Review, 1996, p. 43.

However, in the intervening years, the original conceptualization of the associate degree as both technical and terminal appears to have been abandoned. An increasing number of students begin their education in an associate degree nursing program, intending to continue on to the baccalaureate level. Between 1971 and 1980, total baccalaureate enrollment nearly doubled, but RN enrollment in baccalaureate programs increased 338% (data derived from the NLN Nursing Data Book, 1982). In 1994, more than 40,000 RNs (graduates of associate degree and diploma programs) were enrolled in baccalaureate nursing education programs, comprising almost 28% of the total baccalaureate enrollment (Nursing Data Review, 1996, p. 41).

Graduate Education

By 1996, 9% of RNs were projected to hold master's or higher degrees (National Advisory Council, 1996, p. 45), although approximately one-third of the degrees were not in nursing. The deficit of master's and doctorally prepared nurses is becoming increasingly acute.

The lack of nurses with advanced education in nursing has particularly affected nursing administration and nursing education. In 1995, only 13.7% of all graduates of master's programs in nursing had a concentration in administration, and only 8.3% had a concentration in teaching. However, graduations of nurse practitioners almost doubled between 1993 and 1995, to 43% of the graduations from master's programs in nursing (Nursing Data Review, 1996, p. 33).

Research in nursing has also been handicapped by inadequate levels of support. Between 1971 and 1981, $40 million was awarded for nursing research. During that same period, the National Institutes of Health (NIH) received $1.7 billion for general biomedical research. However, since the National Center for Nursing Research was established within the NIH in

1986, and converted to the National Institute for Nursing Research in 1993, funding has improved to a budget of over $66 million in fiscal year 1996.

RECENT ORGANIZATIONAL DEVELOPMENT

National League for Nursing

The mission of the NLN is "to improve education and health outcomes by linking communities and information" (NLN, 1995–1997). It achieves its mission through collaborating, connecting, creating, serving, and learning. Nine goals clarify the emphases of NLN programs:

1. To provide leadership in redesigning the delivery of nursing education and health care services through community-focused models
2. To develop and advance the educational models most appropriate for emerging health care needs and services
3. To promote and monitor the quality, accessibility, and appropriateness of nursing education programs
4. To transform the teaching–learning environment for nursing and health care
5. To promote access to information and resources that will enhance the positive health status of diverse communities and individuals
6. To expand nursing's research agenda to include innovative nursing educational models, community-focused education, and health outcomes of diverse communities
7. To increase and diversify membership
8. To develop NLN as a knowledge-based educating organization
9. To ensure NLN's economic growth and fiscal soundness

The NLN is recognized in the United States as the national accrediting body for all basic nursing education programs, as well as for master's degree nursing programs. In 1996, the NLN Accrediting Commission was established as an independent entity whose sole purpose is the accreditation of nursing education programs. The NLN also provides a voluntary peer-review accreditation program for home health agencies and community nursing services through the independent subsidiary Community Health Accreditation Program.

In 1996, the NLN was restructured into four centers with 11 membership councils:

Center for Nursing Education and Interdisciplinary Education
    Council of Associate Degree Programs
    Council of Baccalaureate and Higher Degree Programs
    Council of Diploma Programs
    Council of Practical Nursing Programs
Center for Nursing Practice and Interdisciplinary Health Care
    Council of Nursing Practice
    Council of Nursing Centers
    Council of Nurse Executives

Center for Research in Nursing Education and Community Health
   Council of Research in Nursing Education
   Council for Nursing Informatics
   Council for Community Health Sciences
Center for Collaborating Organizations and Community Groups
   Council of Constituent Leagues

In addition to its accreditation activities, the NLN provides consultation services, continuing education programs, analysis of statistical data related to nursing education and manpower resources, various examination and test services, and a variety of information packages to affect recruitment, image, and legislative affairs. *NHC Perspectives on Community* is the official journal of the NLN. Agency membership in the NLN is open to nursing education institutions and providers of nursing and other health care services. Individual membership is open to anyone interested in nursing and the improvement of health care.

American Nurses Association

The ANA is the professional organization for RNs in the United States. It is a federation of constituent nurses associations in each of the 50 states and in the District of Columbia, Guam, and the Virgin Islands. Individual RNs join at the state level.

The purposes of ANA are to "work for the improvement of health standards and the availability of health care services for all people, to foster high standards of nursing, and to stimulate and promote the professional development of nurses and advance their economic and general welfare" (ANA Bylaws, 1995, p. 1).

The ANA does the following:

- Accredits continuing education programs
- Provides for voluntary certification for individual registered nurses through the ANCC
- Supplies data for research and analysis
- Provides public policy analysis and political education and maintains government relations and political action activities
- Implements an economic and general welfare program
- Publishes a variety of publications, including *The American Nurse* and its official journal, *The American Journal of Nursing*
- Holds conferences and a biannual convention

The ANCC has been established by the ANA as a separately incorporated center for credentialing services. Eleven boards on certification are responsible for programs and policies relating to a specialty area of practice. Eight of these boards have been recognized by the ABNS as meeting national standards for certifying organizations. In 1995, certification examinations in 28 specialty areas were offered through the ANCC.

Through the ANA's Congresses on Nursing Economics and Nursing Practice, standards and programs are developed for nursing education, nursing practice, research, organized nursing services, economic security and employment, and priorities for human rights. Through its councils, members of constituent state nurses associations can participate at the national level to discuss and communicate issues and concerns relevant to specialized areas within nursing (eg, computer applications, community health nursing, medical–surgical nursing practice, and so forth). The ANA is the sponsoring organization for *The American Journal of Nursing*, The American Academy of Nursing, and The American Nurses Foundation. As a member of the International Council of Nurses, the ANA represents all U.S. nurses.

Sigma Theta Tau International

Sigma Theta Tau became an international organization in 1985. The organization has grown to more than 220,000 members and over 400 chapters (in 1996), including international chapters in Canada, South Korea, Taiwan, and Australia. It is a member association of the Association of College Honor Societies.

Membership is available by invitation through active chapters, based on demonstrated superior scholastic achievement, evidence of professional leadership potential, or marked achievement in the field of nursing. Students in baccalaureate or higher-degree programs in nursing and nurse leaders in the community with a minimum of a baccalaureate degree are eligible. The organization contributes to the advancement of nursing through research via small grants, conferences, and publication of reports in its professional journal, *Image: The Journal of Nursing Scholarship*, and in the electronic journal, *The Online Journal of Knowledge Synthesis*. In addition, the organization sponsors writers' seminars and a media development program, and gives awards in recognition of outstanding contributions to nursing practice, research, education, creativity, leadership, professional goals, and chapter programming. Individual chapters present educational programs and award scholarships. The Center for Nursing Scholarship and Virginia Henderson International Nursing Library, a state-of-the-art electronic library and resource center information services system, were dedicated in November 1989.

National Student Nurses Association

The mission of the National Student Nurses Association (NSNA) (1994) is to:

- Organize, represent, and mentor students preparing for initial licensure as RNs, as well as those nurses enrolled in baccalaureate completion programs
- Promote development of the skills that students will need as responsible and accountable members of the nursing profession
- Advocate for high-quality health care

"The NSNA is autonomous, student financed, and student run. It is the voice of all nursing students speaking out on issues of concern to nursing students and nursing" (Kelly & Joel, 1995, p. 577). Students are eligible for active membership in NSNA if they are enrolled in state-approved programs leading to licensure as an RN or are RNs enrolled in programs leading to a baccalaureate degree in nursing.

The NSNA has a wide variety of activities, services, and projects to carry out its purpose and functions. The organization participates on committees of the NLN and ANA and is a leading participant in the student assembly of the International Council of Nurses (ICN). The NSNA foundation administers a scholarship program and publishes an official magazine, *Imprint*, a newsletter, *NSNA News*, as well as various reports and handbooks.

ISSUES AND TRENDS

Progress in the development of professional nursing is being affected by:

- The power of knowledge over technical skill
- High acuity and short stays of hospitalized patients
- Emphasis on controlling and constraining costs of hospital care
- Continuing explosion of new technologies
- Continuing inadequate supply of nurses educated at the baccalaureate and master's degree levels, and oversupply of nurses educated at the associate degree level
- Downsizing of acute care positions, especially for associate degree-educated nurses
- Reduction of Medicare hospital pass-through revenues for diploma education
- Hospitals' tendency to use nurses interchangeably, regardless of educational preparation
- Shrinking RN staff coupled with increasing use of UAP for direct patient care
- Increasing opportunities in autonomous settings for baccalaureate-educated nurses
- Societal images and expectations of nurses
- Degree of the nursing profession's control over the quantity and quality of practitioners
- Impact of technology and theory on nursing practice's roles and settings
- Sources of financing for health care services
- Professional self-image of nurses

◎ Conclusion

Modern nursing has been developing in the United States for more than 125 years. The factors that shaped its early formation also limited the development of nursing as a profession for more than 80 years. However, in the past 40 years demonstrable progress can be related to an improving professional self-image and the emergence of a theoretical base for practice. Although residual problems are still associated with factors in nursing's roots, there are numerous indications that nursing is finally emerging into true professional status.

THOUGHT QUESTIONS

1 Why was nursing education within a service-dominated model perpetuated for 80 years?

2 How do levels of nursing education affect nursing practice?

3 Are there advantages to the separation between the ANA and the NLN? Would it be desirable to move toward a combination of their functions?

4 What are the implications of the consolidation of hospitals and the growth of ambulatory and home care for nursing education and practice?

5 What can nursing learn about professional status from medicine?

6 How can changes in the health care delivery system be used to advance nursing's professional development?

7 How can an understanding of nursing history help Martha, Carol, and Joe (see vignette) to understand current issues in nursing?

REFERENCES

American Journal of Nursing. (1903). *3*, 562–564.

ANA board approves a definition of nursing practice. (1955). *American Journal of Nursing, 55*, 1474.

American Nurses Association. (1965). *Educational preparation for nurse practitioners and assistants to nurses: A position paper.* New York: Author.

American Nurses Association. (1995). *Bylaws.* Washington, DC: Author.

Bodenheimer, T., & Grumbach, K. (1995). The reconfiguration of U.S. medicine. *Journal of the American Medical Association, 274*, 85–90.

Bridgman, M. (1953). *Collegiate education for nursing.* New York: Russell Sage Foundation.

Brooten, D., & Naylor, M. D. (1995, Summer). Nurses' effect on changing patient outcomes. *Image, 27*, 95–99.

Brown, E. L. (1948). *Nursing for the future.* New York: Russell Sage Foundation.

Buerhaus, P. I. (1995, May/June). Economic pressures building in the hospital employed RN labor market. *Nursing Economics, 13*, 137–141.

Bullough, V., & Bullough, B. (1978). *The care of the sick: The emergence of modern nursing* (3rd ed.). New York: Prodist.

Burgess, M. A. (1928). *Committee on the grading of nursing schools: Nurses, patients and pocketbooks.* New York: Commonwealth Fund.

Carnegie, M. E. (1986). *The path we tread.* Philadelphia: Lippincott.

Dickens, C. (1910). *Martin Chuzzlewit.* New York: Macmillan.

Dock, L. L., & Stewart, I. M. (1938). *A short history of nursing* (4th ed.). New York: G. P. Putnam's Sons.

Facts about nursing 1982–83. (1983). Kansas City: American Nurses Association.

Fickeissen, J. L. (1990). 56 ways to get certified. *American Journal of Nursing, 90*, 50–57.

Flexner, A. (1910). *Medical education in the United States and Canada.* New York: Carnegie Foundation for the Advancement of Teaching.

Ginsberg, E. (1995). A cautionary note on market reforms in health care. *Journal of the American Medical Association, 274,* 1633–1634.

Ginzberg, E. (1949). *A pattern of hospital care.* New York: Columbia University Press.

Goldmark, J. (Secretary). (1923). *Nursing and nursing education in the United States.* New York: Macmillan.

Greenberg, L. (1994). Work redesign: An overview. *Journal of Emergency Nursing, 20,* 28A–32A.

Herzberg, F. (1966). *Work and nature of man.* New York: World Publishing.

Hicks, E. J. (1938). A crusade for safer nursing. *American Journal of Nursing, 38,* 563–566.

Institute of Medicine. (1983). *Nursing and nursing education: Public policies and private actions.* Washington, DC: National Academy Press.

Kalisch, P. A., & Kalisch, B. J. (1986). *The advance of American nursing* (2nd ed.). Boston, Little, Brown.

Kelly, L. Y. & Joel, L. A. (1995). *Dimensions of professional nursing* (7th ed.). New York: McGraw-Hill.

Kjervik, D. K., & Martinson, I. M. (1979). *Women in stress: A nursing perspective.* New York: Appleton-Century-Crofts.

Maslow, A. (1954). *Motivation and personality.* New York: Harper & Row.

McLaughlin, F. E., Thomas, S. A., & Barter, M. (1995). Changes related to care delivery. *Journal of Nursing Administration, 25,* 35–46.

Montag, M. L. (1951). *The education of nursing technicians.* New York: G. P. Putnam's Sons.

Moore, E. J. (1900). Visiting nursing. *American Journal of Nursing, 1,* 17–21.

National Advisory Council on Nurse Education and Practice. (1996). *Report to the Secretary of the Department of Health and Human Services on the basic registered nurse workforce.* Rockville, MD: Health Resources and Services Administration, Division of Nursing.

National League for Nursing. (1995). *Mission and goals 1995–97 biennium.* New York: Author.

National League for Nursing Education. (1939). More graduate general duty nurses. *American Journal of Nursing, 39,* 898.

National Student Nurses Association. (1994). Getting the pieces to fit. New York: Author.

Nicholas, P. (1995). Issues in certification versus advanced practice licensure. *Nurse Practitioner, 20,* 12.

Nursing data book. (1982). New York: National League for Nursing.

Nursing data review. (1996). New York: National League for Nursing.

Parker, J. (1994). Development of the American Board of Nursing Specialties (1991–1993). *Nursing Management, 25,* 33–35.

Porter-O'Grady, T. (1987). Shared governance and new organizational models. *Nursing Economics, 5,* 281–286.

Roberts, M. M. (1954). *American nursing: History and interpretation.* New York: Macmillan.

School improvement program of the National League for Nursing 1951–1960. (1963). New York: Author.

Spradley, B. W. (1990). *Community health nursing: Concepts and practice.* Glenview, IL: Scott Foresman/Little Brown.

Stevens, R. (1971). *American medicine and the public interest.* New Haven, CT: Yale University Press.

Stillwagon, C. A. (1989). The impact of nurse-managed care on the cost of nurse practice and nurse satisfaction. *Journal of Nursing Administration, 19,* 21–27.

Weber, M. (1964). Theory of social and economic organization (4th ed.). New York: Free Press.

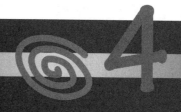

Socialization for Professional Practice

LEARNING OUTCOMES

By the end of this chapter, the student will be able to:

1 Define socialization and understand its scope.

2 Understand differences between adult learning and learning as a child.

3 Differentiate between separatist and integrated philosophies for teaching and learning.

4 Understand the effects of role-related stress.

5 Describe initial socialization processes.

6 Discuss possible effects of experience on resocialization processes.

7 Appreciate the emotions associated with educational resocialization.

8 Discuss issues related to socialization.

9 Apply active strategies toward a positive socialization experience.

Professional socialization is a term used to describe the "formation and internalization of a professional identity congruent with the professional role" (Lynn, McCain, & Boss, 1989, p. 232). Traditionally, the study of socialization has emphasized the ways in which external factors such as family, peers, school, and other institutions affect a person's development. Increasingly, however, socialization is being viewed as an interactive process between individual processes of learning and development and environmental influences. Socialization addresses questions about the *processes* of learning, the *content* learned, what *motivates* the learner, what *outcomes* are desired by the profession and society, and what accounts for *individual differences*.

Professional socialization addresses the processes by which a person develops a professional identity. It is assumed that learners are adults who acquire knowledge, skills, and attitudes for professional roles through teaching and learning in their initial educational programs. Any significant change in the environment, however, such as starting work in the practice setting or changing from a hospital to a community-based position or returning to school, then stimulates a resocialization process. Thus, resocialization is a lifelong occurrence. Although it may be challenging, active involvement with processes of change can reduce discomfort and promote personal and professional growth.

◎ Socialization Processes

Adult Learning

Much of the literature on socialization has focused on the child's development of the values and standards of the social group. Socialization has been viewed as an early and terminal process, with the family exerting primary influence through role modeling and reinforcement of desired behavior. However, increasing attention is now being paid to adult learning as a continuing and recurring process with important implications for the development of attitudes toward a professional career.

How people learn is an important question in socialization. Knowles popularized the term *andragogy* as the "art and science of helping adults learn, in contrast to pedagogy as the art and science of teaching children" (Knowles, 1980, p. 43). Because students of nursing are adults, his proposition that adults learn differently from children in a number of ways is relevant. Table 4-1 compares Knowles's assumptions regarding pedagogy and andragogy.

Knowles assumes that adult learners need to have:

1. A rationale for learning
2. A self-concept of being self-directed in decision-making
3. An accumulated experience that is a rich resource for learning
4. A readiness to learn that is oriented toward the developmental tasks of their social roles

TABLE 4-1

A Comparison of the Assumptions of Pedagogy and Andragogy

Regarding	Pedagogy	Andragogy
The need to know	Must learn what the teacher teaches	Need to know why they should learn something
Concept of the learner	Dependent. Teacher determines when, how, and what is to be learned, and whether it has been learned.	Responsible for own lives. Teachers facilitate self-direction in learning.
Role of learner's experience	Experience is of little worth. Only teacher's experience counts.	Have a rich reservoir of experience that is meaningful to them
Readiness to learn	Become ready to learn what they are told they must learn in order to pass.	Ready to learn what they need to know for real-life situations
Orientation to learning	Subject-centered. Education is a process of gaining knowledge that will be used later.	Life-centered. Education is a process of developing increased competence.
Motivation	External (eg, grades or parental pressure)	Internal (eg, self-esteem or quality of life)

From Knowles M: The Adult Learner: A Neglected Species, 4th ed. San Francisco, Jossey-Bass, 1990

5. An orientation toward learning that is shifted toward immediacy of application in performance, and
6. Motivation by applications to real-life situations (Knowles, 1990, pp. 57–63).

Lawler (1991) identified nine principles of adult learning:

1. Adult education requires a physical and social *climate of respect*
2. A *collaborative mode of learning* is central to adult education
3. Adult education includes and builds on the *experience* of the participant
4. Adult education fosters *critical reflective thinking*
5. *Problem-posing and problem-solving* are fundamental aspects of adult education
6. *Learning for action* is valued in adult education
7. Adult education is best facilitated in a *participative environment*
8. Adult education *empowers* the participant
9. *Self-directed learning* is encouraged and enhanced in adult education

These principles have a number of implications for adult education (Brookfield, 1991, p. 31; Knowles, 1984, pp. 9–18; Knowles, 1990, pp. 57–63; Lawler, 1991; O'Connor, 1986, pp. 32–38; Puetz, 1987, pp. 81–104):

1. The learning climate should be based on an atmosphere of respect and mutuality between the teacher and the learner. The physical environment should be informal and comfortable

2. The learner should be involved in diagnosis of learning needs, planning of the learning process, and self-evaluation of the effectiveness of learning (rediagnosis of needs). The teacher should be a resource and guide

3. Feedback and reasonable time limits for achievement should help the learner overcome fear of failure and a possible perception of not being smart carried over from childhood learning experiences

4. Support from peers and teachers can help the learner overcome personal problems, such as possible guilt at leaving his or her family while studying, or lack of confidence in learning capacity

5. Emphasis should be placed on practical application of information. Content should be relevant to the learner's needs and applicable to real-life problems

6. Participation in learning should be encouraged. Techniques such as discussion, simulation exercises, field experiences, and problem-solving situations should be used

7. Learners should be grouped on the basis of needs rather than content areas. The timing and sequence of material should be congruent with the developmental tasks of the learners

8. Unfreezing (ie, recognizing and accepting the need or benefit of a change) may be needed before the individual is ready to learn. Learning from experience should be encouraged

9. Learners represent different learning styles, orientation toward learning, and readiness to learn. Learning experiences should be individualized as much as possible

10. Teachers should be sensitive to the heavy demands placed on learners by tasks of daily life and personal expectations. At times, resources (physical, intellectual, social, and economic) may not be sufficient to meet these demands and also address the demands imposed by the learning situation

These implications for adult learning are applicable to nursing education and to practice with clients.

MODES OF TEACHING AND LEARNING

Traditional approaches to teaching and learning as socialization processes for both children and adults have been influenced by what can be labeled a *separatist* philosophy. Students have been viewed as basically similar raw material to be shaped by the socialization process. In this outcome-oriented view, the student must prove what has been "learned." Knowledge is first accumulated and then applied, with the assumption that theory-based knowledge exists apart from its application and can therefore be applied in any situation. Because disengaged scientific reasoning is highly valued in this view, thought must be separated from emotion, and cognition from affective responses.

Criticism of this approach has connected a focus on abstract and impersonal thinking with a relationship in which a subservient student defers to the authority of a dominant faculty (Horne, 1993). Lack of respect for previous knowledge and work experience, with consequent repetitiveness of content, has also been criticized as contributing to loss of student self-confidence and decreased instructor credibility (Horne, 1993).

Recently, what could be labeled an *integrated* philosophy for teaching and learning has been promoted (Diekelmann & Rather, 1993). This view emphasizes the interplay of theoretical knowledge and practical know-how. Knowledge and application move back and forth, with reflection on experience serving as one source of knowledge. Knowledge, therefore, is viewed as contextual, with meaning depending on the situation. The learner is a unique individual, whose interaction with the teaching situation is influenced by all past, present, and anticipated future influences. Teacher and learner have a collaborative relationship, promoting empowerment of both. A combination of cognitive and emotional responses, and intuition, contribute to a direct understanding of meaning. The separatist and integrated views of teaching and learning socialization processes are compared in Table 4-2.

ROLE THEORY

Professional socialization has been dominated by role theory from the discipline of sociology. In professional socialization, the emphasis is shifted from preparation for life in society to preparation for particular job expectations or roles. A *role* is defined as "a set of expectations that are associated with a position you hold in society" (Hamilton & Fiefer, 1986, p. 3).

TABLE 4-2
Comparison of Separatist and Integrated Views of Teaching/ Learning as Socialization Processes

Separatist View	Integrated View
Knowledge exists apart from application.	Knowledge exists in context.
Knowledge is first accumulated and then applied (additive).	Interplay of theoretical knowledge and practical know-how (dialogic)
Results oriented—must prove what is known.	Process oriented—knowledge evolves
Students are raw material to be shaped.	Students each have a unique history and future.
Analysis—examine differences between	Synthesis—look at commonalities among
Separation of thought from emotion and cognitive from affective (disengaged reasoning)	Embodied knowing
Education as job preparation	Education for lifelong learning

Adapted from Diekelmann NL, Rather ML: Transforming RN Education: Dialogue and Debate. New York, National League for Nursing, 1993.

Because roles are viewed as separate and discontinuous, it is assumed that stress occurs whenever a person assumes either a new role or new expectations within an existing role (Bradby, 1990). For example, when getting married, a woman assumes the new role of wife. In addition, new expectations might be assumed in an existing homemaker role. As adults, nursing students often "wear many hats," with multiple concurrent roles. These roles may include employee, parent, spouse, and provider for an aging parent. There is concern that multiple roles may contribute to role strain, adversely affecting both health and achievement. Given the current "reengineering" in the acute care environment, role strain is of significant concern.

Role strain may be described as a subjective sense of distress when role-related stress is experienced, related to one or more of the following areas:

Role conflict: the existence of clear but competing or incompatible expectations
Role ambiguity: the degree to which role expectations are unclear
Role overload: perceived inadequacy of time to achieve quantity or quality of expectations
Role incongruity: role expectations differing from the individual's self-perception, disposition, attitudes, or values
Role incompetence: perception of inadequate skills, knowledge, or ability to satisfactorily meet role expectations (Mobily, 1991, p. 74)

Any of these sources of role-related stress may be experienced by the nursing student. Signs of stress may include physical symptoms, depression, anxiety, obsessive–compulsive behavior, discomfort, anger, hostility, dissatisfaction, difficulty concentrating, poor grades, decreased productivity, decreased commitment, and "burnout" (McBride, 1988; Mobily, 1991). Role strain can be influenced by "the structure of an individual's social support network, the person's coping style, the centrality of each role to the self, and self-esteem" (McBride, 1988, p. 43).

However, current data suggest that the benefits of multiple roles far outweigh the strains, resulting in a net gain in well-being. By providing links to other persons and resources, multiple roles bring rewards such as privileges, status, security, self-esteem, personality enrichment, and social relationships. In contrast to the "scarcity hypothesis," which indicates that multiple roles compete for limited energy, the "expansion hypothesis" predicts that human energy reserves expand to meet the challenges of multiple roles, provided the roles are rewarding (Froberg et al., 1986, p. 81).

The ability to organize one's resources of time, money, or helpers (social support) to meet demands is beneficial in avoiding or coping with role overload. Role ambiguity, incongruity, and incompetence usually decrease with experience and the support of peers and faculty. However, role conflict may be of more concern as experience increases. Role conflict may be exacerbated by ethical, moral, and economic concerns, as well as by social and political issues. The extent to which role conflict is related to turnover or lack of satisfaction with clinical nursing is not known, but it is probably significant.

⊚ Initial Socialization Into Nursing

VIGNETTE: AMY

Amy, who is 25 years old, is a divorced mother with two small girls. She works as a secretary but has always dreamed of becoming a nurse. She has saved a little money to pay for tuition, but she worries about whether being older than the other students will feel strange. She also worries about whether she will be able to keep up with school work while caring for her children. But she decides that she has to try—it's now or never!

Most students enter nursing with a service orientation, in which they view themselves as doing things that will help sick people recover. In contrast,

> the professional educational image of the nurse is generally of one who (1) defines clients in terms of health and maintaining health, (2) views the relationship between the nurse and clients therapeutically and analytically, (3) approaches technical mastery of tools and procedures from the viewpoint of knowledge principles that guide their use, (4) uses critical inquiry processes to creatively manipulate knowledge in relation to clients concerns, and (5) accepts responsibility/accountability for patient care decisions (Hinshaw, 1976, p. 5).

Clearly, the socialization process involves changes in knowledge, attitudes, values, and skills. These changes can be associated with conflict and strong emotional reactions.

Davis suggested a six-stage model for the process of educational socialization (Hinshaw, 1976). In *stage one*, initial innocence, individuals enter an educational program. Students have an image of what they expect to become and of how they should behave. However, educational experiences (theory and clinical) are often directed toward behaviors that are different from the students' expectation. For example, in some schools, early learning experiences focus on communication with relatively healthy clients. Students who expect to give bed baths to sick patients may express disappointment and frustration and question the value of the educational experience.

In *stage two*, incongruities between initial images and apparent expectations of the educational system are identified, articulated, and shared among students. At this point, students may question whether or not they wish to continue in the program. Students who do continue then enter *stage three*, in which they identify what behaviors they are expected to exhibit by closely observing and monitoring the behavior of faculty members. In *stage four*, students begin to practice the behaviors through role simulation. Over time, these behaviors become a part of the individual. However, until these behaviors become internalized, the student may have a feeling of playing a game and not being true to self, which can produce guilt and confusion.

In *stage five,* students' behavior reflects vacillation between commitment to the new professional image and familiarity with the old lay image of nursing. It is hoped that both increasing identification with professional role models such as the faculty and increasing ability to use professional language will lead to reinforcement of the professional image. Students then move toward *stage six,* stable internalization of the professionally educationally approved model.

ISSUES REGARDING EDUCATIONAL PREPARATION

The issue of whether or not new graduates from any basic educational program are sufficiently prepared for the work setting has been debated for some time. Educators take the position that students are prepared for beginning practice. Employers charge that new graduates are not competent until they complete an expensive orientation period that may last as long as a year. Data suggest that acquiring competence takes at least 2 to 3 years, regardless of educational background (Benner, 1984).

What are the criteria by which new graduates are judged to be inadequate for the work setting? How do changing client needs and their impact on the delivery of care affect expectations of new graduates? What are the implications of the evolving practice environment for changes in educational preparation? Are psychomotor skills valued above cognitive and affective skills? Do students have sufficient educational practice time for competence in psychomotor skills? Does a perception of psychomotor inadequacy on the part of the new graduate interfere with the professional socialization from the educational program? Are new graduates prepared for autonomous practice in community settings? Nursing educators and service administrators must design collaborative strategies to address these issues, or the impasse will continue to have divisive effects on the profession.

Resocialization in the Work Setting

VIGNETTE: BETTY

Betty has been a surgical staff nurse for a month since her graduation from nursing school. She feels lucky to have this job but has become increasingly upset about the way she feels she is being treated by other nurses and the aides. She feels that they expect her to "hit the floor running," and fears that she is not carrying her share of the workload. Betty feels frustrated and angry. She is seriously thinking about leaving hospital nursing.

Preparation of the student for the work setting is only the initial process in socialization. When the new professional enters the work setting, another socialization process occurs. The nurse is faced with the need to make operational the profession's values in primarily bureaucratic settings, which often are not supportive of professional career development. Thus, the transition from the educational setting to the workplace is difficult for many individuals. Kramer (1974) describes a postgraduate resocialization model for the resolution of value and role conflict between the generalized knowledge and skills acquired in the educational program and the specific behaviors required for successful accomplishment in the work setting.

KRAMER'S POSTGRADUATE RESOCIALIZATION MODEL

Stage one in this model is skill and routine mastery. New graduates arrive in the work setting with principles and are confronted with the need to function in a specific manner. Initially the new graduate feels inadequate and frustrated, and responds by focusing on mastery of specific skills and techniques. Certainly, the development of technical expertise is desirable. However, a potential problem at this stage is that the nurse may fixate on technical skills and be unable to refocus on the other important aspects of nursing care.

Stage two is social integration. The nurse's major concern at this stage is getting along with coworkers and being accepted into the group. This probably requires prior mastery of skills and peer recognition of competence and efficiency. The potential problem at this stage is that the nurse may fear alienating newly acquired colleagues if she begins to apply the knowledge and orientation gained in the educational setting.

Stage three is expressed as moral outrage. Corwin (1961) identified three role conceptions believed held in varying degrees by all nurses:

The bureaucratic role conception, associated with rules and regulations of nursing care delivery within the organization, with primary loyalty to the hospital administration

The professional role conception, associated with principles and standards, with primary loyalty to the profession and commitment to knowledge and continued learning

The service role conception, associated with values such as humanity, compassion, dedication, and understanding, with primary loyalty to the client as an individual

In stage three, the incongruities among these roles in the actual work setting are realized. The new graduate feels frustrated, angry, and inadequately prepared.

In *stage four*, individuals either capitulate their behaviors or values, or integrate the professional and bureaucratic systems by using four types of conflict resolution:

1. Behavioral capitulation: change of behavior but not of values. Individuals usually leave nursing altogether or choose a work situation outside organized service settings
2. Value capitulation: values of the bureaucratic system are accepted and the values gained in the educational program are given up
3. Conformity: both values and behaviors are given up and the individual simply maintains a working position
4. Biculturalism: the healthiest and most successful type (Kramer, 1974, p. 162). Nurses realize that they are not only a target of influence and pressure from others, but also are individuals able to influence others as well. "In essence, these new graduates are able to identify and use the values and behaviors of both the professional and bureaucratic work systems in a politically astute manner" (Hinshaw, 1976, p. 8)

BENNER'S NOVICE TO EXPERT MODEL

Although Kramer's model applies exclusively to graduates from an initial educational program, Benner (1984) and Benner, Tanner, and Chesla (1996) have described a model of stages from novice to expert that is relevant for experienced nurses. Benner (1984, p. 13) describes stages in the progression of patient care expertise that can result from practical nursing experience (Table 4-3). This model, based on work by Dreyfus and Dreyfus (1986), suggests three general aspects of skilled performance:

1. Movement from reliance on abstract principles to use of past concrete experience as paradigms
2. Change in perception of the demand situation from a compilation of equally important bits of information to a more or less complete whole in which only certain parts are relevant
3. Passage from a detached observer to an involved performer who is engaged in the situation

TABLE 4-3

Benner's Stages From Novice to Expert

	Stage I	Stage II	Stage III	Stage IV	Stage V
Title	Novice	Advanced beginner	Competent	Proficient	Expert
Experience level	Graduate	New graduate	2–3 years in same setting	3–5 years	Extensive
Characteristics of performance	Is inflexible Exhibits rule-governed behavior	Formulates principles Needs help with priority setting	Plans Feelings of mastery	Perceives "wholes" Interprets nuances	Has an intuitive grasp

Adapted from Benner P: From Novice to Expert. Menlo Park, CA, Addison-Wesley 1984, pp. 21–34.

Stage one, the novice stage, corresponds to the student experience in nursing school. Because no background understanding exists, the novice depends on context-free rules to guide actions. But although this approach enhances safety, "rule-governed behavior is extremely limited and inflexible" (Benner, 1984, p. 21).

The new nursing graduate demonstrates marginally acceptable performance as an advanced beginner in *stage two*. The advanced beginner relies on basic theory and principles and believes that "clinical situations have a discernible order" (Benner et al., 1996, p. 54). The advanced beginner can formulate principles for actions, but because all actions are viewed as equally important, help is needed for priority setting.

The competent practitioner who has reached *stage three* typically has worked in the same setting for 2 to 3 years. The competent practitioner is consciously aware of long-range goals and can engage in deliberate planning based on abstract and analytical contemplation. As a result of this planning activity, the practitioner has a feeling of mastery and the ability to cope with contingencies and feels efficient and organized.

By *stage four,* which requires 3 to 5 years of experience, the nurse is a proficient practitioner. The proficient nurse perceives situations as wholes rather than as accumulations of aspects, and performance is guided by maxims. Actions do not need to be thought out, and meanings are perceived in relation to long-term goals. In addition, the proficient practitioner can interpret nuances in situations and recognize which aspects of the situation are most significant.

The *fifth stage,* that of expert practitioner, is achieved only after extensive experience. The expert has an intuitive grasp of situations and thus does not have to think through actions analytically. In fact, the expert is so skilled at grasping the situation as a whole that she often is unable to think in terms of steps in thinking.

Benner (1984, p. 46) has suggested that 31 different competencies are evident in actual clinical practice, organized into seven domains of nursing practice:

1. The helping role
2. The teaching–coaching function
3. The diagnostic and patient monitoring function
4. Effective management of rapidly changing situations
5. Administration and monitoring of therapeutic interventions and regimens
6. Monitoring of and ensuring the quality of health care practices
7. Organizational and work role competencies

Benner states that experience is absolutely necessary for the development of professional expertise. In contrast to Kramer, who focused on the role conflict that may occur as "reality" is integrated with "expectations," Benner describes the stimulus to judgment that occurs when "preconceived notions and expectations are challenged, refined, or disconfirmed by the actual situation" (1984, p. 3).

ISSUES IN EDUCATIONAL PREPARATION FOR THE PRACTICE OF NURSING

Within the traditional, separatist model of teaching and learning, the experienced nurse who has returned to school has been viewed as having deficits in knowledge and a technical skill orientation to practice that must be changed. In contrast, Benner's view is of "the advantages of the experience-rich students returning for a period of scholarly development and reflection" (Benner, 1993, p. 3). When practical experience is viewed as a resource instead of a hindrance, reflection on past experience in the light of new theoretical or scientific information provides an opportunity to challenge, test, and refine theoretical knowledge, creates openness for future clinical learning, and facilitates changes in perception and self-concept (Benner, 1993).

Diekelmann and Rather (1993, p. 35) have described a number of issues they believe can be learned from practice:

1. Gaining a sense of self as a nurse
2. Coping with technology and the technology/human interface
3. Developing a sense of future possibilities—learning about trajectories and learning to keep open to the possibilities in the situation
4. Negotiating with physicians, moving from a stance of delegating responsibility "up" to assuming responsibility for making a case for what a patient needs in a particular situation
5. Facing suffering and death
6. Learning the skill of involvement
7. Learning to cope with own anxieties, fears, and concerns
8. Getting situated in the practice—learning timing, the sense of personal, client, and family space, learning the art of watchfulness, and learning the pace of the unit

◎ Resocialization Through Education

VIGNETTE: CLAIRE

Claire works as a staff nurse on a busy medical floor. Over the past few years she has seen how health care reform has decreased staff and allocation of resources. There are continued demands to do more with less. She finds it rewarding to help people, but her frustration is mounting as achieving daily tasks has become increasingly difficult. She has recently been pondering the thought of returning to school for a bachelor's degree.

Many students choose educational mobility as an alternative route to nursing education. This may involve moving from practical nursing into an associate degree program for registered nursing, or it may involve baccalaureate education following initial nursing education at the associate degree or diploma level. At each level, resocialization is needed to help the student synthesize the changed theory base and new role expectations. But the resocialization may not be fully effective, and the student may finish the program with more knowledge but without changes in behavior reflecting an internalized professional self-image.

KELMAN'S PROCESSES OF SOCIAL INFLUENCE

Kelman (1961) has identified three processes of social influence: compliance, identification, and internalization. In the process of *compliance,* the individual has not accepted the values or expectations of the influencing person or group, but behaves in an expected way to get positive responses. In the process of *identification,* there is selective adoption of certain behaviors perceived as acceptable because they are associated with a role relationship that forms a part of the individual's self-image. However, this does not necessarily include an acceptance of values. It is only in the process of *internalization* that an individual accepts the norms and standards of the new role because he or she believes in them and they have become a part of the person's own value system. An area that needs further study is the effect of the degree of opinion and value change on the course and the extent of later resocialization.

SHANE'S RETURNING-TO-SCHOOL SYNDROME

Shane (1980) describes the positive and negative emotional states experienced by RNs who return to school for baccalaureate education. She labels these states the "returning-to-school syndrome." The first phase, the honeymoon, is positive. The nurse is attuned to the similarities between previous education and the present experience, and these similarities tend to reinforce the original role identity as a nurse. Typically, however, during the first nursing theory or practice course, this phase ends.

The next stage, conflict, is characterized by turbulent negative emotions. Nurses feel increasingly inadequate to meet the new professional demands because they can no longer trust previous experience and knowledge to determine appropriate responses. The nursing student is acutely aware that the old rules are no longer valid, but has not yet understood or accepted the new ones. This stage is often associated with depression and bursts of anger, feelings of helplessness, and academic difficulties.

The beginning of reintegration is characterized by a strong rejection of the new culture—the baccalaureate program. The most common behavior expressed during this stage is hostility, which in its extreme form may result in the student leaving the program to return to the more familiar culture. Shane indicates that

the length of time any individual spends in the hostility phase and the mode of resolution probably depends on the overall resiliency of the individual, the intensity of the emotions and experiences she is feeling, and the interpretation and guidance provided by those significant others (faculty, peers, family) surrounding her (Shane, 1980, p. 123).

Achievement of an ability to integrate the original culture of work with the new culture of school is a positive resolution of the returning-to-school syndrome. The student recognizes personal strengths and growth and also recognizes that graduating will mean functioning in a different way than before. The student's sense of "what nursing is" is forever altered, but it contains elements of both the previous and the new conceptions. The student has not denied the original values and orientation, but is now directed toward getting as much as possible from the academic experience.

Unfortunately, there are two maladaptive dead ends in which some individuals become trapped as a resolution of the conflict stage. One is false acceptance, in which the student feigns to the faculty and to herself a belief in the value, worth, or validity of the baccalaureate program just to complete the program. In the other, chronic hostility, the student does not drop out of school, but persists in vigorous fighting to defend the original nursing ego identity. This student resists the opportunity for real growth and positive change.

Throwe and Fought (1987) developed an assessment tool for use by both faculty and students to assess resocialization progress (Table 4-4). Based on Erickson's theory of developmental stages needed to be mastered through life, the tool presents behaviors that can be observed as developmental tasks associated with role identification. (For another application of Erickson's theory of self-development, see Chap. 5). The student can use the tool as a guide for self-evaluation of growth.

ISSUES IN PROFESSIONAL SOCIALIZATION

Diverse Needs of the Learner

Registered nurses who return to school for baccalaureate education in nursing provide unique challenges for professional resocialization. Their personal characteristics of age, gender, psychological needs, habitual ways of thinking, experience, family situations, and orientation toward education are diverse, and these characteristics influence the educational process in complex ways.

Jako (1981) found that RNs have one or more of five dominant purposes or orientations for seeking baccalaureate education:

1. Provision of service: service to clients in inpatient or community settings
2. Care for patients: direct care of needy clients in various settings
3. Attainment of vertical mobility: advancement toward increased power, influence, and authority

4. Acquisition and dissemination of knowledge: "may be less interested in providing patient care than in teaching, conducting research, or perhaps promoting the status and respectability of academic nursing" (Jako, 1981, p. 6)
5. Frontiering: moving into new areas of nursing to enjoy greater independence or to change the profession

Frontiering was the dominant orientation among 28% of the 437 nurses studied, but role expectations became more complex and less unidimensional as the educational experience progressed. The orientation of the learner may have a significant impact on the educational experience, but the degree to which it may influence identification with and internalization of professional roles is unknown.

Registered nurses who return to school for baccalaureate education are adults of varying ages. Diverse experiential backgrounds suggest the need for individualized learning experiences to facilitate professional resocialization. Some educational programs have adjusted their structure to apply principles of adult learning.

King found that RNs "were not just 'older students,' but rather the RNs had advanced further along both the life stage and ego development continuums" (King, 1988, p. 134). Confronted with the need to learn and internalize new information, they must overcome prejudices and habitual ways of thinking. In addition, many have full-time jobs as well as family responsibilities, and some have to overcome resistance by family members to their return to school. Some have been away from school for a long time, and have to deal with the conflict between the psychological dependency of the student role and the need of the adult to be self-directed. In addition, many nurses have to deal with their perception of nursing as a "good job for a woman," rather than as a lifelong career commitment.

Issues Regarding the Resocialization Process

Socialization has been described as "a process that produces attitudes, values, knowledge, and skills required to participate effectively as an individual or group member" (Kozier & Erb, 1988, p. 47). This definition highlights an inherent conflict: Is socialization a process, or is it an outcome? Many authors (Conway, 1984; Hinshaw, 1976; Kozier & Erb, 1988) refer to socialization as a continuing, interactive, lifelong process. They describe socialization as adaptation to the changing roles that characterize human development as well as professional growth. This view emphasizes the longitudinal and fluid nature of socialization and implies that the educational setting should provide the learner with initial skills for professional practice. These skills will be further developed or modified in the course of continuing education and practice in changing roles. *(text continues on page 92)*

TABLE 4-4

Resocialization Assessment Tool

Developmental task	Role-Resisting Behaviors Observed	Role-Accepting Behaviors Observed
Trust/mistrust Learns to trust the worlds of education and work through consistency and repetitive experiences	Physically isolated from peers both in class, clinical Does not initiate interactions with others Responds only if called on	Involved with classmates Readily and quickly forms/joins groups when directed Initiates discussions with others Asks for clarification
Autonomy/doubt Begins to develop independence while under supervision	Delays joining groups for unstructured activities Does not contribute equally Forgets or suppresses assignment dates Does not meet target dates Self-conscious about being evaluated by others	Joins groups for unstructured activities (study groups) Shares information with group, prepares for activities Meets target dates Able to interact in the teaching/learning environment Begins to develop independence with guidance
Initiative/guilt Can independently identify, plan, and implement skills/assignments	Perceives objectives and assignments as not worthwhile Stress-related symptoms increase Has difficulty setting priorities Waits for instructor to initiate priority setting Lacks initiative to deal with conflicts Unaware of available resources	Objectives and assignments take on meaning Applies new skills, content to other work settings Effective in time management Renegotiates deadline extensions when appropriate Takes initiative in resolving conflict situations Aware of and uses available resources
Industry/inferiority Behavior is dominated by performance of tasks and curiosity—individuals need encouragement to attempt and master skills	Elicits performance rewards and feedback from others Needs direct encouragement especially when performing affective and cognitive skills Last to volunteer to demonstrate new behaviors Seeks rewards by performing old familiar skills rather than those in new dimensions Demonstrates disengaging behaviors (late, uninterested, resistive to learning opportunities)	Able to reward self Confidence thrives Eager to try out new skills; takes risks Volunteers to demonstrate new behaviors Profits from guidance and direction of others Applies self beyond family/work setting Curiosity channeled through educational system
Identity/role confusion The individual searches for continuity and structure, is concerned with how he/she is accepted by others; how he/she is accepted by self; each individual struggles to shape or formulate own identity	Needs a structured clinical setting to further develop ego identity Sees old job as ideal and denies need for change Serious about learning (content and clinical practice) Frustrated with nursing as a career choice Too ideological or overly critical of others	Searches for continuity and structure but can adapt to unstructured clinical settings Identifies role models in clinical setting Articulates need for change or for modification of job-related roles and procedures Appears to enjoy learning and performing in clinical settings Idealistic about own achievements and progress in educational system

Intimacy/isolation

Seeks to combine his/her identity with other self-selected individuals

Participates as a member but resists group leader role
Does not participate in professional meetings
Unsupportive of others' educational advancement
Feels no increased esteem in performing new role behaviors
Meets minimal requirements and sees instructor only in evaluative role
Resists using newly developed skills, more comfortable with previous level of performance
Avoids giving feedback to agency personnel

Volunteers to lead work/study groups
Participates in professional organizations
Recruits others and represents school
Demonstrates pride in new role behaviors and shares with others in work settings
Seeks out instructor for additional learning, information, and professional growth opportunities
Values symbols of profession (using assessment tools, RN name tags)
Evaluates ability of clinical agencies to facilitate meeting learner objectives
Provides feedback to agency personnel

Generativity/stagnation

Efforts are made to guide and direct incoming students; assists others

Avoids social interaction and information sharing with incoming students
Provides minimal care, unconcerned about continuity of patient care
Selects patients with common familiar clinical disorders
No increased ease of learning or improved test-taking abilities
Does not elect to test out of course requirements
Stagnates in same job setting

Guides and directs incoming students
Provides quality nursing care to patient, family, and community
Takes calculated risks (questions level of care, seeks multiple learning opportunities, shares level of expertise, elects to test out required/elective courses)
Demonstrates critical problem-solving skills
Attains mastery of test-taking skills
Self-directed learner
Demonstrates clinical problem-solving in own work setting
Uses holistic approach to delivery of health care

Ego integrity/despair

Acceptance of one's own progress, achievement, and goals through realistic self-appraisal

Frustrated with progress and achievement; stagnated in developing new goals
Crisis prone when changing roles
Self appraisal unrealistic
Does not participate in structured educational opportunities
Returns to old job and does not modify role performance
Sees no reward in risk-taking
High risk for dissatisfaction with profession

Accepts progress, achievement and goal attainment
Realistic in self-appraisal
Resets professional goals (graduate school, participation in continuing education, certification)
Joins new perspectives on old job by use of critical thinking
Takes risks (new jobs, different clinical setting, and leadership roles)

*From Throwe AN, & Fought SG: Landmarks in the socialization process from RN to BSN. Nurse Educator 12, 1987, pp. 16–17. Reprinted by permission of Lippincott-Raven Publishers.

The contrasting view stresses professional outcomes as a result of socialization in an educational program. Thus, new graduates are compared for their degree of attainment of attributes considered professional, and employing agencies expect competent practice of a new graduate.

Every role change is associated with conflict and stress. Socialization of the student to practice as it should be, rather than as it is, exacerbates stress and contributes to early burnout. However, internalization of the ideal role, along with knowledge and experience to facilitate change, is necessary to correct the current ambiguity, lack of autonomy, and limits to professional development of the typical institutional work setting.

It is also essential that the student gain skills to function successfully in the practice arena as it currently exists. For many nurses, that will include the need to develop skills for community-based practice, perhaps with limited hospital experience. In other words, baccalaureate education has the difficult task of socializing the student to competent practice as an outcome, as well as providing the basis for the process of continuing professional resocialization.

Professional organizations agree that baccalaureate education is the minimum education necessary for professional nursing practice. There is broad acceptance of the desirability of characteristics of professional practice. In fact, given the trend in hospitals toward reduction of numbers of RNs in the name of cost containment, critical thinking and professional nursing process skills are essential for all nurses.

The absence of agreement within the profession about levels of nursing raises many issues for educational resocialization. If some diploma and associate degree programs socialize their graduates to perceive that they are professional nurses, how is later resocialization in a baccalaureate program affected? Are there measurable qualitative differences between graduates of "generic" 4-year baccalaureate programs compared to graduates of educational mobility pathways? Is one kind of pathway better? What processes and strategies best facilitate a synthesis of professional knowledge and values with prior educational outcomes?

Data are needed about the factors that facilitate the socialization process. How is the resocialization process affected when students concurrently work in a practice arena acknowledged to reinforce technical practice, while attending classes preparing for professional role changes? Lynn and colleagues (1989) found that RN–BSN students did not change significantly in their conceptualization of the professional role during their baccalaureate education, and held significantly lower program-exit professional orientation scores than generic students.

Estok (1977) asks if reinforcement of technical skills and knowledge is a desirable base for professional socialization. Where are the clinical role models to facilitate professional resocialization? Evidence suggests that a group of people who start a program together can facilitate a "collective passage" (Bradby, 1990), supporting each other, and contributing to a sharing of attitudes and beliefs. Is socialization a process vaguely perceived by the faculty to be needed, or is it a content area integrated throughout the curriculum?

Despite these concerns, some research data are available that document the effectiveness of resocialization in baccalaureate programs for RNs (Lawler & Rose, 1987). Brian, in a study of graduates of six programs, found that "the programs seem to have accomplished their goal of improving the professional orientation of their graduates" (1980, p. 51). The programs were associated with a significant ($p = 0.001$) difference in the graduates attending meetings or workshops, acting as a resource person, acting as a leader or coordinator, reading nursing journals, doing nursing research, being interested in nursing organizations, writing nursing articles, and belonging to nursing organizations.

Leddy (1982) found that a baccalaureate degree program for RNs was associated with significant ($p = 0.01$) change in five personality variables: decreased need for abasement and increased need for change, dominance, sentience, and harm avoidance. The personality changes persisted when subjects were retested 2 to 4 years after completing the program.

The educational setting has the potential to contribute to effective resocialization for professional practice. Success is vital to continued progress in the development of the nursing profession.

Active Involvement in Socialization
Shifts in capabilities, interests, priorities, awareness, and professional values are normal in the life cycle of any career. Some of the implications of a lifelong process of change are:

- Expect periods of great satisfaction and challenge to alternate with periods of dissatisfaction and distress. Be prepared for periods of discomfort.
- How you view role change (challenge or crisis) depends on how you choose to respond to the changes. Take control of your career.
- Role changes affect all aspects of personal and professional life. Perception of crisis or challenge may be related to availability of support in at least one area. Develop personal and professional support systems and ask directly for help.
- Do your best but do not try to be perfect. Learn to let go, relax, and allow yourself to be human.
- Avoiding action prolongs and intensifies discomfort.
- Be willing to compromise and make trades. Use delegation and negotiation.
- Identify, respect, and live within the limits of your energy, resources, and time. You can choose to let go of roles that you are unable to fulfill at a given time.
- Take care of yourself. Practice a healthy lifestyle. Make time for your needs. You need stamina and insight.
- Holding on to the past can hinder growth, diminish enjoyment of the present, and block development. Keep the positive and let go of the negative (Hamilton & Kiefer, 1986).

◎ Conclusion

Professional socialization in nursing involves initial socialization in the educational setting, followed by a resocialization process in the work setting. Baccalaureate education for RNs provides educational resocialization experiences, made more complex by the diversity, psychological needs, and multiple roles of adult learners.

THOUGHT QUESTIONS

1 In what ways may "practical experience" enhance or detract from your professional socialization?

2 What resocialization is needed for community-based rather than hospital-based practice?

3 What can the student do to promote adult and integrated approaches to learning?

4 How would you respond to Amy and Betty's concerns in the vignettes?

5 How effective are you in incorporating professional roles into your professional self-identity? What can you do to promote positive socialization experiences?

REFERENCES

Benner, P (1984). *From novice to expert.* Menlo Park, CA: Addison-Wesley.

Benner, P. (1993). Transforming RN education: Clinical learning and clinical knowledge development. In N. L. Diekelmann & M. L. Rather (Eds.). *Transforming RN education: Dialogue and debate* (pp. 3–14). New York: National League for Nursing.

Benner, P., Tanner, C. A., & Chesla, C. A. (1996). *Expertise in nursing practice: Caring, clinical judgment, and ethics.* New York: Springer.

Bradby, M. (1990). Status passage into nursing: Another view of the process of socialization. *Journal of Advanced Nursing, 15,* 1220–1225.

Brian, S. (1980). The bottom line: Graduates and careers. In K. Jako (Ed.). *Proceedings of researching second step nursing education* Vol. 1, 45–54. Rohnert Park, CA: Sonoma State University.

Brookfield, S. D. (1991). *Understanding and facilitating adult learning.* San Francisco: Jossey-Bass.

Conway, M. E. (1984). Socialization and roles in nursing. In H. H. Werley & J. J. Fitzpatrick (Eds.). *Annual review of nursing research* (Vol. 1, pp. 183–208). New York: Springer.

Corwin, R. G. (1961). Role conception and career aspiration: A study of identity in nursing. *Sociology Quarterly, 2,* 69–86.

Diekelmann, N. L., & Rather, M. L. (Eds.). (1993). *Transforming RN education: Dialogue and debate.* New York: National League for Nursing.

Dreyfus, S., & Dreyfus, H. L. (1986). *Mind over machine.* New York: The Free Press.

Estok, P. (1977). Socialization theory and entry into the practice of nursing. *Image, 9,* 8–14.

Froberg, D., Gjerdingen, D., & Preson, M. (1986, Summer). Multiple roles and women's mental and physical health: What have we learned? *Women and Health, II,* 79–96.

Hamilton, J. M., & Keifer, M. E. (1986). *Survival skills for the new nurse.* Philadelphia: Lippincott.

Hinshaw, A. S. (1976, November). *Socialization and resocialization of nurses for professional nursing practice.* (National League for Nursing Publication No. 15-1659, pp. 1–15). New York: National League for Nursing.

Horne, C. D. (1993). Ideological barriers to nursing education for returning RN students. In Diekelmann, N. L. and Rather, M. L. (Eds.). *Transforming RN education: Dialogue and debate.* New York: National League for Nursing.

Jako, K. L. (1981, January). Five professional nursing orientations. In K. L. Jako (Ed.). *Proceedings of researching second step nursing education* Vol. 2, pp. 3–27. Rohnert Park, CA: Sonoma State University.

Kelman, H. (1961). Processes of opinion changes. *Public Opinion Quarterly, 25,* 57–78.

King, J. E. (1988). Differences between RN and generic students and the impact on the educational process. *Journal of Nursing Education, 27,* 131–135.

Knowles, M. (1990). *The adult learner: A neglected species* (4th ed.). Houston: Gulf.

Knowles, M. S. (1980). *The modern practice of adult education: From pedagogy to andragogy.* Chicago: Follett.

Knowles, M. S. (1984). *Andragogy in action.* San Francisco: Jossey-Bass.

Kozier, B., & Erb, G. (1988). *Concepts and issues in nursing practice.* Menlo Park, CA: Addison-Wesley.

Kramer, M. (1974). *Reality shock: Why nurses leave nursing.* St. Louis: Mosby.

Lawler, P. A. (1991). *The keys to adult learning: Theory and practical strategies.* Philadelphia: Research for Better Schools.

Lawler, T. G., & Rose, M. A. (1987, May/June). Professionalization: A comparison among generic baccalaureate. ADN, and RN/BSN nurses. *Nurse Educator, 12,* 19–22.

Leddy, S, (1982, October). Personality changes associated with baccalaureate education for registered nurses [Abstract]. *Journal of Nursing Education, 21,* 45–46.

Lynn, M. R., McCain, N. L., & Bass, B. J. (1989). Socialization of RN to BSN. *Image, 21,* 232–237.

McBride, A. B. (1988). Mental health effects of women's multiple roles. *Image, 20,* 41–47.

Mobily, P. R. (1991, February). An examination of role strain for university nurse faculty and its relation to socialization experiences and personal characteristics. *Journal of Nursing Education, 30,* 73–80.

O'Connor, A. B. (1986). *Nursing staff development and continuing education.* Boston: Little, Brown.

Puetz, B. E. (1987). *Contemporary strategies for continuing education in nursing.* Rockville, MD: Aspen.

Shane, D. L. (1980). The returning-to-school syndrome. In S. Mirin (Ed.). *Teaching tomorrow's nurse* (pp. 119–126). Wakefield, MA: Nursing Resources.

Throwe, A. N., & Fought, S. G. (1987). Landmarks in the socialization process from RN to BSN. *Nurse Educator, 12,* 15–18.

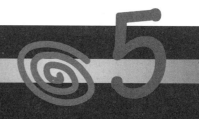

Development and Care of the Professional Self-Concept

LEARNING OUTCOMES

By the end of this chapter, the student will be able to:

1 Identify the characteristics of human systems that influence the development of the personal or professional self.

2 Explain the significance of reflected appraisals to the development of the professional self-concept.

3 Explain the influence of society's image of the profession on the individual nurse's professional self-concept.

4 Identify the goals associated with each stage of development of the professional self.

5 Identify some of the outcomes in the professional self-concept, if the nurse does not view self as an autonomous professional being.

(continued)

6 For female students, appreciate what it means to be socialized as a nurse according to the traditional feminine view of women and how that view affects the achievement of a professional image in society.

7 Identify signs of professional "burnout," and ways to promote "healthy helping."

8 Appreciate ways to promote a healthy lifestyle.

Nursing's primary concern is with human beings (Rogers, 1970, p. 41). Human beings experience the process of life along with other living systems. However, they show the greatest complexity in the sequential development of behavior and possess one attribute believed missing in other living systems: the capacity for conscious awareness of self and the world. This consciousness provides the basis for human rationality, creativity, and humanness. "People are thinking, feeling beings" (Rogers, 1970, p. 41). This awareness of self is the basis for self-concept.

As a person develops patterns of behavior, the self-system becomes organized and strives to actualize itself, although it is continually undergoing change, being repatterned, and affecting the environment in a significant way. These interactional experiences with the environment provide the substance from which a view of the self emerges—the self-concept. As a person, the nurse is continually interacting with the personal environment; as a professional, the nurse is continually interacting with the professional environment. Because human beings develop personal selves first, those personally organized sets of behaviors form the basis of the selves brought into the profession. Thus, the personal self is highly influential on the emerging professional self.

Several assumptions can be made about the development of human self-systems:

1. The human being is an open system, constantly affecting and being affected by other human beings and nonhumans in the environment

2. "Man interacts with his environment in his totality" (Rogers, 1970, p. 44). (Rogers uses the term "man" here in a nonsexist way to mean human being.)

3. As open systems, human beings demonstrate continuous interaction with their surroundings. Energy and materials are constantly being interchanged. The human system both shares with and takes in energy and materials in the environment (Rogers, 1970, p. 49)

4. "Man—environment transactions are characterized by continuous repatterning of both man and environment" (Rogers, 1970, p. 53)

5. "It is in the mutual changing and being changed that evolution proceeds" (Rogers, 1970, p. 54)

6. The evolutionary process is descriptive of or analogous with the development of the self-system, both personal and professional

◎ Theoretical Basis of Self-Concept: Interaction

Known as the father of the interpersonal school of thought in psychiatry, Sullivan attributed great power to the interactional process between the developing person and the "mothering one" (ie, the significant other person in getting needs met). He theorized that the self-system—"the system involved in the maintenance of felt interpersonal security" (Sullivan, 1953, p. 109)—emerges from the interpersonal cooperation in acculturation and the socialization process for the human. "The self-system . . . is an organization of educative experience called into being by the necessity to avoid or to minimize incidents of anxiety" (Sullivan, 1953, p. 165). In humans, anxiety is viewed as "anticipated unfavorable appraisal of one's current activity by someone whose opinion is significant" (Sullivan, 1953, p. 113). The self-concept can be seen as the personal view of oneself developed from interaction with significant others.

Using Sullivan's view of development, Lancaster and Lancaster (1982) stated that the self is formulated through conscious and unconscious perceptions of one's experiences, including achievements, failures, conflicts, embarrassments, and accomplishments. The self is constantly reinforced by feedback responses received from significant persons in one's environment (Lancaster & Lancaster, 1982, pp. 72–77). When the message received is a positive appraisal, the part of the self reinforced is the "good me"; when the message received is a negative appraisal, the part of the self reinforced is the "bad me"; and when the message received is associated with overwhelming anxiety, the part of the self reinforced is the "not me" (Sullivan, 1953, pp. 161–164).

THE SIGNIFICANCE OF REFLECTED APPRAISALS

The view of the personal self is directly related to the appraisals that occur in the personal relationship with significant other persons. As humans develop over the life span, the significant other persons change. In infancy, the parent most directly involved in caregiving is the significant other; that changes to both parents in early childhood, and to other adults next; then to peers of the same sex; then to peers of the opposite sex; and finally to the partners of the mature adult.

In all stages of life, the relationship between a person and her or his significant other is central to acculturation and socialization because learning depends on one's view of self and the existing anxiety level. An inverse relationship exists between one's awareness of self and the anxiety level experienced in the person–significant other relationship. Perceived anxiety in either high dosage or continuous patterns leads to a perception of the self as bad. A person with a bad view of self has learned that view of self through patterns of relatedness established with significant others in circumstances of high anxiety. Positive appraisals result in the perception of self as good. A person with a good view of self has learned that view of self through patterns of relatedness established with significant others in circumstances of low anxiety.

The development of the professional self follows the same path as that of development of the personal self. In every profession, the professional has significant others. Nurses have had different significant others during their various stages of growth and development. These significant others have differed in gender, socioeconomic status, and educational and cultural backgrounds.

Those others who are significant in terms of professional self-development are determined to some degree by the nurse's adjustments to changing situations. The professional nurse moves in and out of new situations. Adjusting to the perceived expectations of the significant other in each situation, the nurse tries to be the kind of person the situation demands. Highly related to how successful the nurse is in moving in and out of changing situations is the nurse's personal self-view, as well as the sensitivity to the professional significant other. The personal self-concept cannot be separated from the professional self-concept, although the professional significant others are different from the personal significant others.

Societal Values of Nursing and Nurses

The nurse's view of self as a professional is greatly influenced by the image of nursing and nurses as portrayed by the public and the profession. People are more reactive to the nurse's personal than professional qualities. The responsibility for the primary focus on personal rather than professional characteristics lies with both the public and nurses. Popular television presents nurses more in terms of their personal qualities and female role expectations than in terms of their professional abilities and responsibilities. Nurses themselves have not marketed their scholarship. Indeed, some nurses still oppose university and college education for nurses. This attitude keeps nursing out of the mainstream of education for the professions.

Nurses will need to deal with the conflicts arising from social oppression before they can exhibit a professional image of pride and expertise. Nursing leaders have recognized that role behavior of the professional nurse is largely related to the image of the nurse held by health care consumers. Thus, the profession has made concerted efforts to influence the mass media to present a scholarly image of the profession and a competent image of the practitioner. The mass media's influence on the consumer perhaps offers the best strategy for changing the professional self-image of nurses. Indeed, the reflected appraisal of the nurse by the consumer plays a vital role in shaping the individual nurse's professional self-concept.

⟳ The Professional Self

To a great extent, the kind of professional a person becomes depends on the person's self-system. The professional self-system emerges from the personal self.

PERSONAL SELF-SYSTEM'S IMPACT ON THE PROFESSIONAL SELF

One's self-concept "results from previous interpersonal relationships" (Simms & Lindberg, 1978, p. 9) and affects one's future relationships. "A person's view of self controls the roles he or she will be able to assume" (Simms & Lindberg, 1978, p. 9). One's self-system determines one's personal characteristics, and these personal qualities enable one to carry out professional roles in more or less successful ways.

Sheehy (1982) cites several qualities of those persons who successfully navigate their roles in life. These qualities are direct outcomes of the development of the self-concept:

1. Willingness to take risks is an outcome of a positive self-concept reflecting the person's ability to trust others, to be confident in assuming responsibilities, and to direct initiative toward changing the self and the environment (pp. 95–97)
2. The sense of right timing is an outcome of a positive self-concept, reflecting the person's ability to anticipate personal needs and the needs of others, as well as the ability to prepare for the future (pp. 130–141)
3. The capacity for loving is an outcome of a positive self-concept, reflecting the person's ability to experience happy or sad emotions by sharing experiences with others and by participating in others' lives (pp. 163–178)
4. Establishment of friendship, kinship, and support systems is the outcome of a positive self-concept, reflecting an ability to establish networks of supportive contacts among friends, family, and other support systems (pp. 206–227)

Simms and Lindberg validate that the professional self is a direct reflection of the personal self-concept. "Responsibility for our own acts—especially toward others—will flourish in an environment which fosters growth of self and independence" (Simms & Lindberg, 1978, p. 7). Understanding self and working to view self positively inevitably leads to more productive professional self-concepts. Negative self-concepts are barriers to the effective independent functioning vital to the successful performance of professional roles.

ACHIEVEMENT OF DEVELOPMENTAL TASKS

The development of the professional self follows the same sequence involved in the development of the personal self-concept. Like personal self-development, professional self-development is based on the achievement of specific tasks in the sequential stages of development. This section describes the stages of professional self-development, using the framework of the developmental tasks associated with the development of the personal self.

The development of the professional self is the process of personal self-transformation arising from the interactions associated with one's education, practice, or research in the nursing profession. The nurse who is ready to enter practice enters the profession with an idealized image of self, clients, coworkers, other workers in the delivery systems, and all others significant to the profession. Nursing is not unlike other professions in developing the professional self from an idealized image of self and others. The maturation of the professional self ensures that the professional does not mistake ideals and illusions for reality.

Table 5-1 outlines the stages of professional development. Each stage, with its associated tasks and goals, is modified from Erikson's stages of the life cycle (Erikson, 1982, pp. 55–82).

The degree of achievement of each goal in each stage of professional development influences what the person as a professional is like. A positive concept of the self as a professional person is essential to the nurse in effectively meeting the health needs of the population that nursing serves.

All developmental theories are based on the assumption that human growth and development is sequential and that successful negotiation of earlier developmental tasks is critical to the negotiation of later developmental tasks. This means that the development of the professional self is greatly influenced by the quality of goal achievement in each of the developmental eras. In the following discussion, the task of each era is stated and is followed by a discussion of the outcomes of either satisfactory or incomplete and unsatisfactory achievement of goals of the era.

The Beginning Professional Nurse During the Orientation Period

Task: Trust
Emerging Strength: Hope

GOALS

The goals of the new nurse entering practice are to trust personal mentors to effectively develop abilities to fulfill professional role requirements; to count on others to assist in the pursuit of professional objectives; to experience gratification in a new role; and to count on recognition from employers and clients for effectively delivering a needed service. These goals require that every professional nurse readily have accessible a number of reliable guides and teachers—relationships characterized by positive appraisals and relationships in which the nurse's professional needs can be satisfied without undue anxiety.

TABLE 5-1

Stages of Professional Development

Stage	Task	Goals
Infancy		
The Beginning Professional—Orientation	Trust	To trust one's own mentors and polestars to effectively guide oneself to develop abilities to fulfill professional role requirements To count on others to assist in the pursuit of professional objectives To experience gratification in a new role To count on recognition from employers and clients for effectively delivering a needed service
Childhood		
The Beginning Professional Nurse—Postorientation	Autonomy	To depend on more mature professionals for guidance some of the time To view self as autonomous in practice some of the time, a professional in one's own right, able to stand on own competence in meeting role responsibilities To view nursing as an independent body, determining its own policies and regulations, effectively using its power, and in control of its own practice
The Young Professional—Moving Into Independence	Initiative	To find rewards in using one's own initiative and imagination to test the realities of nursing roles To independently anticipate professional role responsibilities while being held accountable for own actions
The Growing Professional—Developing Expertise	Industry	To experience competence in independently performing the tasks of the profession To expand one's own knowledge of nursing To integrate a sense of accomplishment in one's own work in the profession
Adolescence		
The Professional With Own Identity	Identity	To feel self-certain in one's role as a professional nurse To feel competent in role experimentation To clearly articulate one's own ideological commitment to the profession
Adulthood		
The Maturing Professional	Intimacy	To develop the capacity to commit oneself to collaborative relationships with clients, professional peers, and other colleagues in the health care delivery system as an interdependent professional
The Productive Professional	Generativity	To be productive for self and others in a professional nursing role, contributing to society through own efforts in nursing education, practice, and research
The Older Professional	Integrity	To find pleasure in the accomplishment of oneself and others in professional pursuits To appreciate the full life cycle of the professional self

Modified from Erikson E: The Life Cycle Completed, pp. 55–82. New York, Norton, 1982.

OUTCOMES OF SATISFACTORY ACHIEVEMENT

Professional nurses who have been able to count on those who have assisted them to develop nursing skills and knowledge most likely will be able to trust their own professional and interdisciplinary peers in their common efforts to assist clients. Such nurses will feel good about their own abilities; will experience satisfaction in relationships with clients, nursing peers, and interdisciplinary team members; and will tend to appreciate the efforts of all concerned in professional experiences.

Nurses who have experienced trusting relationships in professional development will be able to focus their professional energies toward meeting client needs rather than having energies tied up in guarded and nontrusting relationships. They also are giving in their relationships, and are willing to serve as mentors and guides for less-experienced or less-educated nurses. Such nurses, feeling confident about their abilities, welcome accountability and responsibility. These nurses also are optimistic about getting future professional needs met and value lifelong learning as one avenue for professional self-development.

OUTCOMES OF INCOMPLETE OR UNSATISFACTORY ACHIEVEMENT

Professional nurses who have not been able to count on others to assist them to develop skills and knowledge in the professional discipline continue their pursuits until their sense of need is reduced. Unfortunately, however, the pursuit usually is so tinged with anxiety that these nurses are not likely to be very successful. These nurses have entered the work world where abilities are immediately needed.

If nurses do not feel good about their own competence, and if that feeling is at least partially related to their perceptions of their relationships with their teachers and guides, they are unlikely to feel comfortable in future relationships. They will not trust peers or interdisciplinary workers to assist them, and their professional needs will remain unmet. Energies will remain tied up in trying to get their own needs met, thus reducing what they can give to clients, peers, and others.

Indeed, many work environments reward only achievement of short-term tasks rather than value supportive processes. In such an environment, relationships generally need to be calculated rather than open and honest. Relationships with clients are limited to getting the job done, and the pleasures and pains of clients and others are not considered in implementing the nursing process. Nurses working in this environment tend to become task-oriented because they have not integrated the feeling that persons can be counted on when you need them. Rather, they have integrated the feeling that relationships make one vulnerable to negative appraisals more often than to positive appraisals.

Unless professional nurses are successful in finding a significant professional person who offers a relationship in which they can experience positive appraisals as a person while getting professional needs met, these nurses probably will remain untrusting of others throughout professional practice and will not be truly gratified in professional role accomplishments. A work environment that does not recognize professional nurses for effectively implementing the nursing process, but rather recognizes only the quantity of tasks completed, will continue to contribute to the lack of trust existing among its workers.

The Beginning Professional Nurse in the Postorientation Period
Task: Autonomy
Emerging Strength: Will

GOALS
After the nurse has been initiated into the profession, the following goals emerge:

1. To depend on more mature professionals for guidance some of the time
2. To view self as autonomous in practice, a professional in one's own right, and able to stand on one's own competence in meeting role responsibilities
3. To view nursing as an independent body determining its own policies and regulations, effectively using its power, and in control of its own practice

OUTCOMES OF SATISFACTORY ACHIEVEMENT
Nurses who have learned to trust professional leaders, to trust that clients are able to assume responsibility in their own care, and most of all to trust their own selves as being competent and knowledgeable, will move into the work world with an excellent potential for feeling autonomous as a professional person. As beginning practitioners, these nurses:

1. Base practice on nursing theory perceived to be valid
2. Sense that nursing offers a needed professional service that incorporates a high level of technical competency, judgment, and decision making
3. Require effective interpersonal relationships characterized by an ability to collaborate

To view self as autonomous requires that the trusting new professional nurse experience a work environment in which nurses are encouraged to make judgments, to participate in policy-making for nursing, and to establish and pursue their own professional goals. Autonomous beginning professional nurses will feel comfortable trying to put into practice what has been learned. Perhaps even more important, autonomous nurses can appreciate the unique roles of others, as well as feeling competent in their own roles.

OUTCOMES OF INCOMPLETE OR UNSATISFACTORY ACHIEVEMENT
At best, nurses who do not trust others and do not have a sense of existing in their own right can view themselves only as helpmates rather than as autonomous professional persons. The handmaiden image is perpetuated

if both nurses and nursing are perceived to lack the right to exist autonomously. If nursing is viewed only as a subordinate part of medical care, rather than as a partner in health care, then nurses cannot justify the need to be autonomous. In this situation, nurses exist only as assistants on medical teams, nursing is limited to restorative care of sick people under the primary care of physicians, and nurses spend most of their time carrying out the "orders" of others. These nurses cannot feel like real professional persons because primary criteria for any profession are that the profession offer a unique and needed service to people and is based on its own body of knowledge.

Beginning nurses who come to the work environment without a strong sense of professional autonomy (or even with a fledgling sense of professional autonomy) need the help of significant others in the nursing environment. Assistance is needed to:

1. Enable them to feel in control of what they are doing (providing for some successes)
2. Provide orientation and resources for developing essential competencies as professional persons
3. Enable them to participate on nursing teams as they assume responsibility for policies and regulations (providing for a democratic process in decision making)

The beginning professional whose leader is not an advocate may indeed question the belief that nursing is autonomous rather than dependent and will rapidly fall into caring for rather than advocating for clients. One who does not feel autonomous tends not to perceive others as autonomous persons existing in their own right. Without perceiving others as autonomous, the nurse cannot effectively implement nursing in a professional way. At best, this nurse can implement only a technical process.

The Young Professional Who Is Moving Into Independence
Task: Initiative
Emerging Strength: Purpose

GOALS

As nurses grow and become more independent, they try to find rewards in using their own initiative and imagination to test the realities of nursing roles, and to independently anticipate professional role responsibilities while being held accountable for their actions. Clearly, the nurse needs to have achieved a sense of trust and a sense of autonomy as a professional person before truly experiencing pleasure in behaviors reflecting initiative. In addition, the young nurse needs professional leaders who encourage the achievement of mutually agreed-on goals by various means to assist the nurse to develop initiative. Leaders who insist on singular methods and procedures for achieving goals do not support the professional nurse's development of initiative and creativity.

OUTCOMES OF SATISFACTORY ACHIEVEMENT

Implementing the nursing process in various settings with a diverse client population requires competence in critical thinking and the ability to make valid decisions. Protocols and procedures cannot organize all professional behavior. Thus, the nurse needs to be able to demonstrate initiative and creativity in effectively participating as the professional in relationships with clients. The professional who has achieved a sense of initiative can:

> Readily gather the data needed to assess client needs
> Permit the client to participate in the planning for how to best meet that need
> Offer creative ideas for the development of alternatives for problem-solving
> Take risks in carrying out the advocacy role for clients

The nurse with initiative will be:

1. Challenged by the potential or need for change
2. Able to help the health care delivery system respond in a dynamic fashion to meet clients' health needs
3. Willing to explore and assume new roles as a professional person if those roles are indicated for the improvement of health care (Initiative is a prerequisite for role accomplishment as change agent, client advocate, and contributor to the profession.)
4. Able to acknowledge the importance of roles played by other health professionals rather than feeling oppressed or suppressed by others in the system

Finally, nurses who have felt actively involved in planning and implementing the nursing process with clients will assume responsibility for their nursing actions. Accountability for nursing actions is readily accepted if nurses feel responsible for the decisions that determined those actions.

OUTCOMES FOR INCOMPLETE OR UNSATISFACTORY ACHIEVEMENT

A nurse who does not feel a high degree of independent and interdependent abilities or opportunities will have difficulty integrating initiative as a real functional part of the professional self. This nurse may develop a sense of shame in being a nurse and may not perceive nursing as deserving of pride. Many perceive nurses as low-status workers certainly not equal to other professionals, such as physicians, lawyers, and engineers.

A nurse without initiative needs to find rewards in carrying out the directives of others—being appraised positively for following directions that involve little nurse-initiated decision-making. Such a nurse has difficulty keeping clients as the central focus of the nursing process. Employers and agency policies assume paramount importance. Conflict arises when client needs cannot be met by procedures and policies or when critical thinking and active participation in decision-making are needed to solve problems. In this conflict situation, the nurse without initiative can only feel guilty when client needs cannot be met.

Thus, it is clear that professional nurses without initiative are extraordinarily limited in the professional services they can offer clients. They may be skillful in carrying out medical and nursing protocols in the restorative activities that are part of the nursing process, while being limited in carrying out the less prescribed promotional and preventive activities of professional processes. They may be able to react well to the client's illness but not so well to the client's response to illness. They may be effective in dealing with parts of the client but not with the client as a whole human being.

Dealing with the client as a whole, integrated human being requires the abilities to describe, analyze and compare, and evaluate and synthesize the complex relationships that exist within and among human beings. Because these relationships are continuously changing, nurses must have the ability to use initiative to test the realities of the situation at any given moment.

Nurses who have not achieved a sense of initiative will feel overwhelmed by demands to make independent judgments and will feel more comfortable fulfilling prescribed roles and passing on the accountability for the nursing actions to the persons prescribing the nursing role behaviors. What should be professional behaviors become occupational behaviors in which the workers assume primary responsibility for carrying out the directives of employers. From this perspective, one is rewarded for efficiency with skills and for quantitative outcomes rather than for knowledgeable judgments and qualitative outcomes. Nurses without initiative feel accountable to employers primarily and to clients secondarily and perhaps even incidentally.

The Growing Professional Who is Developing Expertise
Task: Industry
Emerging Strength: Competence

GOALS

As nurses develop professional abilities, they desire to experience competence in independently performing the tasks of the profession as well as to expand their own knowledge of nursing and to integrate a sense of accomplishment in their own work in the profession. A professional nurse who has developed a feeling of trust in others, a sense of autonomy in practice, and initiative in the nursing process is ready to practice in an independent role, to feel accomplished in the profession, and to continue a lifelong learning process.

Along with facilitating professional growth, support systems for growing professional persons must value and reward professional accomplishments and must support continued acquisition of knowledge as a primary goal. New and young professionals need to use the knowledge they bring to practice while developing trusting relationships and promoting a sense of competence in their abilities.

It is exciting to see staff development programs tailored to the developmental needs of different staff members. Such programs are organized around the professional's strengths rather than needs, promoting initiative rather than conformity. In such a setting, professional role achievement assumes priority over bureaucratic structure and function. During this period, it is essential that the nurse expand and use professional networks.

OUTCOMES OF SATISFACTORY ACHIEVEMENT

The professional nurse who integrates well a sense of industry—that is, who feels comfortable and competent to carry out the tasks of the nursing process—is able to identify and carry out the duties inherent in particular roles. The consequent sense of obligation to clients and to society creates the desire to know more.

Acting on the motivation to know more inevitably translates into improved quality of nursing care for clients. This professional nurse experiences both pleasure in providing competent nursing care and satisfaction in learning more. Accomplishments with clients and ongoing learning form the basis for the nurse's real feeling of being a true professional who has either the ability or the potential for meeting all professional obligations. Continuing education is viewed as a pleasurable professional responsibility rather than a job or a requirement for relicensure.

OUTCOMES OF INCOMPLETE OR UNSATISFACTORY ACHIEVEMENT

The nurse who for any reason does not feel comfortable and competent in carrying out professional responsibilities cannot develop a pleasurable sense of industry. Rather, the nurse feels inferior and thus incompetent and unable to carry out the nursing activities previously identified as professional expectations. It is not uncommon for the nurse who feels other-directed rather than self-directed to experience conflict rather than satisfaction in the work role.

For example, the nurse who says "I know I'm not doing what I need to do as a professional person because I don't have the time" reflects an inability to negotiate the task of industry. The nurse indeed feels that she or he has worked hard and is industrious, but clearly does not feel in control of professional practice. Someone else is in control, and the nurse develops a feeling of inferiority. This nurse may feel competent in fulfilling the assigned tasks but incompetent in fulfilling the real professional tasks. In this situation, continued learning is commonly viewed as a mandate and another assigned task rather than a pleasure.

Certainly, the nurse who does not feel competent in meeting professional obligations and is not motivated to expand knowledge is limited as to the goals that can be achieved with clients. At this stage of professional development, the nurse who has not achieved the developmental task of industry inevitably must find some way to receive satisfaction from work. Unmet professional needs must be negotiated or defended against. Obviously, the profession and the public can only profit from a nurse who has satisfactorily achieved a sense of industry.

The Professional With Own Identity

Task: Identity
Emerging Strength: Fidelity

GOALS

To integrate professional identities, nurses set the following goals:

To feel self-certain in their roles as professional nurses
To feel competent in role experimentation
To clearly articulate their own ideological commitments to the profession

One does not develop a professional identity by completing the assigned tasks of a discipline. Rather, one develops a professional identity by assuming the responsibilities of a role that is perceived appropriate for accomplishing the goals of the profession. We believe that the profession's goal is to facilitate health of clients, that the nurse plays a leadership role in society for promoting health, and that the significant emerging leadership roles for the nurse are change agent, client advocate, and contributor to the profession.

OUTCOMES OF SATISFACTORY ACHIEVEMENT

The most significant outcome of the successful achievement of a professional identity is that identity enables the person to carry out role responsibilities. The nurse who feels self-certain in the change agent role clearly is able to implement all the activities involved in a planned change process. Planned change is much more likely than accidental change to result in improved client health habits.

The nurse who assists clients to take necessary steps to change health behavior often is more effective when also carrying out the advocate role. Finally, the nurse influences other nurses to facilitate change in clients toward better health through responsibly implementing the contributor to the profession role. The person who has a personal sense of a professional identity:

Knows what the roles involve
Is willing to experiment with role implementation
Is able to begin to articulate a personal belief system about the discipline

OUTCOMES OF INCOMPLETE OR UNSATISFACTORY ACHIEVEMENT

The obvious outcome of unsuccessful achievement of a professional identity is confusion about role responsibilities and behaviors. A common indictment of nursing today is that the profession is not clear about what it should be doing; its identity is vague in terms of professional criteria. In terms of occupational tasks derived from employer expectations, the occupational identity of the nurse may be clearer. The most significant outcome of the professional nurse not achieving professional identity is that the health care needs of the public will be incompletely or ineffectively met.

Nursing is the only health discipline that clearly states that its primary goal is to facilitate health by responding to the human being's whole response to health and illness. Because humans respond holistically, some health care discipline must serve that purpose if health care delivery is to be adequate. Otherwise, the public will perceive even more strongly that health care is fragmented or inaccessible in this era of high technology. Without a professional identity, the nurse cannot implement nursing processes that respond to the whole person, and thus human needs will be incompletely or ineffectively met.

The Maturing Professional

Task: Intimacy
Emerging Strength: Love

GOALS

For the maturing nurse, the goal is to develop the capacity to commit to collaborative relationships with clients, professional peers, and other colleagues in the health care delivery system as interdependent professionals. A professional person who has a clearly developed professional identity is able to function interdependently as well as independently. Being secure in the professional self and professional role responsibilities, the nurse can share some energy within collaborative relationships. Nursing and other health care disciplines thus mutually agree on their common goal: the well-being of the client. They can mutually:

1. Assess the client's total health care needs
2. Respect the specific contributions of each discipline
3. Determine who is best qualified to help meet specific aspects of the client's health care needs

Nursing can share experiences with other disciplines and contribute to the evaluation of health care delivery, keeping the client as the central focus throughout the collaborative process.

OUTCOMES OF SATISFACTORY ACHIEVEMENT

Intimacy reflects the ability to value someone else's needs as much as one's own. The nurse who can be intimate in professional relationships offers the greatest opportunity for affecting change in others. Influence and vulnerability are greatest in intimate relationships. Although nurses are more vulnerable in such relationships, they also have learned to trust, to feel confident, and to take risks to enhance effectiveness.

By virtue of their needs in the nurse–client relationship, clients are considerably more vulnerable than nurses. Thus, it is extremely important that the nurse value clients as people in their own right, deserving of respect and unconditional acceptance. Use of the client's abilities is much more likely to occur in this accepting relationship. If the client has been valued and has actively participated in the nursing process, achievement of mutually agreed-on goals is more likely and, perhaps more important, is more likely to endure. The achievement of the optimum level of health is enhanced. In the same manner, the nurse who can value professional peers and other health care workers in their own right clearly will be more effective in advocacy efforts for clients. Energy can be directed toward collaboration for the benefit of all rather than toward competition for the benefit of self only.

OUTCOMES OF INCOMPLETE OR UNSATISFACTORY ACHIEVEMENT

A nurse who has achieved a clear professional self-identity but cannot express intimacy has a limited ability to influence clients, peers, and others. If unable to value others' beliefs, rights, abilities, and responsibilities as much as their own, nurses cannot maximize the positive outcomes of the nurse–client relationships. Without such respect for others, nurses cannot participate effectively in collaborative relationships, which have been demonstrated the most effective in producing positive changes. Lacking collaborative abilities, the nurse practices in isolation in either competitive or, at best, cooperative relationships. Thus, professional influence is limited.

Although expert in nursing knowledge and skill, the nurse is not the expert in experiencing the client's human responses or determining what the client must or can do. In this, the client is the expert. Nurses (or any health care worker) who feel that their expertise includes all factors related to achieving health tends to respond in ways that clients perceive as dehumanizing. The nurse who has not integrated intimacy and thus cannot fully understand the value of other human beings will tend to distort professional expertise and behave in ways that dehumanize clients rather than maximize their abilities in collaborative relationships. One can readily understand that a nurse who has not felt respected as an equal on the health care team will have more difficulty developing collaborative abilities with clients, peers, and others.

The Productive Professional

Task: Generativity
Emerging Strength: Care

GOALS

The mature professional nurse develops the goals of being productive for self and others in professional nursing roles and contributing to society through personal efforts in nursing education, practice, and research. Nurses who have developed the ability to collaborate consistently with all persons with whom they are professionally involved moves forward to a developmental stage of maximum productivity. Professional contributions peak, and the nurse experiences the greatest return for investment in professional activities.

Nurses who do well in this stage of professional life influence society's image of nursing most positively. Their activities are viewed as real contributions to society through practice of the profession with clients, education of future professional persons, and research that substantiates the significance of nursing in health care delivery.

OUTCOMES OF SATISFACTORY ACHIEVEMENT

If the nurse achieves the task of professional generativity, the public and the professional self are greatly enriched. To feel productive—to feel absolutely essential to the world one knows—is a personal and professional need of every nurse. "Leaving one's legacy" is a human need. As a change agent and an advocate, the mature professional nurse provides the highest quality of professional nursing practice. This nurse appreciates:

1. The value of practice with clients, acting as a mentor for other nurses
2. The value of nursing education, acting as a continuing consumer as well as a contributor in some manner
3. The significance of nursing research, acting as a consumer of research findings in practice and education and as a participant in research at some level

Society's image of the professional nurse depends on the productivity of nurses in this generative stage of professional development.

Outcomes of Incomplete or Unsatisfactory Achievement

The nurse who does not reach the maturity stage in the profession characterized by productivity nevertheless leaves a mark on the professional world. However, this legacy in all likelihood contributes to a societal image of nursing as something less than professional. At best, this image may be of a person who has technical expertise or competent restorative care abilities. At worst, it could be of a person who primarily serves as a helpmate to all other health workers and secondarily is an attendant to clients.

The image of the nurse as a real professional person depends on the majority of nurses reaching a mature level of professional development. The professional who does not experience productivity and generativity will experience perhaps long periods of feeling stagnant, even burned out—unsatisfied with opportunities and personal performance in a fast-moving, highly technologic environment.

The Older Professional

Task: Integrity
Emerging Strength: Wisdom

GOALS

As a professional grows older, goals change to finding pleasure in the accomplishments of oneself and others in professional pursuits and appreciating the full life cycle of one's professional self. To paraphrase a concept made real by Elisabeth Kübler-Ross (1981) in her work with people in the terminal stage of life, the older professional has opportunities and obligations to complete unfinished business and to reflect on and to cherish significant contributions and relationships. If this is done successfully, these professionals feel well-integrated in the profession as long as they live. This achievement requires an environment that values its older members, permits task adjustments to enable older professionals to continue to contribute, and includes professional peers who call on older members for sage counsel.

OUTCOMES OF SATISFACTORY ACHIEVEMENT

The professional who achieves a sense of integrity while growing older in the profession wields an extraordinarily strong influence on shaping future directions for the profession. For example, the six founders of Sigma Theta Tau, all of whom probably were successful in achieving the developmental tasks of each professional era, exerted the most influence on the profession as older professionals. In their later years, they espoused the integrity of the profession. They never despaired about the potential for nursing to offer a vitally needed service to society. They expressed great pleasure in their own professional achievements and, perhaps more importantly, in the achievements of those who followed them in the organization they founded.

In an environment that truly treasures them, as expressed in the ongoing founders' awards program, the remaining founders create the most dramatic moments at the biennial conventions. Their dreams and accomplishments are passed on in the most memorable way, through interaction among younger professionals and older professionals who have achieved the highest level developmental task: integrity.

OUTCOMES OF INCOMPLETE OR UNSATISFACTORY ACHIEVEMENT

An older professional who cannot find pleasure in personal accomplishments or is dissatisfied with the professional practice of others cannot achieve a sense of integrity as a professional person. Rather, just as it occurs in personal self-development, the professional self-development is characterized by a sense of despair. This person cannot complete unfinished business and recount the accomplishments of self or others in the profession. This nurse cannot appreciate ongoing change and development.

The inability to achieve integrity in older professional life, although understandable, usually leaves the older nurse alone and unsupported. The sense of despair creates a vicious cycle of alienation. As a result, this nurse cannot yield a positive influence on health care and generally is viewed by society in a stereotypical way, characterized by such axioms as "You can't teach an old dog new tricks."

CHALLENGING THE PERSONAL SELF-SYSTEM IN THE DEVELOPMENT OF A PROFESSIONAL IDENTITY

A parallel has been drawn between developmental tasks of the personal self and the professional self. The professional tasks to be achieved for full professional development have been suggested to be identical to the personal tasks identified by social scientists. Thus, it is logical to conclude that those persons with the greatest achievement of personal tasks in the development of the personal self-system have the best potential to achieve the professional tasks more fully.

Simms and Lindberg (1978, p. 9) state that the personal self-concept "results from previous interpersonal relationships" and that the resultant self-concept "affects future interactions." They conclude that "a person's view of self controls the roles he or she will be able to assume." They view the self-concept as an internal barrier or support for the professional self. During the developmental process that occurs between developing professionals and their significant professional others, it is entirely possible that the established self-system will be challenged.

Given the assumption that the person always has the potential to change in a positive way, the developmental professional experience can be used as a corrective growth experience. Arthur (1992, p. 718) suggested that there were "seven dimensions of the professional self-concept of nurses":

Flexibility/creativity
Knowledge
Skill/competence
Caring
Communication
Leadership
Satisfaction

Just as an individual's personal characteristics influence the professional characteristics she or he can exhibit, so can professional experiences have an impact on the personal self. Thus, the personal self-system and the professional self-system demonstrate a reciprocal relationship in which both are always open to change in relation to constraints or opportunities experienced by the person.

Essentially, the nurse who has achieved the tasks of personal self-development can use that personal strength to achieve professional tasks. Stein (1995, p. 192) indicates that "rather than striving to change an existing negative aspect of the self, an important means to bring about change may be to help a person elaborate an unacknowledged strength, and diminish the importance of one's vulnerabilities." The nurse who has not done as well in achieving personal tasks in previous developmental eras can use professional significant others to further develop the professional self.

◎ Professional Identity and Image

Nursing has struggled with its identity for at least a century (Strasen, 1992). During this struggle, society has perceived nurses as they have practiced in reality and as they are portrayed by the various communication media. Because most people receive far more information about nurses from the mass media than from actual nurse–client relationships, it is essential to understand the media portrayal of nurses.

Consider the following example. On November 1, 1991, *The Wall Street Journal* ran a lead article titled "Danger In White: The Shadowy World of 'Temp' Nurses," that portrayed nursing in a negative light. The journalist uncovered the unethical behavior of agency executives as well as the unethical and illegal behavior of nursing personnel (mostly practical nurses and health care aides) during the nursing shortage situation in Florida in the early 1990s (Bogdanich, 1991). Clearly, these women behaved as oppressed people seeking to get ahead any way they could. Publicizing this scandal reinforces any negative images of the nurse that the public may have.

Investigating the current public image of nursing, Kaler, Levy, and Schall (1989) found that sex-role stereotyping of nurses continues. The sample of 110 predominantly middle-class, mixed ethnic, and stratified gender persons selected characteristics validated as feminine and nurturant to describe the nurse. Findings revealed the need for increased public awareness that nurses are scholars and leaders.

CHALLENGING THE IMAGE

Because the current status of the profession relates in some ways to the images of nursing reflected by society, as well as to the origins of the group, it is important to challenge the distorted images and to differentiate the professional self of nursing. Nurses can decide to maintain, modify, or overcome the status problems of nursing. With a clear professional self-concept, the nurse can challenge the myths and assumptions from previous generations. However, two of nursing's major problems in articulating a clear professional self are nurses' relationships to the hospital (employer–employee) and socialization in the traditional female role.

One of the positive challenges to the stereotypical image of the nurse has occurred in the relationships between medicine and nursing. Stein, Watts, and Howell (1990) have described the changes that have occurred in the doctor–nurse relationship since 1967, when most agreed that doctors were superior to nurses, that nurses had to appear passive when they took initiative or made recommendations, and that open disagreements were to be avoided at all costs. Today, nurses, struggling for respectability, have decided to stop playing the "doctor–nurse game" and enter into truly collaborative relationships with physicians and other health care workers. Nurses are rebelling against oppression. Maybe someday all health care professionals will "see the benefits to patients and themselves when the relationship between medicine and nursing is one of mutual respect and interdependence" (Stein et al., 1990, p. 264).

Muff (1988, p. 197) agrees that the socialization in the traditional female role is a problem. "The dual socialization of female nurses—as women and as nurses—to traditional 'feminine' identifications contributes to the status and power inequities in nursing." Muff further observes that nursing schools not only admit traditionally oriented women, but also reinforce that orientation through isolationism, authoritarianism, and perfectionism. She describes the isolationism both physically and academically, with the educational settings often existing out of the mainstream of higher education and with the science courses often being less rigorous.

Hughes (1990) further elaborates the dual socialization of female nurses. The duality she describes is the ideology of domesticity and the ideology of professionalism. Much of nursing's history comprises its efforts to deal with the "constraints that the ideology of domesticity has imposed on the lives of women" (Hughes, 1990, p. 25). Hughes also describes how nursing's efforts to professionalize have been limited by the fact that nursing is seen as an occupation uniquely defined as women's work.

Social identity theory, which originated in social psychology, provides a way to address status relations between different groups in society and individual responses to low status (Breinlinger & Kelly, 1994). Because the theory assumes that people will strive for a positively valued sense of social identity, "it is assumed that women will be motivated to acquire a positive social identity by following one of three strategies" (p. 2):

1. Individual mobility—involves a change for the individual
2. Social creativity—"emphasizes the positive value of traditional 'female' characteristics of sensitivity, intuition, and ability to nurture" (p. 2); changes the comparison group and avoids comparisons with the high-status group (men); and emphasizes dimensions (interpersonal skills, relationships, negotiation) by which women may argue that they compare more favorably with men
3. Social competition—involves a direct challenge to the higher status group through use of collective action

The use of collective action through influence of public policy is discussed in Chapter 12.

Muff (1988) describes authoritarianism in terms of the continuing faculty belief in obedience rather than assertiveness and the continuing focus on protocols and procedures rather than on the inquisitive risk-taking behaviors necessary in today's world of business. She describes perfectionism as the hallmark of authoritarian faculty, who supervise large and small details (even the mundane details) and organize learning experiences toward the goal to practice until perfect. Muff concurs that one useful way to consider the socialization problems of nurses is to analyze the developmental milestones that occur. She suggests that nurses need to address the developmental image problems by recognizing:

1. Women's issues as being nurses' issues
2. Identity problems and definitions of boundaries and roles

3. Dependence–independence problems
4. Perceptual distortions and interpersonal problems
5. The need for business acumen
6. Propaganda, stereotypes, sexism, and professional issues (Muff, 1988, pp. 217–218)

CONVEYING THE PROFESSIONAL IMAGE

Professional nurses can successfully challenge distorted images of nursing by differentiating their desired professional selves through the following behaviors (Winstead-Fry 1977):

1. Say something directly to persons distorting the professional image
2. Understand the group's generational linkages to hospitals and the productive and nonproductive outcomes of this linkage
3. Address the issue of reasonable relationships to hospitals
4. "Come to grips with what we want to be as a young profession peopled primarily by women" (p. 1454), which involves dealing with issues of women's liberation that are significant to the profession and differentiating today's professionals from previous generations and from those aspects of nursing's history that interfere with independence and professional autonomy

All of these actions directed toward conveying the professional image of nursing need to occur within the peer group of nursing, the larger health care delivery team, and societal groups that influence the image of the profession. The information sharing that could grow from these actions could act as a strong determinant for nursing to achieve its rightful place in society as a valuable professional discipline offering an essential service to the society it serves.

◎ The Professional Self-System and Career Development

How one views one's profession and feels about oneself as a professional influences how one thinks and acts in professional relationships. Nursing has some inherent difficulties in clearly differentiating a professional self that meets all the criteria for a legitimate profession. Jordan has suggested that all professions extensively peopled by women have a common problem: Women do not really act out the equality that they say they feel.

> The problem remains that we fail to define ourselves in terms of whole human beings, full human beings. We reduce the definition of our lives just a little bit because somewhere in the back of our minds is the thought that we are really not quite equal. So what are women going to do about it? How are we going to change all that? It is going to take long, hard, slow, tedious work. And we begin with our own self-concept. We begin to try to internalize how we really feel about ourselves, and proceed to actualize the thinking that we finally evolve from the look inward and the projection outward. (Jordan & Hearon, 1979, pp. 218–219)

Jordan believes that the true professionalization of women's groups can occur only when women have clearly dealt with their personal self-concepts.

Regardless of the dynamics of the nursing profession's evolution, it has been assumed that the kind of professional self each nurse becomes makes a substantial difference in what each client can gain from the nursing process. If most nurses achieve mature professional self-concepts (in terms of the professional tasks that need to be negotiated), nursing will be a constructive force for health in society. The nursing process will then be both educative and therapeutic, and the nurse and the client will be able to know and respect each other, "as persons who are alike, and yet, different, as persons who share in the solution of problems" (Peplau, 1952, p. 9) and the enhancement of strengths. Building on these strengths serves as the basis for career development as a professional nurse.

Clifford (1990) notes that career development must become a planned "articulated pathway" in reorganized health care delivery systems and states that this will "necessitate the reorganization of experienced and advanced nursing practice to provide clinical leadership for the novice nurse, as well as to direct patient services" (p. 620). Nurses must become careerists. Clifford envisions self-managed work groups of nurses who provide autonomous care of clients and consultative services for novices. She believes that such a career model will serve as an incentive for young professional nurses to purposefully pursue their own career development.

Labich (1991) advises a professional to take control of his or her career and manage it as if it were a business. He describes three stages in a career:

1. First stage (20s to middle-to-late 30s)—focused on assembling a repertoire of basic skills and gaining exposure to as many leadership opportunities as possible
2. Second stage (late 30s to 40s)—focused on becoming a key player in strategic planning, asking important questions, and leading in getting things done in the profession
3. Third stage (late 40s and older)—focused on being valued and productive until it is time to retire. The extent to which one is valued and productive is directly related to the degree to which one imparts accumulated wisdom to novices

Diers (1990, p. 66) advises nursing novices that

> to work as an apprentice alongside the master is to learn not only the craft but also the experience of doing the craft. Learning by doing shores up the novice nurse, who can believe that the work is not only possible but fulfilling as the master shows it to be.

It is interesting to note that there are now assertions that women are ideally suited for the leadership in the 1990s because "teamwork and a free flow of information are paramount" (Fierman, 1990, p. 115). Clifford

(1990) reminds all mature professionals of their responsibilities in assisting novices to grow and achieve satisfaction in their careers.

 ## Care of the Professional Self-System

PROFESSIONAL STRESS AND BURNOUT

VIGNETTE

Karen has been working in a staff nurse position for the past 2 years. For awhile she has noticed that she is frustrated and anxious at work, and she has had difficulty sleeping. Her coworkers have begun to avoid her because of her short temper and negative attitude. Karen wonders, "What happened to me? I used to love nursing."

Environmental and Personal Factors in Burnout

In the current health care environment, nurses experience significant pressure and stress from four system levels. The health care system contributes stress through its multiple regulations, reimbursement issues, and mandates (Cullen, 1995). For example, given the short length of hospital stays, nurses rarely see evidence of a positive impact, and eligibility criteria force nurses to deny care to uninsured families. The institutional system creates obstacles in the workplace, such as short staffing, mandatory overtime, insufficient or faulty equipment, and having to lower standards because of "cost containment." As Cullen (1995, p. 24) says, "you can't give quality care in a structural environment that's consistently understaffed, underequipped, and taxing on caregivers." The societal system often devalues the work that nurses perform, and the nursing system itself does not prepare nurses for the extraordinary responsibility they will encounter in their professional roles. All of these forces contribute to "a toxic work environment" (Cullen, 1995).

Personal characteristics also contribute to stress. Low self-esteem and limited confidence are associated with feelings of vulnerability and powerlessness. This nurse, who experiences obstacles rather than challenges, may direct aggression at peers because it cannot be taken out on those with power; may undermine peers with passive-aggressive behavior; or may "keep trying to achieve more in order to prove her worth" (Cullen, 1995, p. 25). Kahn and Saulo (1994) identify several additional personal characteristics that contribute to work stress:

■ Not establishing realistic limits. You can easily overextend yourself by believing "only I can do it."
■ Seeking to meet needs for approval, affection, and intimacy from one's career

- Avoiding fears, such as of death and personal loss
- Overconscientiousness; needing to give your very best all the time
- Emotional empathy rather than compassion, or cognitive (detached) empathy

Healthy Helping

A number of strategies have been proposed to help the nurse avoid burnout and promote health of the professional self (Avoiding burnout, 1994; Cullen, 1995; Kahn & Saulo, 1994):

- Love yourself. "You need to give to yourself in order to continue to be able to give to others" (Kahn & Saulo, 1994, p. 56).
- Get your priorities straight. You are not your job. Know where nursing belongs within the larger context of your life.
- Recognize that you cannot rescue. Even with your best efforts, some patients get sicker or die.
- Set goals for yourself. Acknowledge to yourself that you have done a good job.
- Develop a solid social support system. Make sure you are receiving as well as giving.
- Find outlets for creativity. Learn new skills and continue to grow as a professional.
- Do not assume responsibility where you have none. You are not "on duty" 24 hours a day.
- Create and enjoy work breaks.
- Try thought control. Try approaching each task as a challenge.
- Heal your own wounds. Work on your own unhealthy patterns.
- Do not stay in a situation that consistently fails to meet your needs. Give yourself permission to leave.
- Take care of yourself.

HEALTH OF THE PROFESSIONAL SELF

Promoting a Healthy Lifestyle

The choice of healthy lifestyle behaviors can be thought of as a way that nurses can promote their own healing. Scandrett-Hibdon (1996, pp. 18–21) describes six elements in what she calls the "endogenous healing process":

Awareness—the alerting mechanism
Appraisal—exploration, evaluation, and assigning of meaning to what is now conscious
Choosing—setting goals, avoiding, or continuing previous behaviors
Acceptance—"letting go"
Alignment—"integration of the internal and external actions that support the movement toward harmony" (p. 21)
Outcome—being in harmony and experiencing a sense of wholeness (p. 21)

Using this process, the nurse can gradually move to develop the personal strength of a healthier lifestyle to promote the self's ability to heal itself.

NUTRITION AND DIET

Kahn and Saulo (1994) and Weil (1995) suggest that a healthy diet is high in fruits and vegetables, whole grains, and the right kinds of fish, and low in:

Fat, especially saturated
Protein, especially from animal sources
Calories in excess of need
Sugars
Chemical additives
Caffeine
Alcohol
Salt

"Foods rich in vitamins C, E, A, beta carotene, B_6, B_{12}, and folic acid support optimal immune function. Adequate intake of zinc, selenium, iron, calcium, magnesium, and manganese is also important" (Kahn & Saulo, 1994, p. 179). Garlic, ginger, and soy protein are also recommended (Weil, 1995).

LIFESTYLE EXERCISE

Pender (1996) describes lifestyle exercise as the integration of numerous bouts of exercise into daily living. A number of benefits of exercise have been proposed (Pender, 1996), including:

- Reduction of blood pressure and total cholesterol
- Decrease in body fat
- Increased metabolic rate
- Maintenance of bone mass
- Increased muscle strength and endurance
- Decreased chronic back and joint pain
- Improved self-concept
- Improved body image
- Decreased anxiety and depression
- Enhanced general mood and well-being

Gradually increasing walking to 45 minutes a day, 5 days a week has been highly recommended as part of a healthy lifestyle (Weil, 1996).

STRESS REDUCTION

Relaxation is an important method of reducing stress. Various ways can be used to promote relaxation (Clark, 1996), including:

- Abdominal breathing
- Meditation
- Biofeedback
- Self-hypnosis

- Imagery
- Time management
- Coping affirmations
- Exercise
- Prayer
- Therapeutic touch
- Massage
- Reflexology

Far from a waste of time, relaxation is an active, creative, and dynamic process that involves intention and practice, and it influences all other coping skills (Kolkmeier, 1995).

In addition to relaxation, examples of other mechanisms to promote stress reduction include:

Enjoying nature
Creating purpose in life through meaning, commitments, and goals
Being interested and keeping a sense of curiosity (Gardner, 1996)
Promoting community through relationships with colleagues and peers

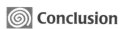 ## Conclusion

Relationships and conditions of the workplace environment provide the framework for determining both the positive and negative outcomes that can occur in each stage of professional development. Nurses must be proactive in creating healthy helping skills and in adopting a healthy lifestyle, to thrive on stress, and take care of themselves.

THOUGHT QUESTIONS

1 What is your stage of professional development in your career? What tasks are appropriate for this stage?

2 Can you identify a mentor? How might you start the mentoring process?

3 How healthy is your lifestyle? Are you ready to make changes toward increased health?

4 What has happened to Karen (in the vignette)? What can she do about it?

REFERENCES

Arthur, D. (1992). Measuring the professional self-concept of nurses: A critical review. *Journal of Advanced Nursing, 17,* 712–719.
Avoiding burnout. (1994). *Nursing94,* 101–103.
Bogdanich, W. (1991, November 1). Danger in white: The shadowy world of "temp" nurses. *The Wall Street Journal,* pp. B1, B4.

Breinlinger, S., & Kelly, C. (1994). Women's responses to status inequality: A test of social identity theory. *Psychology of Women Quarterly, 18,* 1–16.

Clark, C. C. (1996). Stress management. *Nursing Spectrum, 5,* 65–68.

Clifford, J. C. (1990). The future of nursing practice. In N. L. Chaska (Ed.). *The nursing profession: Turning points* (pp. 617–623). St. Louis: Mosby-Year Book.

Cullen, A. (1995). Burnout: Why do we blame the nurse? *American Journal of Nursing, 95,* 23–27.

Diers, D. (1990). Learning the art and craft of nursing. *American Journal of Nursing, 90,* 64–66.

Erikson, E. (1982). *The life cycle completed.* New York: Norton.

Fierman, J. (1990, December 17). Do women manage differently? *Fortune,* pp. 115–118.

Gardner, J. W. (1996). Self-renewal. *The Futurist, 30,* 9–12.

Hughes, L. (1990). Professionalizing domesticity: A synthesis of selected nursing historiography. *Advances in Nursing Science, 12,* 25–31.

Jordan, B., & Hearon, S. (1979). *Barbara Jordan—a self portrait.* Garden City, NY: Doubleday.

Kahn, S., & Saulo, M. (1994). *Healing: A nurse's guide to self-care and renewal.* Albany NY: Delmar.

Kaler, S. R., Levy, D. A., & Schall, M. (1989). Stereotypes of professional roles. *Image, 21,* 85–89.

Kolkmeier, L. G. (1995). Relaxation. In B. M. Dossey, L. Keegan, C. E. Guzzetta, & L. G. Kolkmeier (Eds.). *Holistic nursing: A handbook for practice* (2nd ed.). Gaithersburg, MD: Aspen.

Kubler-Ross, E. (1981). *Living with death and dying.* New York: Collier.

Labich, K. (1991, November 18). Take control of your career. *Fortune,* pp. 87–96.

Lancaster, J., & Lancaster, W. (1982). *The nurse as change agent.* St. Louis: Mosby.

Muff, J. (1988). Of images and ideals: A look at socialization and sexism in nursing. In A. H. Jones (Ed.). *Images of nurses: Perspectives from history, art, and literature* (pp. 197–220). Philadelphia: University of Pennsylvania Press.

Pender, N. J. (1996). *Health promotion in nursing practice* (3rd ed.). Stamford, CT: Appleton & Lange.

Peplau, H. E. (1952). *Interpersonal relations in nursing.* New York: G. P. Putnam's Sons.

Rogers, M. E. (1970). *An introduction to the theoretical basis of nursing.* Philadelphia: Davis.

Scandrett-Hibdon, S. (1996). The history of energy-oriented healing. u D. Hover-Kramer (Ed.). *Healing touch: A resource for health care professionals.* Albany, NY: Delmar.

Sheehy, G. (1982). *Pathfinders.* New York: Bantam.

Simms, L. M., & Lindberg, J. (1978). *The nurse person.* New York: Harper & Row.

Stein, K. F. (1995). Schema model of the self-concept. *Image, 27,* 187–193.

Stein, L. I., Watts, D. T., & Howell, T. (1990). The doctor-nurse game revisited. *Nursing Outlook, 38,*:264–268.

Strasen, L. L. (1992). *The image of professional nursing: Strategies for action.* Philadelphia: Lippincott.

Sullivan, H. S. (1953). *The interpersonal theory of psychiatry.* New York: Norton.

Weil, A. (1995). *Spontaneous healing.* New York: Knopf.

Winstead-Fry, P. (1977). The need to differentiate a nursing self. *American Journal of Nursing, 77,* 1452–1454.

The Knowledge Bases of Professional Practice

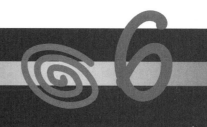

Patterns of Knowing and Nursing Science

LEARNING OUTCOMES

By the end of this chapter, the student will be able to:

1 Discuss the evolution of three systems of thought about how to organize developing knowledge in science.

2 Understand the differences between logical empiricism and historicism in their philosophic approach to the development of knowledge.

3 Appreciate the differences among the four patterns of nursing knowledge.

4 Know the four central concepts of nursing that identify the focus for scientific inquiry.

5 Appreciate why theory is essential to the practice of nursing.

VIGNETTE: PAUL

Paul, an RN for 7 years, just completed a BSN degree program. He believes that knowledge from "hard science" is the only way nursing will achieve respect. He also believes that research looks good on a resume, and is a good way to "get ahead." He wants to do "practical" research, "none of that conceptual stuff for me."

Understanding a body of knowledge is essential for competent professional practice. Knowledge can be obtained from a number of sources, including experience, reflection, and values. Science is "a unified body of knowledge about phenomena that is supported by agreed-upon evidence" (Meleis, 1997, p. 10). "Since nursing is a learned profession, it is both a science and an art." The practice of nurses is the creative use of knowledge in human service (Rogers, 1992, pp. 28–29).

The science of nursing incorporates the study of relationships among nurses, clients, and environments within the context of health. It is also the result of interrelationships among theory, practice, research, and education. Theory provides the tools to direct nursing practice. Practice provides the professional individual with the setting to apply and test nursing knowledge and develop theories. Research provides the means to test theories, and education provides the means to shape belief systems and to synthesize and disseminate knowledge.

Nursing science is emerging as an autonomous, distinctive professional discipline that is valued by society. As an emerging science, nursing uses and builds on knowledge developed in many disciplines through centuries of evolution.

The Evolution of Scientific Thought

Science, which has changed the face of the earth and our knowledge about the boundaries of the universe, has evolved since prehistoric humans. To a large degree, science accounts for humankind's progress. Because it is not possible within the scope of this book to discuss every era of human history, we have chosen to highlight the evolution of three systems of thought about organizing developing human knowledge (Spradlin & Porterfield, 1984).

At first, ancient humans were characterized by a *belief in magic* and in being controlled by forces beyond human understanding or control. A second way of trying to know about the world began during the first *scientific revolution* (around 1500) and continued until recently. This view emphasized measurement and quantification of observable data as the means of understanding the world. Increasingly, however, both an acceptance of *uncertainty and a focus on processes* have influenced human thought since Einstein's discovery of relativity early in the 20th century.

ANCIENT HUMANS

Early humans differentiated the world into two parts: me (internal) and not me (external). The external world was viewed as being populated by spirits, demons, and gods, who assumed both good and evil characteristics of humans. Because gods were believed to be nonrational and to be moved by whims and passions, humans tried to influence the gods' behavior instead of trying to figure out rational causes of events.

Through trial and error, humans discovered that some patterns of action led to predictable outcomes, which could be reproduced as long as the procedure was followed exactly (like a cookbook). Thus, humans did in an elementary way study and observe phenomena sufficiently to gather many isolated facts. However, the facts remained isolated, rather than being organized into a body of data that could form the basis for scientific conclusions. To the extent that nursing functioned primarily from protocols and procedures for many years, it somewhat followed the methods of science that existed until approximately two centuries ago.

Because disease, aches, and pains were assumed to be caused by gods and evil spirits, early medicine was associated with religion or magical beliefs. However, over time, attention to cause and effect led to practical approaches and logical sequencing of steps of treatment. Hippocrates (460–377 BCE) was followed by Aristotle (384–322 BCE), who emphasized classification of signs and symptoms. Increasingly, attention was paid to exploring the mechanisms of the human body (Spradlin & Porterfield, 1984).

THE SEARCH FOR CERTAINTY

By the 1500s, the development of mathematics coincided with increasing interest in scientific study of humans and nature. The ability to count made relationships appear more logical and the world more predictable. The philosophy of logical positivism drove the search for certainty. This was based on a belief that the world was like a simple machine, but that only God understood the laws by which it operated. Time and space were absolute. Time flowed smoothly and uniformly. A reductionistic approach was used to identify causes to predict effects.

> Scientific scholars became engulfed in a spiral of logic and increasing certainty about quantification of relationships among absolute entities that lead to concepts of truths that could be validated. . . . We could, with the use of observation, measurement, and logical reasoning, know the laws of nature. . . . All the entities that composed the whole of nature could be reduced to their smallest parts, studied and understood, and rebuilt (Spradlin & Porterfield, 1984, p. 106).

Reduction of humans into separate psyche and soma (Cartesian dualism), both of which could be measured physically, was advanced by Descartes (1596–1650), who saw the human being as a machine ruled by the same laws as all of nature (Spradlin & Porterfield, 1984, p. 108). The separation of mind from matter (body) and the emphasis on the human being as the sum of minute parts has dominated medical and nursing science ever since.

Four basic assumptions about humans and the universe are inherent in this kind of a mechanistic world view: determinism, quantity, continuity, and impersonality. Leaving no room for uncertainty, the *principle of determinism* reflects the belief that "nature proceeds by a strict chain of events from cause to effect, the configuration of causes at any instant fully determining the event in the next instant, and so on forever" (Ware, Panikaar, & Romein, 1966, p. 127). The ability to predict comes out of this principle, while lack of predictability and the presence of uncertainty represent ignorance.

The *quantitative principle* expresses the exact nature of science. It reflects the belief that science consists of "measuring things and setting up precise relations between the measurements" (Ware et al., 1966, p. 129). In this view, humans and the universe are described by numbers (eg, spatial coordinates, time, position, amounts, and locations) that quantify physical properties and by relations among these quantitative characteristics.

Continuity, the third principle, is concerned with the "transitions of nature from one state to another [and] express[es] the sense, deeply engrained in the outlook of the age, that the movements of nature are gradual" (Ware et al., 1966, p. 129). This principle reflects the belief that the processes involving humans and the universe are continuous.

In the fourth principle, *impersonality*, the scientist is viewed as an instrument, not a person. The scientist

1. uses observation rather than imagination;
2. passively finds order in phenomena rather than creating it; and
3. does not permit personal influence on the phenomena under observation (Ware et al., 1966, p. 129).

Belief in these principles led Galileo (1564–1642) and Newton (1642–1727) to develop the scientific method, based on a particular method of reasoning: logic. Logic encompasses principles of reasoning applicable to any branch of knowledge. Because logic is based on reason and sound judgment, it can be convincing.

Inquiry is a technique of science. It seeks truth, information, or knowledge to meet the goal of problem-solving. A problem is any question or matter involving doubt, uncertainty, or difficulty that needs solution. Solution is the act of solving a problem by finding the answer or explanation. The most extensive investigative process of science is the systematic inquiry of research.

THE RELATIVE WORLD OF PROCESS

By the 20th century, scientists realized that the physical world consisted of matter and forces that interact with matter, such as gravity, magnetism, and electricity. By exploring the cell, genetic mechanisms and mechanisms that influenced cellular structure and function were explained. It appeared that "the immutable laws which governed the world" were being discovered.

Then, in the early 20th century, Einstein demonstrated that the world was composed not of events, but of observations, which were relative to the place and velocity of the observer. "Any absolutes or cause and effect sequences (are) illusions . . . testable only in a retrospect organization of events" (Spradlin, 1984, p. vi). Heisenberg's (1971) and von Bertalanffy's (1968) work in quantum physics led to postulation that mass, energy, time, and space coordinates are interchangeable. All systems are considered interrelated and interdependent, on a continuum of relativity and probability, and thus uncertainty.

The implications of this different conceptual system are enormous. Continuity is replaced by discontinuity, and probability (determined statistically) replaces certainty. Emphasis is placed on patterning rather than on discrete entities and on interactions rather than on isolated events. The scientist is no longer an isolated objective observer of "events." "Man came to be seen not as a detached observer but as an irremovable part of his observations" (Ware et al., 1966, p. 148). In addition, awareness of the limitations and biases of individual perception has increased, implying that truth and meaning are not absolute but are relative to history and context.

Nonetheless, "while physicists have become increasingly concerned with . . . a relative world of process, biologists have until recently tended to be even more involved in the reductionistic approach to life" (Spradlin & Porterfield, 1984, p. 189). Because one's belief system is critical to determining sources and methods of discovering knowledge, the following section discusses differing approaches to the philosophy of science that are currently influencing nursing science.

◎ Philosophy of Knowledge

Based on Plato's concepts, knowledge is considered to be belief that has been justified through reason (Stumpf, 1993). What constitutes adequate justification is the concern of the discipline of philosophy. This discipline considers questions such as whether there is such a thing as truth and how one can be certain that something is true. It is necessary to accept that some things can be true to question the truth or falseness of any particular thing. But must certainty be beyond all possible doubt, or is certainty sufficient if it is beyond logical and reasonable doubt? How does an individual acquire knowledge? What are the roles of intellect, perception, and intuition in the process of knowing?

PROCESSES OF KNOWING

The three primary processes of knowing are rationalism, empiricism, and intuition. *Rationalism* involves belief in the possibility of knowing truth by thinking and by use of reason that is *a priori*, or independent of experience. *Empiricism* involves belief that the only source of certainty about knowledge is immediate experience. However, because raw experience is subject to individual perception, the emphasis must be on verification and on either confirmation or refutation of observations. *Intuition* is sometimes described as "just knowing." The source of the knowing is internal to the individual and often is perceived as occurring independently of experience or reason. It is subjective and personal in origin although it can be validated through experience and interaction with others.

APPROACHES TO KNOWING

Logical Empiricism

Logical empiricism, a philosophic approach to the development of knowledge accepted since the 16th century, is based on the following assumptions:

1. A body of facts and principles that explain the way the world operates is waiting to be discovered. These include abstract, general, and universal principles. Theories provide alternative explanations of how the body of facts is ordered and systematically unified.
2. Cause and effect (linear) relationships can be established by using deductive processes and experimental methodology. The results are context-free generalizations that can be applied to all individuals. Truth is achieved through sensory data and controlled experiments.
3. It is necessary to control values and biases to achieve "objective" knowledge; therefore, the observer must be separated from the observed world. Science is value free. Social relevance is unimportant.
4. Theoretical reduction is an important scientific goal. It is assumed that the ultimate character of reality will be best explained using the logic and simplicity of the fewest possible theoretical concepts and laws.
5. The whole is the sum of its parts. Circumscribing (reducing) observations to small parts of the whole gives better control of the data and stronger explanatory power.

Historicism

Historicism, advanced since the 1930s under the influence of concepts such as relativity and process, is based on the following assumptions:

1. Because "truth" is dynamic and constantly changing, what is important is the effectiveness of a theory for solving problems.
2. The whole is more than the sum of its parts. Reducing the whole to parts is counterproductive. Interrelationships and interactions are part of what must be studied.
3. An individual or a phenomenon must be studied as a whole in a natural setting. The observer is part of the setting, and, therefore, interactions between the observer and the setting should be described rather than controlled. Emphasis is on process rather than fact.
4. Multiple research traditions are desirable (eg, theories from psychology, physiology, education, and so forth) to explain different dimensions of the same phenomenon. Synthesis and development of multiple theories are encouraged.
5. Knowledge is related to context. Values, subjectivity, intuition, history, and tradition are useful for discovery.

Until recently, nursing research and theory were dominated completely by empiricism and logical positivistic philosophy. However, beginning with Rogers (1970) and increasing in the 1980s, nurse scientists incorporated principles of historicism and process into theory, research, and practice.

Currently, a debate about appropriate methods for developing nursing knowledge is being waged in the nursing literature. Some authors in support of qualitative methods maintain that "human behaviors cannot be isolated and quantified and that the attempt to do so results in misleading and dehumanizing outcomes rather than in knowledge that is useful for nursing practice" (Campbell & Bunting, 1991, p. 2). Others suggest that quantitative and qualitative methods can be used at different times to serve different purposes. Meleis advocates development of a

> world view [Weltanschauung] that includes an integration of norms emanating from different theories of truth. It combines rigor and intuition, sensory data as they exist and as they appear, perceptions of the subject and of the theoretician, and logic with observable clinical data (1997, p. 87).

Such a synthesis of philosophical approaches would encourage various methods for development of nursing science.

The next section discusses patterns (ways) of knowing and methods for their utilization.

Patterns of Nursing Knowledge

Chinn and Kramer describe knowing as

> interrelated processes that arise from the whole of experience. . . . Each of the patterns of knowing is an aspect of the whole . . . makes a unique contribution. . . [is] equally vital and must be integrated with other patterns as knowledge is developed and applied (1995, pp. 4–5).

Gender differences have been identified in the ways in which men and women may develop frameworks for the organization of knowledge. Perry (1970) identified four positions through which men make sense of their educational experiences:

1. Basic dualism: Authorities hand down the truth, and the learner is passive. Choices are perceived as either right or wrong, black or white, good or bad, we or they.
2. Multiplicity: The teacher may not have the right answer. A personal opinion is acceptable and may be valid.
3. Relative subordinate position: Evidence is sought for opinions. The emphasis is on analysis and evaluation of information.
4. Full relativism: Truth is relative. The meaning of knowledge depends on its context.

Perry suggested that the positions occurred in a linear sequence, with each position an advance over the previous.

In a study of women's perceptions, Belenky, Clinchy, Goldberger, and Torule (1986) described five major categories used for the organization of knowledge:

1. Silence: The individual is subject to the whims of an external authority and perceives herself to be mindless and voiceless.
2. Received knowledge: External authority is all-knowing. The individual is capable of receiving and even reproducing knowledge, but not of creating it.
3. Subjective knowledge: Truth and knowledge are personal, private, and subjectively known or intuited.
4. Procedural knowledge: The individual is invested in learning and in applying objective procedures for obtaining and communicating knowledge.
5. Constructed knowledge: The individual experiences herself as a creator of knowledge. She views knowledge as contextual and values both objective and subjective strategies for knowing.

Further study is needed to identify whether these categories develop sequentially.

Gender has been linked to the distribution of power and privilege in society (Marecek, 1995). Doering (1992) states that knowledge reinforces and supports existing power relations that "subtly support male dominance and reinforce female submissiveness" (p. 26). "When the male model is assumed to be the human model, women are viewed as the 'other,' deviant from the male norm or prototype" (p. 31). However, Doering continues, "since power is always exercised in relation to a resistance" (p. 31), ways of knowing (such as intuititive knowing, and contextual, phenomena-centered knowledge), that are not based on a male world view, "may alter the balance of the nursing–medicine power relation" (p. 32).

Carper (1992), in "an effort to understand the kinds of knowledge comprising the discipline of nursing," (p. 73) analyzed the nursing literature published between 1964 and 1975. Her results, which were published in a seminal 1978 article, identified four fundamental patterns, or ways, of knowing in nursing: empiricism, aesthetics, personal knowledge, and ethics. These ways of knowing have been extended by Chinn and Kramer (1995) and White (1995).

EMPIRICAL KNOWLEDGE

"Empirical data, obtained by either direct or indirect observation and measurement . . . are formulated as scientific principles, generalizations, laws, and theories that provide explanation and prediction" (Carper, 1992, p. 76), or enrich understanding through interpretation or description (White, 1995). Empirical knowledge is obtained through the senses, can be verified, is credible, and is used to impart understanding. "The processes related to creating empiric knowledge are describing, explaining, or predicting" (Chinn & Kramer, 1995, p. 7).

AESTHETIC KNOWLEDGE

Aesthetics, the art of nursing, is an integrative pattern (Chinn, 1994). It contributes to an understanding of how nursing, as an expression of personal qualities and skill, makes a difference in client health. Because it is based on the "direct apprehension of a situation . . . that arises from the practice of nursing" (Chinn, 1994, p. 24), this knowledge is not universal but is unique and has subjective meaning. "Esthetic knowing involves the creative processes of engaging, intuiting, and envisioning" (Chinn & Kramer, 1995, p. 10).

"Art begins with the assumption of a common, generalizable human experience . . . and seeks expression of the infinite creative possibilities for experiencing or responding to the human experience" (Chinn, 1994, p. 30). Intuition, defined as "an immediate apprehension, or the power of gaining knowledge without evidence of rational thought" (Mitchell, 1994, p. 2), can be an important component of aesthetic knowledge in nursing practice.

Benner and Tanner (1987) discuss six aspects of intuitive judgment previously identified by Dreyfus (1985). These aspects are not sequential, but rather are used in combination by the practitioner.

1. Pattern recognition is the ability to recognize patterns and relationships without prior consideration of the separate components.
2. Similarity recognition is the ability to see similarities and parallels among patient situations, even when there are marked dissimilarities in objective features.
3. Common sense understanding is "a deep grasp of the culture and language, so that flexible understanding in diverse situations is possible. It is the basis for understanding the illness experience, in contrast to knowing the disease" (Benner & Tanner, 1987, p. 25). It is a way of "tuning in" to the patient and grasping the patient's experience.
4. Skilled know-how is based on a combination of knowledge and experience that permits flexibility of actions and judgment.
5. A sense of salience makes it possible to differentiate what is particularly significant in a situation.
6. Deliberative rationality involves the use of analysis and past experience to consider alternative interpretations of a clinical situation.

Carper emphasizes the importance of integrating aesthetic knowledge into the nursing process. The experience of helping and caring "must be perceived and designed as an integral component of its desired result rather than conceived separately as an independent action imposed on an independent subject" (Carper, 1978, p. 17). The result is a richness and appreciation of the practice of nursing as an art as well as a science.

PERSONAL KNOWLEDGE

Personal knowledge involves a "person's individualized and subjective ways of learning, storing, and retrieving information about the world" (Rew, 1996, p. 96). It is a "discovery of self-and-other arrived at through reflection, synthesis of perceptions, and connecting with what is known" (Moch, 1990, p. 155). Both the nurse and the client are considered to be "integrated, open system(s) incorporating movement toward growth and fulfillment of human potential" (Carper, 1978, p. 19). In the process of mutually establishing a nurse–client relationship, there must be efforts toward "receptive attending" (Moch, 1990, p. 155), engagement and authenticity, rather than detachment and a manipulative impersonal orientation. The result is an authentic knowing of an individual apart from the category of nurse or client. "The creative processes of personal knowing are opening, centering, and realizing" (Chinn & Kramer, 1995, p. 9).

Because personal knowing "concerns the inner experience of becoming a whole, aware self" (Chinn & Kramer, 1995, p. 9), the individual needs to accept ambiguity, vagueness, and discrepancies in what is essentially a subjective and existential process. There is no specific methodology that can be used consistently. The individual must be open to experience and intuitive feelings, be honest with self, and make efforts to acknowledge the responses of others. This is an ongoing process, as the self is constantly changing.

Belenky and colleagues state that

> educators can help women develop their own authentic voices if they emphasize connection over separation, understanding and acceptance over assessment, and collaboration over debate; if they accord respect to and allow time for the knowledge that emerges from firsthand experience; if instead of imposing their own expectations and arbitrary requirements, they encourage students to evolve their own patterns of work based on the problems they are pursuing (1986, p. 229).

Moch (1990, pp. 156–159) describes three overlapping components of personal knowing:

1. Experiential knowing involves becoming aware through participation in which the knower learns through self-observation, by observing others, through feeling, and through sensing.
2. Interpersonal knowing is increased awareness through connectedness or interaction, which can involve intense attending, opening oneself to another, and conveying feelings to another.
3. Intuitive knowing involves the immediate knowing of something without the use of reason. The knower often describes this as a "hunch" or as a "feeling about something."

Moch believes that personal knowing can be viewed only from within a context of wholeness; includes a process of encountering, passion, commitment, and integrity; and entails a shift in connectedness at the conscious or unconscious level (1990, p. 159).

In identifying implications for research and knowledge development, Moch (1990, p. 162) suggests the following assumptions for capturing and transmitting personal knowing:

1. All perceptions are involved in data gathering
2. The process of the experience may take precedence over the product
3. The product of knowing is validated by the knower with both internal and external validation criteria
4. No attempts are made to reproduce the process or the product because each situation is unique

"The processing may consist of any combination of human and environmental interaction, rational intuiting, appraisal, active comprehension, and personal judgment" (Sweeney, 1994, p. 917).

ETHICAL KNOWLEDGE

Sarvimaki (1995) describes four aspects that represent different ways of organizing and expressing moral knowledge. *Theoretical/ethical knowledge* "stands for an intellectual conception of what is good and right. It is organized into concepts and propositions that are formulated into judgments, rules, principles, and theories" (p. 344). *Moral action knowledge* means "having the skill necessary for performing the act as well as having good judgment . . . . Values and principles are manifested in action" (p. 345). *Personal moral knowledge* "refers to the way in which morality is organized in the person, that is, in his motives, inclinations, emotions and commitments" (p. 346). *Situational knowledge* "means being aware of the moral significance of the situation and being able to identify its morally significant traits" (p. 347).

Biomedical ethics are derived from models of patient good, rights-based notions of autonomy, or the social contract of medical practice (Fry, 1989). However, it has been argued (Fry, 1989; Sarvimaki, 1995; White, 1995) that nursing ethics should be based on an ethic of caring and must consider the nature of the nurse–client relationship. A caring orientation is based on the moral ideal of doing what is good rather than that which is just. Mutuality, not autonomy, is foundational (White, 1995). "Creative processes of ethical knowing in nursing are clarifying, valuing, and advocating" (Chinn & Kramer, 1995, p. 8).

White (1995) proposes that a fifth way of knowing, sociopolitical knowing, needs to be added to the original patterns identified by Carper. "The pattern of sociopolitical knowing addresses the 'wherein'" (White, 1995, p. 83), a broader context that includes the context of nurse and client (including cultural identity), and the context of nursing as a practice profession. White (1995) states, "a sociopolitical understanding in which to frame all other patterns of knowing is an essential part of nursing's future in an increasingly economically driven world" (p. 85).

In addition, Munhall (1993) proposes "unknowing" as another pattern of knowing in nursing. She argues that the state of mind of unknowing is a condition of openness, and "a de-centering process from one's own organizing principles of the world" (p. 125). The intent is to "come to know the patient's world" (p. 126), and "lead to a much deeper knowledge of another being, of different meanings, and interpretations of all our various perceptions of experience" (p. 128).

Three different perspectives, each described as reflecting a different point of view (paradigm) of the way to develop nursing knowledge, have been identified (Newman, Sime, & Corcoran-Perry, 1991, p. 4):

1. Particulate–deterministic perspective: Phenomena are viewed as "isolatable, reducible entities having definable properties that can be measured." Knowledge includes facts and universal laws that can be used to predict and control change.
2. Interactive–integrative perspective: Phenomena are viewed as having multiple, interrelated parts. Reality is assumed to be multidimensional and contextual. Relationships may be reciprocal (rather than linear and causal) and knowledge may be context dependent.
3. Unitary–transformative perspective: Each phenomenon is viewed as a "unitary, self-organizing field embedded in a larger self-organizing field. It is identified by pattern and by interaction with the larger whole." Change is unpredictable. Knowledge is personal and involves pattern recognition. Both the viewer and the phenomenon are involved in a process of "mutuality and creative unfolding."

Patterns as ways of knowing are not mutually exclusive. "Different ways of knowing are not judged against one another. Rather, different ways of knowing and of creating knowledge are each, in their own right, useful for some purpose" (Chinn & Kramer, 1995, p. 4). Because each pattern adds only one specific component, none alone is a sufficient source of knowledge for nursing science. Comprehensive nursing knowledge must be based on an integration of all the ways of knowing. "Nursing depends on the specific knowledge of human behavior in health and in illness, the aesthetic perception of significant human experience, a personal understanding of the unique individuality of the self and the capacity to make choices within concrete situations involving particular judgments" (Carper, 1978, p. 22).

◎ The Development of Nursing Science

CONCEPTS

For a discipline to have growth of knowledge, the concepts—highly abstract and general "words describing mental images of phenomena" (Fawcett, 1995, p. 2)—that are important for the discipline must be identified, and there must be a shared acceptance of conceptual definitions. Four concepts have been commonly accepted as central to the discipline of nursing:

The human being (who may be a nurse or client individual, a family, group, or community)

The environment (which may be alive or inanimate)

Health (which may include well-being and illness), and

Nursing actions (which include all the interactions among nurse, client, and the environment in the pursuit of health)

In addition, there recently has been renewed interest in the concept of *caring*. Newman and coworkers even assert that "nursing is the study of caring in the human health experience" (1991, p. 3). However, others have expressed concern that "caring is relatively underdeveloped as a concept, has not been clearly explicated and often lacks relevance for nursing practice" (Morse, Bottorff, Neander, & Solberg, 1991, p. 119).

At least five conceptualizations of caring have been identified: a human trait, a moral imperative, an affect, an interpersonal interaction, and a therapeutic intervention (Morse et al., 1991, p. 122). Caring seems to be part of content and relationship (Knowlden, 1991, p. 202) and associated with varying outcomes such as the client's physical response and the client's or the nurse's subjective experience (Morse et al., 1991, p. 122).

At present, in the absence of consensus on definitions for these concepts, multiple definitions coexist (see Chap. 8).

THEORIES

Theories are generally introduced when scientists have studied a class of phenomena and have found a system of uniformities that can be expressed in the form of laws. A theory is a "creative and rigorous structuring of ideas that project a tentative, purposeful, and systematic view of phenomena" (Chinn & Kramer, 1995, p. 72). All theories include relationships among defined concepts, have structure that gives it a systematic nature, and is tentative because it is based on assumptions, values, and judgments as well as on empirical observations. Theories help nurses understand how and why the phenomena of nursing are associated with one another.

Meleis has elaborated on two types of theory (1991, pp. 19–20):

Descriptive theory "describes a phenomenon, an event, a situation, or a relationship; identifies its properties and its components; and identifies some of the circumstances under which it occurs."

Prescriptive theory "addresses nursing therapeutics and the consequences of interventions."

Effectiveness in practice is directly related to the ability to understand, describe, explain, and anticipate human responses in regard to health.

THEORETICAL FRAMEWORKS

A theoretical or conceptual framework has been defined as "a structure composed of concepts related to form a whole" (Chinn & Kramer, 1995, p. 212). A model is composed of abstract and general concepts and propositions that are linked together in a distinctive way. Fawcett states that a conceptual model "provides a unique focus that has a profound influence on our perceptions" (1995, p. 3). Developing theoretical frameworks for nursing ensures practice that is effective in achieving the overall goal of the profession: improving quality of health.

MODELS FOR NURSING

Several nurse scientists have proposed individual and distinctive models about the interrelationships of concepts that form the nature and processes of nursing. Each nurse scholar who has proposed a conceptual model has based the model on empirical observation, intuitive insights, or deductive reasoning (Fawcett, 1995, p. 3). Although they may present diverse views of nursing phenomena, each conceptual model is useful for professional nursing because of the organization it provides for thinking, observing, and interpreting in nursing practice. Each provides principles from which guidelines for practice can be derived. See Chapter 8 for a discussion of selected conceptual models.

◎ Conclusion

There is growing agreement on the central concepts of the discipline of nursing. Those central concepts that could be used as parameters of the science of nursing are:

1. The client or consumer of nursing actions
2. The nurse and the accompanying nursing actions
3. The environment
4. The processes of health of the consumer and the nurse

The science of nursing evolves from these four components and their inseparable interrelationships. Indices for observing and understanding the phenomena and their interrelationships are emerging as the true scientific study of nursing evolves.

THOUGHT QUESTIONS

1 How can nursing scholars resolve empiricism/historicism debates to advance knowledge development through research?

2 How do issues of power and privilege affect client needs and nursing practice?

3 Can you envision integrating the ways of knowing holistically? What are the implications for knowledge development?

4 How would you respond to Paul in the vignette at the beginning of the chapter?

REFERENCES

Belenky, M. F., Clinchy, B. M., Goldberger, N. R., & Torule, J. M. (1986). *Women's ways of knowing: The development of self, voice and mind.* New York: Basic Books.

Benner, P., & Tanner, C. (1987). Clinical judgment. How expert nurses use intuition. *American Journal of Nursing, 87,* 23–31.

Bertalanffy, L. V. (1968). *General system theory.* New York: Braziller.

Campbell, J. C., & Bunting, S. (1991). Voices and paradigms: Perspectives on critical and feminist theory in nursing. *Advances in Nursing Science, 13,* 1–5.

Carper, B. A. (1978). Fundamental patterns of knowing in nursing. *Advances in Nursing Science, 1,* 13–23.

Carper, B. A. (1992). Philosophical inquiry in nursing: An application. In J. F. Kikuchi & H. Simmons (Eds.). *Philosophic inquiry in nursing* (pp. 71–80). Newbury Park, CA: Sage.

Chinn, P. L. (1994). Developing a method for aesthetic knowing in nursing. In P. L. Chinn & J. Watson (Eds.). *Art and aesthetics in nursing* (pp. 19–40). New York: National League for Nursing.

Chinn, P. L., & Kramer, M. K. (1995). *Theory and nursing—A systematic approach* (3rd ed.). St. Louis: Mosby-Year Book.

Doering, L: Power and knowledge in nursing: A feminist poststructuralist view. *Advances in Nursing Science, 14,* 24–33.

Dreyfus, H., & Dreyfus, S. (1985). *Mind over machine. The power of human intuition and expertise in the era of the computer.* New York: Free Press.

Fawcett, J. (1995). *Analysis and evaluation of conceptual models of nursing* (3rd ed.). Philadelphia: Davis.

Fry, S. T. (1989). Toward a theory of nursing ethics. *Advances in Nursing Science, 11,* 9–22.

Heisenberg, W. (1971). *Physics and beyond.* New York: Harper and Row.

Knowlden, V. (1991). Nurse caring as constructed knowledge. In R. M. Neil & R. Watts (Eds.). *Caring and nursing: Explorations in feminist perspectives.* New York: National League for Nursing.

Marecek, J. (1995). Gender, politics, and psychology's ways of knowing. *American Psychologist, 50,* 162–163.

Meleis, A. (1997). *Theoretical nursing: Development and progress* (3rd ed.). Philadelphia: Lippincott.

Mitchell, G. J. (1994). Intuitive knowing: Exposing a myth in theory development. *Nursing Science Quarterly, 7,* 2–3.

Moch, S. D. (1990, Summer). Personal knowing: Evolving research and practice. *Scholarly Inquiry for Nursing Practice, 4,* 155–170.

Morse, J. M., Bottorff, J., Neander, W., & Solberg S. (1991, Summer). Comparative analysis of conceptualizations and theories of caring. *Image, 23,* 119–126.

Munhall, P. L. (1993). 'Unknowing': Toward another pattern of knowing in nursing. *Nursing Outlook, 41,* 125–128.

Newman, M. A., Sime, A. M., & Corcoran-Perry, S. A. (1991). The focus of the discipline of nursing. *Advances in Nursing Science, 14,* 1-6.

Perry, W. G. (1970). *Forms of intellectual and ethical development in the college years.* New York: Holt, Rinehart and Winston.

Rew, L. (1996). *Awareness in healing.* Albany, NY: Delmar.

Rogers, M. E. (1970). *An introduction to the theoretical basis of nursing.* Philadelphia: Lippincott.

Rogers, M. E. (1992). Nursing science and the space age. *Nursing Science Quarterly, 5,* 27–34.

Sarvimaki, A. (1995). Aspects of moral knowledge in nursing. *Scholarly Inquiry for Nursing Practice, 9,* 343–358.

Spradlin, W. W., & Porterfield, P. B. (1984). *The search for certainty.* New York: Springer-Verlag.

Stumpf, S. E. (1993). *Socrates to Sartre: A history of philosophy* (5th ed.). New York: McGraw-Hill.

Sweeney, N. M. (1994). A concept analysis of personal knowledge: Application to nursing education. *Journal of Advanced Nursing, 20,* 917–924.

Ware, C. F., Panikaar, K. M., & Romein, J. M. (1996). *History of mankind, cultural and scientific development: Volume 6, the twentieth century.* New York: Harper & Row, 1966.

White, J. (1995). Patterns of knowing: Review, critique, and update. *Advances in Nursing Science, 17,* 73–86.

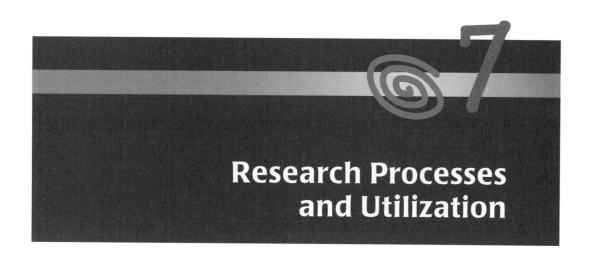

Research Processes and Utilization

LEARNING OUTCOMES

By the end of this chapter, the student will be able to:

1 Describe how professional nurses can contribute to research in nursing.

2 Discuss the sequential steps in nursing research.

3 Appreciate why the researcher needs an understanding of ethics to conduct research.

4 Compare and contrast theories of research utilization.

5 Identify barriers to research utilization by the nurse clinician.

6 Identify strategies to facilitate clinical research utilization.

7 Discuss how the increase in nursing research and researchers can affect the public image of nursing.

VIGNETTE: SANDY

Sandy has been a practicing nurse for a number of years. She is proud of her experience and practices "the way I was taught." She has only scorn for new college graduates "who talk a good game about research, but don't know anything about the real world."

Central to the growth and development of any profession is research to develop and validate the knowledge base on which the profession is built. Also essential to any practice discipline is research to validate principles and techniques of practice. Thus nursing, which is viewed as a practice discipline, critically needs nursing research to establish the knowledge base for the profession and develop recommendations for direct application of knowledge in nursing practice.

Serious efforts to conduct nursing research and develop theory to guide practice began 35 to 40 years ago, in pursuit of the professional goal of basing the practice of nursing on theory and fact rather than on opinion and prescribed protocols from other disciplines. As Martha Rogers said more than 30 years ago, "Only the most uninformed and those endeavoring to maintain a long obsolete hierarchal control would propose that in today's world society is better served by ignorance than by knowledge." (Rogers, 1967). However, a study of medical–surgical nurses found that they rely on information from individual patients, personal experience, and information gained during nursing school far more than on facts from journal articles (Baessler et al., 1994). Clinicians must appreciate that incorporation of research findings into practice is not an optional activity for when there is time, but a critical component of professional practice.

"Research is diligent, systematic inquiry or investigation to validate and refine existing knowledge and generate new knowledge" (Burns & Grove, 1993, p. 3). That knowledge must be applied to practice to "improve client outcomes, enhance the professional practice environment, and contain costs of health care" (Titler et al., 1994, p. 307). In fact, Heater, Becker, and Olson (1988) have found that research-based nursing interventions lead to improved patient care outcomes. In turn, practice generates new ideas for research.

The baccalaureate-prepared nurse can contribute to nursing research in several ways, including:

1. Using nursing research findings to guide nursing practice
2. Valuing a sense of inquiry about the phenomena of nursing
3. Participating in research projects as opportunity allows
4. Refining the ability to collect, organize, categorize, and analyze data
5. Suggesting nursing research questions that need to be addressed to improve practice

To participate in these ways, the nurse must have an understanding of the research process and of strategies to overcome barriers and facilitate research utilization.

Research Processes in Nursing

This section serves as an overview to facilitate understanding of the components of the research process. The logical steps of inquiry can be developed in greater detail as one continues to develop abilities as a nurse researcher.

Beginning with the nurse's query about some aspect of nursing, the research process structures the systematic investigation of that question and the reporting of the answers and new questions about that aspect of nursing. The research process follows the methods of science, which essentially means that the process:

- Has an identifiable order
- Includes controls over factors not being investigated
- Includes the gathering of evidence about the question
- Is built on a theoretical framework
- Operates for the purpose of applying results to improve nursing practice

RAISING QUESTIONS

The most significant step in the nursing research process may be the first one—the nurse's articulation of a question that must be answered to increase professional understanding and better serve the public. Nurses are accountable for asking questions that reflect sensitivity to the need to better understand all that is within the domain of nursing. These domains include the client in terms of the experience of health, the nurse in terms of professional characteristics and responsibilities, the environment of the client and nurse, the dynamics of health, and the interactions among all these factors.

QUANTITATIVE AND QUALITATIVE APPROACHES

Two research approaches to developing nursing knowledge have emerged in recent years: the quantitative approach and the qualitative approach. In the earliest years of nursing research, valuing of the scientific method led to the use of quantitative approaches to develop objective information. Currently, however, nurse researchers are open to using qualitative approaches to develop subjective information while also remaining open to using quantitative approaches. According to Mariano (1990, p. 354), qualitative research has, "as its foci, perspectives, meaning, uniqueness, and subjective lived experiences . . . . Its aim is understanding." It is the quality of individual experience that is important.

According to Haase and Myers (1988, pp. 130–131), quantitative and qualitative research approaches have a common purpose: to gain understanding. The difference between the approaches is one of emphasis. Quantitative approaches focus on the "confirmation of theory by explaining," demonstrating an empirical analytical emphasis. Qualitative approaches focus on "discovery and meaning of theory by describing," demonstrating a human science emphasis (Haase & Myers, 1988, p. 131).

According to Guba and Lincoln (reported by Haase & Myers, 1988, pp. 131–134), the differences between the two approaches can be categorized in three ways, according to the assumptions made by each approach: (1) the nature of reality, (2) the nature of relationships, and (3) the nature of truth. The following comparison of quantitative and qualitative assumptions according to the three categories is presented from the work of Haase and Myers (1988, pp. 130–134):

1. View of reality
   Quantitative: Researcher focuses on objective reality seen as singular; the process for discovering reality is reductionistic; and it is believed that knowledge of the whole can be gained through knowledge of the parts.
   Qualitative: Researcher focuses on subjective realities seen as multiple and related; the process for understanding reality is ecologic; and it is believed that "the whole is greater than the sum of its parts" (p. 132).
2. View of relationships
   Quantitative: Researcher objectively distances self from subjects and believes that boundaries must exist to ensure objectivity.
   Qualitative: Researcher interacts with the subject and believes that a unity exists between them and that both are integral to the research process.
3. View of truth
   Quantitative: Researcher sees the world as stable and predictable and believes that the truth is discovered in common laws, principles, and norms. Thus, the researcher's goal is generalizability.
   Qualitative: Researcher sees the world as dynamic and believes that truth is discovered in the changing patterns of the world. Thus, the researcher's goal is to discover uniqueness, valuing differences as well as similarities.

Appreciating the complexity of nursing phenomena and valuing subjective experiences as legitimate foci of nursing research, Artinian (1988) notes that nurses are now open to trying qualitative approaches, all of which use participant observation and in-depth interviewing. Cohen and Tripp-Reimer (1988, p. 226) support ethnography as a significant qualitative research approach to help nurses understand cultural differences, stating that "ethnography is a method designed to describe a culture. The ethnographer seeks to understand another way of life from the native's point of view" (p. 226).

Using grounded theory methodology, Artinian (1988, pp. 138–149) describes four modes of inquiry the qualitative researcher can use:

1. *Descriptive mode*, which "presents rich detail that allows the reader to understand what it would be like to be in a setting or to be experiencing the life situation of a person or group" (p. 139)
2. *Discovery mode*, which "enables the researcher both to identify patterns in the life experiences of the subjects and to relate the patterns to each other" (p. 141)
3. *Emergent fit mode*, which is "used when a substantive theory has already been developed about the phenomenon under study" from which a research question "is formulated to extend or refine the previously developed theory" (p. 142)
4. *Intervention mode*, in which the researcher tries to answer the fundamental question of how to make something happen after the "phenomenon has been adequately conceptualized so that the conditions under which the basic social process takes place are understood" (p. 139)

The researcher can decide which of the four modes of inquiry to use only after clarifying the purpose of the research and evaluating knowledge that is currently available on the topic.

STEPS IN THE RESEARCH PROCESS

Whether the nurse researcher chooses the qualitative or the quantitative approach, the overall steps in the research process remain the same. Knowledge of the research steps discussed in the following sections will facilitate the nurse's use of findings in practice.

Focus on the Problem Area

From where do the questions that need to be answered about nursing arise? Of these questions, which ones require research for adequate response? Which ones have sufficient data already available for effective problem-solving? Polit and Hungler (1995) suggest that the experience of the professional person can be used to raise questions because that experience requires the nurse to make decisions, some of which may have little support in theory or research findings.

Nurses can also focus on a problem area by reviewing the current research and other information in the literature on a topic of interest; by deriving questions from the theories or conceptual model used to guide practice in the nurses' practice setting or educational program; or by getting ideas from external sources such as faculty, peers, or priorities established for practice.

For example, Riegel and colleagues (1993) reviewed the research done in the 10 years since the American Association of Critical Care Nurses (AACN) priorities for clinical research were published in 1980. Although several areas have been studied extensively (eg, pain, vascular line infection, and ventilator weaning), "few studies have been conducted in several of the priority areas" (p. 420).

The development of the research problem, according to Polit and Hungler (1995), incorporates the following sequential steps:

1. Note a general area of interest about which you have some questions.
2. Narrow the topic through critical evaluation of ideas with a mentor or expert. That evaluation must address feasibility and worth.
3. Establish the benefit of the investigation of the selected problem to nursing by addressing who will benefit, what are the applications, what is the potential for the results to be relevant to theoretical basis of practice, and whether anyone cares about the potential findings (how important is it to nursing practice or education?).
4. Establish that the problem selected is amenable to scientific methodology and is not chiefly a moral issue.
5. Critique the feasibility of the problem in terms of time factors, availability of subjects, cooperation required, necessary facilities and equipment, and costs.

The initial review of the literature will help to accomplish these steps in the early development of the problem.

Initial Review of the Literature

"The primary purpose for reviewing relevant literature is to gain a broad background or understanding of the information that is available related to a problem" (Burns & Grove, 1993, p. 141). Once the researcher has raised a question, an initial review of the literature is helpful in:

1. Identifying the major variables in the area of interest
2. Finding out what is already known
3. Gathering feasibility data on the needs for investigation of that question
4. Refining the focus of the problem to be investigated

A review of the literature should make the researcher aware of all the possible relevant material available about a problem of interest. Helpful sources for locating resource materials include indexes from nursing, related disciplines, and popular literature; abstracting services from nursing and related disciplines; computer searches of appropriate data bases; dictionaries; encyclopedias; guides; and directories. Reference librarians in most libraries can help the beginning nurse researcher locate and use these materials.

In summary, the initial review of the literature should answer some questions about the topic of interest, describe other people's interests in the topic, and develop a strong knowledge base of what has been written and reported on the topic. Such a knowledge base makes it possible for the researcher to move on to the next stage of research: specifying the problem and defining the variables.

Specification of the Problem and the Defining Variables

Once the initial review of the literature is completed and the researcher has gained a general understanding of the research topic and a sense of what is known about the topic, the researcher can more clearly delineate the problem to be investigated. A decision is made about exactly what is to be investigated—that is, what part of the nursing domain is to be studied. The nurse researcher may be investigating some client aspect that is clearly important to understand in the nursing process, some client health phenomenon, some client outcomes associated with particular nursing interventions, some aspect of the nurse–client relationship, some aspect of the delivery of nursing care services, some aspect of the environment that affects the health status, or any combination of these factors in the nursing domain.

Clear articulation of the problem incorporates the identification of the phenomenon to be investigated. This research phenomenon is generally called a "variable." A *variable* is a characteristic, a trait, a property, or a condition. If the variable is purposefully manipulated by the researcher to observe and measure another variable, it is an *independent variable*. The variable that is observed and measured and is presumed to be influenced by or related in some special way to the independent variable is the *dependent variable*.

An example of a investigative problem with one variable that is manipulated and another that is observed and measured is: what is the relationship between specific parenting guidance by the professional nurse and the development of positive nutritional habits of the toddler? In this investigation the independent variable is the specific parenting guidance, the dependent variable is the toddler's nutritional habits, and the approach to studying the variables is quantitative.

To make these variables measurable, the researcher must determine exactly what is meant by each variable—what constitutes parenting guidance and what constitutes positive nutritional habits in the toddler. The statement of the problem may be in the form of either a question or a declaration. In both cases, this problem statement must also clearly identify who is to be studied as well as what is to be studied.

Establishment of Tentative Propositions—Hypotheses and the Second Review of the Literature

After the nurse researcher has clarified the problem under investigation, studied the available data, and recalled observations from professional experience, he or she may formulate a hypothesis, "a tentative prediction or explanation of the relationship between two or more variables" (Polit &

Hungler, 1995, p. 51). Not all studies require that the researcher state a hypothesis; for example, surveys, historic studies, and studies of an exploratory nature do not need hypotheses. But for studies requiring manipulation of an independent variable and measurement of a dependent variable, hypotheses must be stated and tested.

Nurses have excellent opportunities to form some hunches about the relationships among variables they observe in practice. Thought of as bridges, hypotheses connect theory with observation and are derived from observations, reasoning, and theoretical bases.

Hypotheses in quantitative studies are tested statistically in relation to the laws of chance. Thus, they are based on statistical probability and incur an element of risk of reaching an incorrect conclusion. How much risk can be afforded is a judgment of the investigator, but when permanent or serious consequences are involved, the investigator cannot afford to take too many risks. Because hypotheses sometimes force the investigator to infer from the sample findings to an interpretation about the population, the researcher uses probability statistics (level of significance) to determine the likelihood that the relationship between the variables results from something other than chance.

At the stage in research when the researcher is determining hypotheses, further review of the literature is used to evaluate testing procedures and to project a research design appropriate for investigating the variable(s). The review of the literature can be used to learn what investigative methods have been used, how data have been collected and analyzed, and what has and has not been successful in previous research.

In summary, in quantitative studies, hypotheses may be stated to declare the researcher's proposition about the relationship between variables, and then serve as the means for testing the proposed relationship.

Determination of a Suitable Research Design

The nurse researcher selects the type of research design suitable for the study on the basis of the appropriate approach to inquiry: descriptive, experimental, or historical. The descriptive design is based on describing the ongoing events of the present. The experimental design is based on the need to manipulate one or more specific variables to measure the effect on other variables. The historical design is based on the desire to describe or evaluate past events.

Development of Measurement Methods and Instruments

After the approach is selected for a particular study, the nurse researcher must decide on the appropriate method for gathering data about the variables. Depending on the purpose of the research, the investigator then selects instruments for data collection. Those instruments generally are categorized under three methods: observation, questioning, and measurement.

Examples of data collection instruments from these categories include critical incidents, tests, interviews, questionnaires, checklists, records, scales, and physical measurement techniques. The researcher strives to select a measurement tool that is appropriate to answer the research question; that is not biased; and that has precision in measuring the variables under study.

Knafl and Webster (1988, pp. 196–203) have pointed out how the researcher's data collection, analysis of those data, and reporting are likely to vary, according to the purpose of the study. They describe four purposes of qualitative research:

1. *Illustration*, in which the researcher aims to identify qualitative examples of specific quantitative variables
2. *Instrumentation*, in which the researcher aims to collect data that serve as the basis for developing an instrument to describe and measure perceptions of some phenomenon of interest to nursing
3. *Description*, in which the researcher aims to "translate the data into a form that would facilitate an accurate, complete description" (p. 200) of a phenomenon of interest to nursing by identifying and delineating the major themes
4. *Theory building*, in which the researcher aims to conceptually explain the phenomenon under study

Knafl, Pettengill, Bevis, and Kirschoff (1988) reported that, although debate continues about the credibility of using either qualitative or quantitative approaches to study particular nursing phenomena, some nurse researchers are beginning to use both qualitative and quantitative methods in single studies. It is believed that integrating the two approaches could "maximize the strengths and minimize the weaknesses of each" (p. 30).

In addition to selecting instruments for data collection during this stage of research, the nurse must also determine the composition of the sample, establish a process for collecting data from the sample, and prepare a format for data collection (which may include designing specific forms), data classification, and data storage for later analysis. The sample subjects must be clearly described, and the method for choosing the subjects must be appropriate. The number of sample subjects must meet statistical requirements for the nurse to draw appropriate conclusions about the findings.

Assurance of an Ethical Process

Essential to the conduct of scientific inquiry in any discipline is the assurance of an ethical process for the subjects. Protection of human rights must be ensured. This protection is provided primarily through informed consent and freedom from harm.

Informed consent means that the subjects are provided with a clear description of what the study is about and how they fit into it. The subjects must understand and consent to their role in the study. Having given informed consent does not keep any subject from changing his or her mind anytime during the study and withdrawing from the study.

Protection from harm means just that—the investigator will not knowingly do anything that will harm or abuse the subjects.

Collection of Data

After protection of human rights for all subjects is ensured, data can be collected. Before any subject associated with an institution can even be approached, however, the researcher must have approval from appropriate agency personnel.

The researcher or a specified data collector orients each subject clearly and concisely to the data collection method, then administers the data collection instrument to each subject in the same manner. Throughout this implementation stage, the researcher follows the written proposal (in the methodology) as closely as possible. While collecting data, the researcher records the data on the prepared forms developed earlier. Then the data are ready to be classified and organized for analysis.

Analysis of Data and Report of Findings

The researcher should organize data in a manner that make them amenable to analysis. If the researcher's goal is simply to display the data collected, no analysis other than the narrative description of the displayed data is needed. If, however, the researcher aims to infer some characteristics about a population or to evaluate some relationship among variables, the organized data must be subjected to statistical analysis. Computations are done. If hypotheses have been stated, statistical testing, by hand or by computer, of those hypotheses must be done.

On the basis of accurate data analysis, the researcher must report the findings exactly as they occurred. Summaries of the data must reflect the individual subjects' findings exactly. All data collected for purposes of testing the hypotheses must be reported. Tables, charts, and graphs used to present data should be pertinent, clear, and well labeled, and they should be discussed in the text of the research report. The reports of the findings are then used to draw conclusions.

Conclusions and Implications

Using the theoretical framework on which the study is based and the analysis of the data collected, the researcher must then determine the meaning of those findings and their value to nursing. Findings are analyzed first by inspecting the statistical tests performed, to test the hypotheses or evaluate data. Then the researcher interprets what the numerical analysis means. The findings may support the predicted relationship with demonstrated statistical significance (findings were not due to chance alone); the findings may not be in the predicted direction; the findings may be contradictory; or the findings may indicate an unpredicted relationship.

Based on the analysis and interpretation of data, the researcher might make generalizations about what the data mean and whether the data can be applied to groups different from the sample. Generalizations should emerge only from the findings, and the researcher should not go beyond the data as a result of the excitement generated by scientific discovery.

The implications of the study are usually related to one of the three aspects of professional nursing: practice with clients; education of the professional; and further research in nursing. Implications are generally reported in the section of a research study called "recommendations." The implications for practice—ie, how they affect the nursing process with clients—are spelled out. Recommendations for the education of practitioners and on future research are usually given. If the recommendations are clearly and concisely stated and derived logically, they are the power of the study.

The Written Report

Research completed but not written up is wasted. It can be argued that the research process is really not complete until it is shared in writing or some other public medium. Characteristics of an effective research report are brevity, clarity, and complete objectivity.

Although there are variations on the form of the report that may be determined by faculty, a particular style manual, or other institutional requirements, the usual report follows the outline of the research process presented in this chapter. Most outlines include the problem statement, review of literature, methods of investigation, presentation of findings, discussion of the analyses and conclusions, bibliographic data, and appendixes. The reader is directed to either a nursing research book or a writing style manual for specific guidance in developing each part of the written research report.

Utilization of Nursing Research

VIGNETTE: JOAN

Joan is an experienced staff nurse on a general surgical unit. She prides herself on giving prompt medication to patients in pain. She has seen several published research articles about noninvasive nursing interventions that could reduce the need for narcotic analgesia. But Joan is unsure of how to decide whether to use the research findings in her practice.

New knowledge is being generated rapidly. What is learned in an academic program is unlikely to be current within a few years, and the professional nurse cannot plead ignorance of new knowledge and practices.

Professional accountability requires keeping up with the literature and applying new knowledge appropriately in practice.

The utilization of a scientific base for clinical practice has a number of benefits, including:

- A sound foundation for practice
- Enhanced self-confidence, autonomy, critical thinking skills, and professional self-concept
- Cost-effective patient care
- Increased patient and job satisfaction and quality of care
- Improved patient outcomes
- A stimulus for collaborative practice, retention, and recruitment
- An improved image of nursing
- An ever-increasing scientific nursing knowledge base (Goode et al., 1991, pp. 8–9)

Research utilization may be as simple as one nurse changing the way in which care is given (Gennaro, 1994). However, despite the significant amount of available nursing research, there is a well-documented gap in the use of research findings to improve practice. This section describes two major theories of research utilization, discusses possible barriers, and describes strategies to facilitate the use of research findings in practice.

THEORIES OF RESEARCH UTILIZATION

Rogers's Theory of Diffusion of Innovations

According to Rogers (1983), "*Diffusion* is the process by which an innovation is communicated through certain channels over time among the members of a social system" (p. 5). Rogers defines an *innovation* as "an idea, practice, or object that is perceived as new" (p. 11). In the vignette above, noninvasive nursing interventions would be considered an innovation.

Rogers (1983) suggests that a five-stage process is used for deciding whether to adopt an innovation (something perceived as new by those who are considering adoption). The *knowledge stage* is the first awareness of the existence of the innovation. The *persuasion stage* occurs when the individual forms an attitude toward the innovation. A *decision* occurs when the individual makes the choice for adoption or rejection of the innovation. In the *implementation* stage, the individual uses the innovation, and in the *confirmation* stage, the individual seeks reinforcement of the decision. Reversal of the decision can occur at any time during the implementation and confirmation stages.

For an individual to consider adoption of an innovation, the person must be aware of the innovation. Rogers (1983) used the term diffusion to describe the dissemination of an innovation. His theory proposes that diffusion of an innovation is enhanced by face to face and mass media communication channels, time, and interaction within the social system. Adoption of an innovation is enhanced by persuasion by a peer colleague or by influence from opinion leaders within the social system. An outside change agent may also facilitate diffusion and adoption of an innovation.

The perceived characteristics of the innovation affect favorable or unfavorable attitudes toward the adoption. The probability and speed of adoption are enhanced if the innovation is perceived to be better than current practice; is consistent with current values, past experience, and priority of needs; is not difficult to understand or use, or require learning new skills; can be tried out on a limited basis with the option of returning to previous practices; and has highly visible results (Burns & Grove, 1993).

The Stetler/Marram Decision-Making Model

While Rogers's theory addresses the structure of diffusion of any innovation, including research findings, the revised Stetler/Marram model (Stetler, 1994), refers to a six-phase critical thinking and decision-making process to assist the individual practitioner in using published research.

In phase I, *preparation,* the nurse determines the purpose for the research review. For example, the purpose might be to solve a difficult problem, stay current in a clinical specialty, or revise a procedure or policy. Does some aspect of client care need to be improved? The purpose will influence the development of measurable outcomes later in the process. In phase II, *validation,* the strengths and weaknesses of a research study are assessed to accept or reject findings based on their potential for applicability.

Phase III, *comparative evaluation,* determines whether it is desirable or feasible to apply findings in practice. Criteria include similarity of the study sample and environment to the population and setting of the nurse; assessment of the effectiveness of current practice and whether or not theory would be an improvement; assessment of risk, need for resources, and readiness; and substantiating evidence. Multiple research articles with congruent findings or a meta-analysis are, of course, more desirable than one study. Liehr and Houston (1993) describe an outline for examining the fit, flow, and feasibility of reported research that fits with phases II and III (Table 7-1).

Phase IV, *decision-making,* may result in the decision to use the new knowledge to change practice or modify a way of thinking without waiting for additional data. Another alternative is to consider use but continue to collect additional data. A third option might be to delay use until further research has been conducted. A fourth alternative might be to reject or not use the information because of the risks or costs involved, lack of consistent, strong findings, or the strength of current practice (Stetler, 1993).

Phase V, *translation/application,* involves generalization of the similarities or differences in the sources that were reviewed and identification of implications for practice (the "so what"). In phase VI, evaluation, the expected outcomes are compared with the purpose that was defined in the preparation phase. Following this decision-making process, the nurse would implement a planned change model (see Chap. 17) to actually in-

TABLE 7-1	
Fit, Flow, and Feasibility: Markers and Tips for Preliminary Evaluation of Nursing Research	

Title and Abstract . . . are you interested? If yes, proceed	
Markers	**Tips**
FIT	
Does the purpose of the study fit with your area of clinical interest or work?	Adopt a broad view.
Is the sample appropriate and representative?	Look for a representative sample from a homogeneous group.
FLOW	
Do the questions/hypotheses flow from the purpose?	Find the researcher's statement of intent to compare and contrast study variables.
Is a logical system of ideas presented as a basis for the research?	Look for the underlying conceptual support (eg, nursing, psychosocial).
Do the measures for the variables make sense?	Yes or no, based on your knowledge and experience.
Is the reliability and validity (R & V) of selected measures discussed?	Evaluate how R & V "test" subjects compare with sample of paper you are reviewing.
Does the researcher control factors that may influence results?	List factors from knowledge and experience; are they controlled?
Are appropriate statistics used for each research question/hypothesis?	If a relationship study: Pearson's correlation or multiple regression; if difference study: t test or analysis of variance.
Is the sample size adequate for selected analysis?	If no significant effect, sample size may be too small.
Do the study conclusions accurately reflect findings?	Make a list of findings and compare to conclusions.
FEASIBILITY	
Is it ethical and legal to apply the study findings?	Yes or No
If there is a cost to the patient or institution (money and time), is it within acceptable limits?	Yes or No
If a change in practice is required, is it congruent with the nursing philosophy of the institution?	Yes or No
FOCUSED OBSERVATION	

From Liehr, P., Houston, S. (1993). Critiquing and using nursing research: Guidelines for the critical care nurse. *American Journal of Critical Care, 2,* 407–412.

corporate the new knowledge into practice. The Stetler model is presented in Figure 7-1.

BARRIERS TO RESEARCH UTILIZATION

"It has been found that although the majority of nurses are aware of research-based interventions, few use them even sometimes" (Miller, 1996, p. 175). Goode and colleagues (1991, pp. 7–8) and Funk, Champagne,

Wiese, & Tornquist (1991) identified a number of barriers to research utilization, including barriers from the research, the clinician, the researcher, and the administration. Barriers from the research include:

Insufficient current research with solutions to complex clinical problems

Research findings that have not been replicated and cannot be generalized to settings beyond the study site

Research reports that are difficult to read

Much research (eg, theses, dissertations) unpublished and difficult to access

Lack of compilation of research in one place

Barriers from the clinician include:

A majority of entry-level and experienced practitioners who lack education in how to read, conduct, and use research

Attitude among practicing nurses that using research findings is more trouble than it is worth

Practitioners unaccustomed to reading research journals

Clinicians not able to understand statistical analyses

Dependence on tradition, which is difficult to change even if it is ineffective

Difficulty determining if studies are well designed and scientifically sound

Practitioners isolated from knowledgeable colleagues who could help

Barriers from the researcher include:

Communicate primarily in journals that are not read by clinicians

Use language that is not understood by clinicians

Often lack direct patient care experience

Findings often not presented in a form that is usable for clinical implementation

Barriers from the administration include:

Minimal value placed on research by many administrators and managers

No provision made for resources such as time, financial support, and education

Lack of nursing autonomy within a bureaucratic structure to implement data-based solutions to problems

Lack of incentives for nurses to participate in research utilization activities

Reliance on policy and procedure, rather than openness to change

Lack of support for implementation of research findings by physicians and other staff

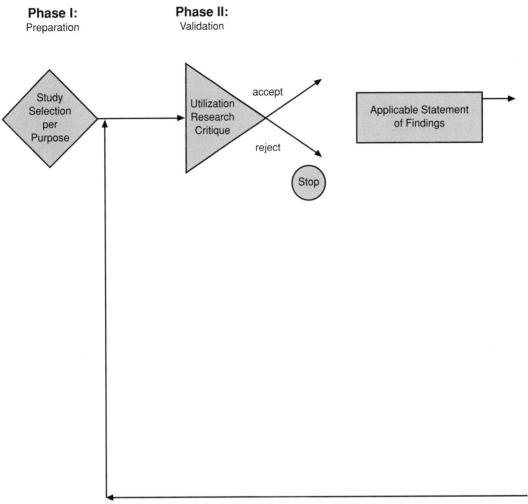

FIGURE 7-1 The Stetler model for research utilization. (Stetler, C. B. [1994]. Refinement of the Stetler/Marram model for application of research findings to practice. *Nursing Outlook, 42,* 18–19. Used with permission.)

Unfortunately most clinicians are not familiar with research methods, language, and statistical methods because "almost half of the practitioners never had a research course" (Cronenwett, 1995, p. 429). However, baccalaureate-educated clinicians should be able to raise questions during practice and recognize effective and ineffective interventions from experience. Strategies to address barriers and facilitate the utilization of research must build on basic professional education. Some strategies to facilitate research utilization are discussed in the next section.

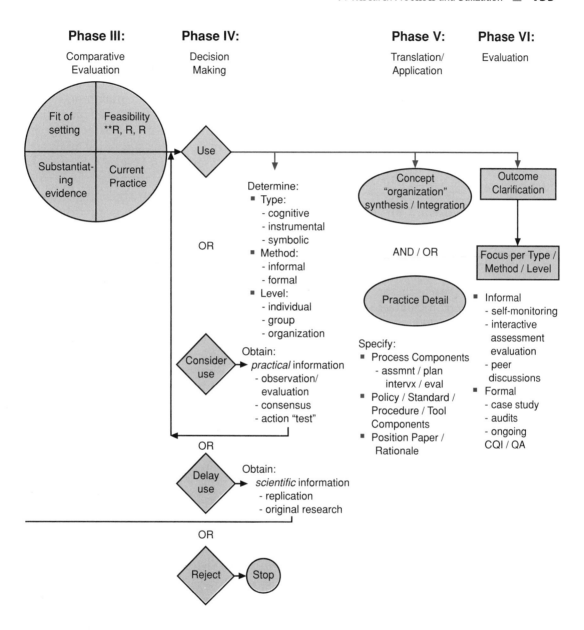

STRATEGIES TO FACILITATE RESEARCH UTILIZATION

"Prior research instruction, awareness of support for research, and positive attitudes toward research were predictive of nurses' participation in research activities" (Rizzuto, Bostrom, Suter, & Chenitz, 1994, p. 193). In the baccalaureate degree program, the student is exposed to the basics of the process of conducting research. This content is intended to help the student understand research terminology and will facilitate reading published research reports with basic statistical analysis. However, many baccalaureate-educated nurses still feel that they cannot truly understand much published research.

Researchers need to make the effort to write for a clinician audience and to emphasize the meaning of the findings for practice in language that is understandable by most clinicians. Consultation with a master's degree-educated nurse will be helpful in interpreting complex statistical analyses. The clinical setting may employ a master's-prepared research facilitator who is available for consultation. Another source might be graduate students or faculty from a local school of nursing. Possibly a group of nurses could work together with a consultant in locating and interpreting relevant literature.

To use research findings, practicing nurses must read professional journals, including research journals. A number of journals, including *Applied Nursing Research* and *Clinical Nursing Research*, now focus on use of the research for practice. The literature has to be accessible by way of electronic data bases such as Medline or CINAHL. Many hospitals have a basic medical library that includes a core collection of nursing journals. Another source might be a nearby college or university library. Library privileges and a prepaid photocopying card should be requested by the nurse if they are not provided automatically. Nurses should look for integrative reviews or meta-analyses that review a number of studies and provide information about the quality of the results.

Other ways of gaining access to research findings might include a research bulletin board, newsletters, or research grand rounds, but these strategies need to be organized and maintained. Many institutions have a research committee that could take responsibility for coordinating the review of literature, exploration of ideas, pilot testing of innovations, and the development and dissemination of protocols and policies.

Another resource might be the in-service education department. Master's-prepared clinical educators could evaluate and synthesize knowledge across studies and provide direction for clinicians. Practitioners need continuing in-service education to help with identifying and locating appropriate literature, evaluating the quality of research, understanding data analysis, and determining the relevance of research findings for practice modifications.

An atmosphere where questioning and evaluating of practice and supporting and valuing of research use by managers and administrators is crucial. Ideally, the valuing of research as a way of knowing would be demonstrated by a positive attitude and by providing tangible resources for research utilization such as time and consultation. Incentives and rewards for risk-taking and creativity are desirable. Collaboration with peers and other colleagues is a strategy that can be productive. Most of all, the atmosphere must be one of respect and encouragement for professional practice and delegation of authority so that nurses control nursing practice.

However, in the final analysis, the clinician has to value the use of research as the basis for practice enough to provide the effort and make the time for research utilization activities. When a significant number of nurses value scholarship enough to participate in its creation, dissemination, and utilization, then, and only then, nursing will truly be viewed as a profession.

◎ Creating a Public Image of the Nurse as Scholar

A visit to a college or university today reveals the strides that nursing has made in developing research and researchers. Among the many nursing journals are several major nursing research journals, including an online electronic journal published by Sigma Theta Tau International. These journals reflect important strengths of an emerging profession.

Advanced technology offers great support for the nurse researcher today. The storage, retrieval, and analysis of data afforded by computer support makes the time factor much more appealing and possible for many nurses to conduct research. In most educational and practice settings, a researcher should not have to manually manage data. As another great help to research, the computer's ability to manipulate numbers allows almost unlimited analysis of data and the ability to use research findings to a fuller capacity.

Further, it is anticipated that the word processing supports and electronic transmission of information offered by computers will be helpful in sharing more research findings with clinicians in practice. Thus, nursing is moving into a period of valuing and conducting research at a time when technology is greatly supportive to many aspects of the research process.

Traditionally, nurses have not been viewed as scholars. As a result, their higher education and research productivity have been extremely limited. What the public continues to see is a group in which approximately 70% possess less-than-baccalaureate preparation in the discipline. That lack of credentialing alone probably explains the tiny proportion of researchers in nursing.

As nursing has developed its own theory base over the last 35 years, nurses have begun to value the scholarship role of the nurse. Most nurses today would probably agree that a practice based on research is desirable. Capitalizing on that consensus, the profession can begin to present a different image to the public. To help actualize the motivation to base nursing practice on research, educational programs need to prepare students in scientific inquiry while also preparing them to apply theory in the conduct of professional roles.

As nurses begin to feel and act like scholars, the public will begin to see a scholarly side of nursing. If the profession nourishes this scholarship in nurses, it will undoubtedly help change the image of the nurse. Because scholars accept that research is a vital component of nursing, the development of scholars will increase the supply of researchers to better serve the profession and the public.

◎ Conclusion

In the 1960s through the 1990s, many researchers and scholars provided a beginning theory base for nursing. As we approach the 21st century, researchers and scholars will be even more important to the emergence of nursing as an autonomous profession and to the provision of better nursing services to the public.

THOUGHT QUESTIONS

1 What are the relative merits of quantitative and qualitative methods in nursing research? How does a researcher decide which methods to use?

2 How can nurses promote research utilization in their practice? How would you respond to Sandy in the vignette at the beginning of the chapter?

3 What is the public image of nursing? Does the public respect nursing's knowledge base?

REFERENCES

Artinian, B. A. (1988). Qualitative modes of inquiry. *Western Journal of Nursing Research, 10,* 138–149.

Baessler, C. A., Blumberg, M., Cunningham, J. S., Curran, J. A., Fennessay, A. G., Jacobs, J. M., McGrath, P., Perrong, M. T., & Wolf, Z. R. (1994). Medical-surgical nurses' utilization of research methods and products. *MEDSURG Nursing, 3,* 113–121.

Burns, N., & Grove, S. K. (1993). *The practice of nursing research: Conduct, critique, and utilization* (2nd ed.). Philadelphia: Saunders.

Cohen, M. Z., & Tripp-Reimer, T. (1988). Research in cultural diversity: Qualitative methods in cultural research. *Western Journal of Nursing Research, 10,* 226–228.

Cronenwett, L. R. (1995). Effective methods for disseminating research findings to nurses in practice. *Nursing Clinics of North America, 30,* 429–438.

Funk, S. G., Champagne, M. T., & Wiese, R. A., & Tornquist, E. M. (1991). Barriers to using research findings in practice: The clinician's perspective. *Applied Nursing Research, 4,* 90–95.

Gennaro, S. (1994). Research utilization: An overview. *Journal of Obstetric, Gynecologic, and Neonatal Nursing, 23,* 313–319.

Goode, C. J., Butcher, L. A., Cipperley, J. A., Ekstrom, J., Gosch, B. A., Hayes, J. E., Lovett, M. K., & Wellendorf, S. A. (1991). *Research utilization: A study guide.* Ida Grove, IA: Horn Video Productions.

Haase, J. E., & Myers, S. T. (1988). Reconciling paradigm assumptions of qualitative and quantitative research. *Western Journal of Nursing Research, 10,* 128–137.

Heater, B. S., Becker, A. M., & Olson, R. K. (1988). Nursing interventions and patient outcomes: A meta-analysis of studies. *Nursing Research, 37,* 303–307.

Knafl, K. A., Pettengill, M. M., Bevis, M. E., & Kirschoff, K. T. (1988). Blending qualitative and quantitative approaches to instrument development and data collection. *Journal of Professional Nursing, 4,* 30–37.

Knafl, K. A., & Webster, D. C. (1988). Managing and analyzing qualitative data: A description of tasks, techniques, and materials. *Western Journal of Nursing Research, 10,* 195–218.

Liehr, P., & Houston, S. (1993). Critiquing and using nursing research: Guidelines for the critical care nurse. *American Journal of Critical Care, 2,* 407–412.

Mariano, C. (1990). Qualitative research: Instructional strategies and curricular considerations. *Nursing and Health Care, 11,* 3354–3359.

Miller, S. P. (1996). Dissemination and utilization of research: Outcome behaviors at the baccalaureate level. *Journal of Nursing Education, 35,* 175–177.

Polit, D. F., & Hungler, B. (1995). *Nursing research: Principles and methods* (5th ed.). Philadelphia: Lippincott.

Riegel, B., Banasik, J. L., Barnsteiner, J., Beecroft, P., Kern, L., Lindquist, R., Prevost, S., & Titler, M. (1993). Reviews and summaries of research related to AACN 1980 research priorities: Clinical topics. *American Journal of Critical Care, 2,* 413–425.

Rizzuto, C., Bostrom, J., Suter, W. N., & Chenitz, W. C. (1994). Predictors of nurses' involvement in research activities. *Western Journal of Nursing Research, 16,* 193–204.

Rogers, E. (1983). *Diffusion of innovations* (3rd ed.). New York: Free Press.

Rogers, M. E. (1967, February 3). *Nursing science: Research and researcher.* Presented at the Annual Conference on Research and Nursing, Teachers College, Columbia University, New York.

Stetler, C. B. (1994). Refinement of the Stetler/Marram model for application of research findings to practice. *Nursing Outlook, 42,* 15–25.

Titler, M. G., Kleiber, C., Steelman, V., Goode, C., Rakel, B., Walker, J. B., Small, S., & Buckwalter, K. (1994). Infusing research into practice to promote quality care. *Nursing Research, 43,* 307–313.

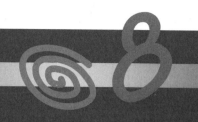

Nursing Models and Theories

LEARNING OUTCOMES

By the end of the chapter, the student will be able to:

1 Know the critical elements of systems, adaptation, caring, and complexity theories.

2 Understand how nursing's metaparadigm concepts are defined in each of the various models.

3 Appreciate how multiple models of nursing can be of value to nursing practice.

VIGNETTE

Peter works evenings in an intensive care unit in a large metropolitan city. He has always been interested in conceptual models, but his coworkers say they "don't have time," "there isn't enough staff," and "models don't really make any difference in care anyway." Peter wonders if his colleagues are right.

Value of Theories for Nursing

Nurses traditionally have based their practice on intuition, experience, or the "way I was taught." These methods lead to rote and stereotypical practice. Practice based on theories, however, allows for hypotheses about practice, which make it possible to derive a rationale for nursing actions. Testable theories provide a knowledge base for the science of nursing. As the science of nursing develops, nurses will be able to (1) more accurately understand and explain past events, and (2) provide a basis for predicting and controlling future events. In addition, practice based on science will support the image of nursing as a professional discipline.

CHARACTERISTICS OF THEORIES

Theory is "a creative and rigorous structuring of ideas that project a tentative, purposeful, and systematic view of phenomena" (Chinn & Kramer, 1995, p. 72). By taking individual concepts such as humans, society, health, and nursing and developing statements of possible relationships among them, a theory makes it possible to "organize the relationship among the concepts to describe, explain, predict, and control practice" (Torres, 1986, p. 21). Torres (1990, p. 6–9) suggested the following characteristics of theories:

1. Theories can interrelate concepts in such a way as to create a different way of looking at a particular phenomenon
2. Theories must be logical in nature
3. Theories should be relatively simple yet generalizable
4. Theories can be the bases for hypotheses that can be tested
5. Theories contribute to and assist in increasing the general body of knowledge within the discipline through the research implemented to validate them
6. Theories can be used by the practitioners to guide and improve their practice
7. Theories must be consistent with other validated theories, laws, and principles but will leave open unanswered questions that need to be investigated

Models of Nursing

Until fairly recently, nursing science was derived principally from social, biologic, and medical science theories. However, from the 1950s to the present, an increasing number of nursing theorists have developed models of nursing that provide bases for the development of nursing theories and nursing knowledge.

A *model*, as an abstraction of reality, provides a way to visualize reality to simplify thinking. For example, an airplane model provides a representation of a real airplane. A conceptual model shows how various concepts are interrelated and applies theories to predict or evaluate consequences of alternative actions. According to Fawcett (1995), each conceptual model provides a systematic structure and a rationale for scholarly activities. A conceptual model "gives direction to the search for relevant questions about phenomena and suggests solutions to practical problems" (p. 3).

A conceptual model describes the concepts that compose it. Four concepts are generally considered central to the discipline of nursing:

The person who receives nursing care (the patient or client)
The environment (society)
Nursing (goals, roles, functions)
Health

All existing models of nursing describe these four concepts. But the models vary in the amount of emphasis placed on each concept, as well as in the kinds of theories that might explain the interrelationships among the concepts.

GROWTH AND STABILITY MODELS OF CHANGE

There are two major differences in philosophical beliefs, or "world views," about the nature of change. "The world view of change uses the growth metaphor, and the persistence view focuses on stability" (Fawcett, 1989, p. 12). Within the change world view, change and growth are continual and desirable, "progress is valued, and realization of one's potential is emphasized" (Fawcett, 1989, p. 12). In contrast, "the persistence world view maintains that stability is natural and normal . . . . Persistence is endurance in time and is produced by a synthesis of growth and stability. The focus is on continuation and maintenance of patterns and routines" (Fawcett, 1989, p. 12). This persistence world view emphasizes equilibrium and balance.

CATEGORIES OF CONCEPTUAL MODELS

Ten conceptual models of nursing have been classified according to two criteria:

- The world view of change reflected by the model (growth or stability)
- The major theoretical conceptual classification with which the model seems most consistent (systems, stress/adaptation, caring, or growth/development)

It is hoped that this structure for grouping nursing models will give the reader a basis for understanding how these models compare and contrast conceptually.

The following discussions indicate the essence of each model, from original sources as much as possible, so that the reader can appreciate the similarities and differences among them and the points of congruence with the theoretical perspective on which the model is based. The intent is to clarify the models, rather than to analyze strengths or weaknesses, critique the models, or to select the best model. Interpretations of the nursing process based on these models are presented in Chapter 9.

⊚ The Stability Model of Change

SYSTEMS THEORY AS A FRAMEWORK

Systems theory is concerned with changes due to interactions among all the factors (variables) in a situation. Interactions between the person and the environment occur continuously; thus, the situation is complex and constantly changing. General systems theory will be emphasized because this theory has influenced several conceptual models in nursing. Systems theory provides a way to understand the many influences on the whole person, as well as the possible impact of change of any part on the whole. This theory can be useful in nursing to understand, predict, and control the possible effects of nursing care on the client system and the concurrent effects of the interaction on the nurse system.

A *system* is defined as "a whole with interrelated parts, in which the parts have a function and the system as a totality has a function" (Auger, 1976, p. 21). Systems are organized into hierarchical levels of complexity, with subsystems and suprasystems. Single systems may be subsystems of more complex systems, although each system also has a suprasystem.

A person is composed of cells, organs, and physiologic systems—the subsystems of humans. These subsystems are continuously interacting and changing. For example, as a person eats, the blood supply to the gastrointestinal organs increases. Absorption of carbohydrates increases the blood glucose level, which results in increased insulin secretion. Simultaneously, changes in the blood circulation and blood glucose level affect the attention level and the feeling of hunger. The person may feel satisfied and contented.

The gastrointestinal, endocrine, cardiovascular, and emotional systems are subsystems of the person, and the whole person is the suprasystem for each physiologic or psychological system. The person's internal environment is composed of interacting subsystems.

The person is a subsystem of the family system (which is a suprasystem of the person), which is a subsystem of the community system, and so on. Subsystems may be isolated for study, but human beings are more than and different from the sum of their parts (Rogers, 1970, p. 46). Thus, a person cannot be characterized by describing physiologic, psychological, and sociocultural subsystems. A person's behavior is holistic, a reflection of the person as a whole. The focus of systems theory is on understanding the interaction among the various parts of the system rather than on describing the function of the parts themselves (Auger, 1976, p. 20).

All persons are open systems, which means that they exchange matter, energy, and information across their boundaries with the environment (Sills & Hall, 1977, p. 20). A person's internal environment is in constant interaction with a changing external environment. Changes occurring in one affect the other. For example, walking into a cold room (change in the external environment) affects various physiologic and psychological subsystems of the internal environment, which in turn will change blood flow, ability to concentrate, feeling of comfort, and so on. Similarly, a person's angry outburst (change in the internal environment) can have a demonstrable effect on the moods of others. It is this openness of human systems that makes nursing intervention possible.

> A general systems approach allows for consideration of the subsystems levels of the human being, as a total human being, and as a social creature who networks himself with others in hierarchically arranged human systems of increasing complexity. Thus the human being, from the level of the individual to the level of society, can be conceptualized as client and becomes the target system for nursing intervention. (Sills & Hall, 1977, pp. 24–25).

Systems analysis assumes that structure and stability can be measured during a arbitrarily frozen time period. The system is conceptualized as seeking equilibrium or a steady state, in which a balance exists among the various forces operating within and on the system. Factors from the environment impinge on the system across the system boundary. These factors cause tension, stress, strain, or conflict and can upset the balance of the system. Change is a process of tension reduction and dynamic equilibrium, which restores a new position of system balance after a disturbance (Chin, 1976).

Energy, information, or matter provide input for the system. The system "transforms, creates, and organizes input in the process known as throughput, which results in a reorganization of the input" (Sills & Hall, 1977, p. 21). Thus, each system modifies its input. Simultaneously, energy, information, or matter is given off into the environment as output. When output is returned to the system as input, the process is known as feedback.

For example, information about a therapeutic diet given to the client by the nurse is system input for the client system. What the client eats would be one type of system output, based on the throughput related to assimilation and acceptance of the information originally given. The nurse, using the client's reported food intake as feedback, can help either reinforce or modify the client's future behavior (Fig. 8-1).

A person can be viewed as "an interrelated, interdependent, interacting, complex organism, constantly influencing and being influenced by [the] environment" (Sills & Hall, 1977, p. 24). Because the person is in constant interaction with the environment, a number of interrelated factors, including the influence of the nurse, will affect the person's health status. The person's response, in turn, then will result in change in the

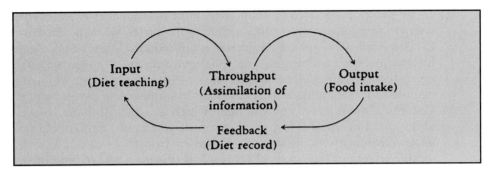

FIGURE 8-1 An example of systems interaction.

environment. Because of these interactions, a change in any part affects the whole human–environment system.

Using systems theory to guide nursing process directs assessment of the relationships among all variables that affect the client–environment interaction, including the influence of the nurse. In intervention, the nurse must anticipate the system-wide impact from change in any part of the system and appreciate the simultaneous, rather than cause and effect, nature of change in open systems.

The following section describes two nursing models based on systems theory:

Imogene King's systems interaction model
Betty Neuman's health care systems model

Imogene King's Systems Interaction Model
In this model, the purpose of nursing is to help people attain, maintain, or restore health.

TERMS
   Transaction: observable behavior of human beings interacting with their environment

The focus of King's model is on "individuals whose interactions in groups within social systems influence behavior within the systems" (King, 1989, p. 152). As humans interact with their environment, their perceptions influence their behavior and their health. Nurses can interact with clients to facilitate achievement of health-related goals, as can other persons in the environment.

Perception is the comprehensive concept in personal systems. It is "a characteristic of a human process of interaction, and along with communication provides a channel for passage of information from one person to another" (King, 1989, p. 153). Concepts of self, growth and development, learning, body image, time, and space also relate to individuals as personal systems.

Interaction is the comprehensive concept in interpersonal systems. Related concepts include communication, transactions, roles, stress, and all the concepts identified in personal systems. Organization is the comprehensive concept in social systems, with related concepts of power, authority, status, decision-making, and control (King, 1989, pp. 152–153).

Humans are "open systems interacting with environment" (King, 1981, p. 10) They are seen as "rational, sentient, reacting, social, controlling, purposeful, time-oriented, and action-oriented" (King, 1987, p. 107). The human "perceives the world as a total person" (King, 1981, p. 141). As the person interacts with the environment, he or she must continuously adjust to stressors in the internal and external environment (King, 1981, p. 5).

Health assumes achievement of maximum potential for daily living and an ability to function in social roles. It is the "dynamic life experiences of a human being, which implies continuous adjustment to stressors in the internal and external environment through optimum use of one's resources to achieve maximum potential for daily living" (King, 1981, p. 5). "Illness is a deviation from normal, that is, an imbalance in a person's biological structure or in his psychological makeup, or a conflict in a person's social relationships" (King, 1989, p. 5).

"The goal of nursing is to help individuals and groups attain, maintain, and restore health" (King, 1981, p. 13). "Nursing's domain involves human beings, families, and communities as a framework within which nurses make transactions in multiple environments with health as a goal" (King, 1996, p. 61). Nursing care is accomplished within goal-oriented nurse–client interactions "whereby each perceives the other and the situation, and through communications, they set goals, explore the means to achieve them, agree to the means, and their actions indicate movement toward goal achievement" (King, 1987, p. 113).

King's model conceptualizes three levels of dynamic interacting systems:

Individuals are called "personal systems."
Groups (two or more persons) form "interpersonal systems."
Society is composed of "social systems."

King originally selected 15 concepts relevant to an understanding of these systems, but more recently she defined and discussed 10 concepts that relate to the personal and interpersonal systems (King, 1987, pp. 109–110):

1. *Interaction*: "a process of perception and communication between person and environment and between person and person, represented by verbal and non-verbal behaviors that are goal-directed"
2. *Perception*: "each person's representation of reality"
3. *Communication*: "a process whereby information is given from one person to another"
4. *Transaction*: "an observable behavior of human beings interacting with their environment . . . [in which] valuation is a component of human interaction"

5. *Role*: "a set of behaviors expected of persons occupying a position in a social system"
6. *Stress*: "a dynamic state whereby a human being interacts with the environment to maintain balance for growth, development, and performance"
7. *Growth and development*: "continuous changes in individuals at the cellular, molecular, and behavioral levels of activities"
8. *Time*: "a continuous flow of events in successive order that implies change, a past, and a future"
9. *Self*: "a personal system defined as a unified, complex whole"
10. *Space*: "existing in all directions and the same everywhere"

King has proposed the theory of goal attainment in which these concepts are interrelated in a number of propositions and hypotheses which "identifies the nature of nurse–client interactions that lead to goal attainment" (King, 1995, p. 27). Decision-making is "a shared collaborative process in which client and nurse give information to each other, identify goals, and explore means to attain goals; each moves forward to attain goals. This is identified in the theory as a critical independent variable called mutual goal setting" (King, 1989, p. 155).

Examples of testable hypotheses generated from King's theory include the following (King, 1987, p. 111):

Mutual goal-setting will increase functional abilities in performing activities of daily living.
Goal attainment will be greater in clients who participate in mutual goal-setting than in clients who do not participate.
Role conflict between nurse and client may increase stress in the nursing situation.

King's model and the theory of goal attainment provide a "theoretical base for applying the traditional nursing process . . . aimed at maintaining or restoring health" (Magan, 1987, pp. 129, 132). Major concepts as defined in this model are summarized in Table 8-1.

Betty Neuman's Health Care Systems Model
In this model, the purpose of nursing is to facilitate optimal client system stability.

TABLE 8-1	
Major Concepts as Defined in King's Model	
Person	Open system interacting with the environment
Environment	That with which or whom the person interacts
Health	A dynamic state of well-being
Illness	An imbalance in biologic structure, psychological makeup, or social relationships
Nursing	Process of human interaction

TERMS
    Lines of defense: normal range of responses through which a person deals with stressors to maintain equilibrium of the system

Lines of resistance: protection from stressors
Neuman's model, organized around stress reduction, is primarily concerned with how stress and the reactions to stress affect the development and maintenance of health. The person is described as an open system that interacts with the environment to promote "harmony and balance between his internal and external environment" (Neuman, 1982, p. 14). The person is a composite of physiologic, psychological, sociocultural, developmental, and spiritual variables viewed as a whole. According to Newman (1982, p. 14), "No one part can be looked at in isolation . . . . Just as the single part influences perception of the whole, the patterns of the whole influence awareness of the part." Thus, the functioning of any subsystem or part of a system must be evaluated in the context of the entire system.

The environment includes "all internal and external factors or influences surrounding the identified client or client system" (Neuman, 1989, p. 31). Client and environment have a reciprocal relationship.

A person is constantly affected by stressors from the internal or external environment. Stressors are tension-producing stimuli that have the potential to disturb a person's equilibrium or normal line of defense. This normal line of defense is the person's "usual steady state." It is the way in which an individual usually deals with stressors. Stressors may be of three types:

Intrapersonal: forces arising from within the person
Interpersonal: forces arising between persons
Extrapersonal: forces arising from outside the person

Resistance to stressors is provided by a flexible line of defense, a dynamic protective buffer made up of all variables affecting a person at any given moment. These variables may include a person's physiologic structure and condition, sociocultural background, spiritual beliefs, developmental state, cognitive skills, age, sex, and so forth. The interrelationships among these variables determine the person's resistance to any given stressor or stressors.

If the flexible line of defense is no longer able to protect the person against a stressor, the stressor breaks through, disturbs the person's equilibrium, and triggers a reaction. The reaction may lead toward restoration of balance or toward death, depending on the internal lines of resistance that attempt to restore balance. The reaction to the stressor and the prognosis are influenced by:

The number and strength of the stressors affecting the person
The length of time that the person is affected
The meaningfulness of the stressor to the person

Neuman intends for the nurse to "assist clients to retain, attain, or maintain optimal system stability" (Neuman, 1996, p. 69). Thus, health (wellness) seems to be related to dynamic equilibrium of the normal line of defense, where stressors are successfully overcome or avoided by the flexible line of defense. Neuman defines illness as "a state of insufficiency—disrupting needs are yet to be satisfied" (Neuman, 1982, p. 10). Illness appears to be a separate state when a stressor breaks through the normal line of defense and causes a reaction with the person's lines of resistance.

> The major concern for nursing is in keeping the client system stable through accuracy both in assessing the effects and possible effects of environmental stressors and in assisting client adjustments required for an optimal wellness level. Optimal means the best possible health state achievable at a given point in time (Neuman, 1995, p. 33).

Nursing intervention is accomplished through primary, secondary, or tertiary prevention. *Primary prevention* is appropriate before the person comes in contact with a stressor. *Secondary prevention* is appropriate after the stressor has penetrated the normal line of defense. *Tertiary prevention* accompanies restoration of balance, moving in a circular manner toward primary prevention.

This model suggests various primary, secondary, and tertiary prevention nursing activities to reduce stress factors and strengthen the person's resistance. As an example of a systems model compatible with the medical model, it has been applied in a number of practice and education settings. The major concepts defined in Neuman's model are summarized in Table 8-2.

TABLE 8-2	
Major Concepts as Defined in Neuman's Model	
Person	Open system seeking balance and harmony; a composite of physiologic, psychological, sociocultural, and developmental variables viewed as a whole
Health	A dynamic equilibrium of the normal line of defense
Illness	Reaction of stressors with lines of resistance
Environment	Internal and external stressors and resistance factors
Nursing	Reduction of stressors through primary, secondary, or tertiary prevention

STRESS/ADAPTATION THEORY AS A FRAMEWORK

In contrast to systems theory, stress and adaptation theories view change due to person–environment interaction in terms of cause and effect. The person must adjust to environmental changes to avoid disturbing a balanced existence. Adaptation theory provides a way to understand both how the balance is maintained and the possible effects of disturbed equilibrium. This theory has been widely applied to explain, predict, and control biologic (physiologic and psychological) responses of persons. It is the basis for much current medical therapy.

The human body functions as a whole. All body cells are affected by the activities of other cells. This communication is made possible because all cells are surrounded by the same fluids (ie, blood, lymph, interstitial fluid), which form an internal environment for the entire body. The internal environment provides a medium for the exchange of nutrients and wastes and provides a stable physiochemical environment for cell function.

Normal physiologic cell function requires that the constancy of the internal environment be maintained within relatively narrow limits, even though the body is constantly changing in response to interactions between the internal and external environments. The necessary stability of the internal environment is maintained through feedback among regulatory mechanisms. As changes occur in the internal environment, regulatory systems such as the nervous system and the endocrine system respond to keep these changes within well defined limits.

The word homeostasis (*homeo:* like, similar; *stasis:* stay) was originally used by Cannon (1932) to describe relative constancy of the internal environment due to the action of regulatory mechanisms. Constancy does not mean that the internal environment is static. It is constantly changing, but a relative equilibrium is maintained, called by some theorists "homeodynamics."

The regulatory systems operate by way of compensation. Any change in the internal environment automatically initiates a response to minimize or counteract the change. For example, when the blood glucose level drops, the endocrine system responds with increased cortisol secretion, which decreases the rate at which cells use glucose and stimulates the conversion of amino acids into glucose. These compensatory actions cause the blood glucose level to rise. If it should increase above acceptable limits, insulin secretion would increase the rate of glucose uptake by cells, tending to reduce the blood glucose level.

Compensation occurs constantly as the body adjusts to stimuli that tend to disturb equilibrium. These stressors may be anything that creates change in the internal environment and thus places demands on the body to compensate. Examples of potential stressors include changes in external environmental temperature or sleep pattern, hunger, joy, and infection. Stressors may be beneficial or harmful, but they all require the body to respond with adaptation.

A person's ability to adapt to changes in life events may be synonymous with health or may be a major factor in determining the potential for health or disease. One way that a person adapts is through coping mechanisms that aim "to master conditions of harm, threat, or challenge when a routine or automatic response is not readily available" (Monat & Lazarus, 1977, p. 8). Some regard coping methods primarily as psychological barriers when stressors are perceived as threats. Thus, a person's reaction to stress involves cognitive appraisal and psychological coping methods, in addition to physiologic reactions.

One of the best known nursing models is the model developed by Sister Callista Roy, which combines elements of both systems and stress/adaptation theories.

Callista Roy's Adaptation Model

In this model, the purpose of nursing is to promote a person's adaptation.

> TERMS
> Stressors: stimuli from the environment that require a person to adapt
> Adaptive modes: ways that a person adapts (eg, through physiologic needs, self-concept, role function, or interdependence relations)
> Classes of stimuli: focal (immediately confronting the person), contextual (all other stimuli present), and residual (nonspecific stimuli such as beliefs or attitudes)
> Adaptation level: range of a person's ability to respond to and cope with stimuli
> Coping: ways of responding to stressors

The philosophic assumptions of the Roy adaptation model are based on the principles of humanism and veritivity (Roy, 1988). In *humanism*, it is believed that the individual:

- Shares in creative power
- Behaves purposefully, not in a sequence of cause and effect
- Possesses intrinsic holism
- Strives to maintain integrity and to realize the need for relationships (Barone & Roy, 1996, p. 66)

In *veritivity*, it is believed that the individual in society is viewed in the context of the:

- Purposefulness of human existence
- Unity of purpose of humankind
- Activity and creativity for the common good
- Value and meaning of life (Barone & Roy, 1996, p. 66)

The essence of Roy's model, organized around adaptive behaviors, is the set of processes by which a person adapts to environmental stressors. The person as a unified system is viewed as a biopsychosocial being. The person is in constant interaction with a changing environment. The transaction between the environmental demand of adaptation and the person's response is stress (Roy & Roberts, 1981, p. 56).

The person is affected by stressors described as "focal stimuli." The focal stimulus is a change immediately confronting the person, which requires an adaptive response. Accompanying the focal stimulus are contextual (all other stimuli present) and residual stimuli (other relevant factors such as nonspecific stimuli), which mediate and contribute to the effect of the stressor to produce the interaction called stress.

The pooled effect of the three classes of stimuli result in the person's adaptation level. The person's adaptation level determines a zone that indicates the range of further stimulation that will have a positive or adaptive response. If further stimuli fall outside of the zone, the person cannot respond positively, and ineffective coping occurs.

According to Roy and Roberts (1981, p. 56), "Coping refers to routine, accustomed patterns of behaviors to deal with daily situations as well as to the production of new ways of behaving when drastic changes defy the familiar responses." The two major coping mechanisms are the regulator subsystem, comprised mainly of automatic neural, endocrine, and chemical activity, and the cognator subsystem, which includes cognitive–emotive channels and provides for perceptual/information processing, learning, judgment, and emotion (Andrews & Roy, 1986, p. 7).

Persons are conceptualized by Roy as having four adaptive modes, or categories of behavior resulting from coping: physiologic, self-concept, role function, and interdependence relations. The desired end result is a state in which conditions promote the person's goals, including survival, growth, reproduction, and mastery.

Recently Roy (1997, p. 44) redefined adaptation as the "process and outcome whereby the thinking and feeling person uses conscious awareness and choice to create human and environmental integration." "When coping mechanisms are effective in dealing with stress, a dynamic state of equilibrium results that fosters goal achievement. When unusual stresses or weakened coping mechanisms make the person's usual attempts to cope ineffective, then nursing care is needed" (Roy & Roberts, 1981, p. 45). The client may be a family, a community, or society, but Roy emphasizes adaptation of the person (Roy & Roberts, 1981, p. 42).

Health had previously been described as "a continuum from death to high-level wellness" (Galbreath, 1990, p. 240). However, in more recent writings, Roy (1987, p. 42) states that "health is a process of responding positively to environmental changes." Thus, health is now viewed as both "a state and a process of being and becoming an integrated and whole person" (p. 42).

The goal of nursing is "to promote adaptation by the use of the nursing process, in each of the adaptive modes, thus contributing to health, quality of life, and dying with dignity" (Roy, 1987, p. 43). "The criterion for judging when the goal has been reached is generally any positive response made by the recipient to the stimuli present that frees energy for responses to other stimuli" (Riehl & Roy, 1980, p. 183). The goal of adaptation is fostered through nursing assessment and intervention, with the client as an active participant.

Roy's model provides a classification system for stressors that may affect adaptation, as well as a system for classifying nursing assessment. The model "has been useful in supporting the traditional concept of nurs-

TABLE 8-3	
Major Concepts as Defined in Roy's Model	
Person	A biopsychosocial being forming a unified system that seeks equilibrium
Health	As a state—adaptation resulting from successful coping with stressors; as a process—responding positively to environmental changes
Illness	Ineffective coping on a continuum from death toward adaptation
Environment	External conditions and influences that affect the development of the person
Nursing	Manipulation of stimuli to foster successful coping

ing practice within the medical model perspective" (Huch, 1987, p. 63). A widely used model, it is the basis for a growing body of research. Major concepts defined in Roy's model are summarized in Table 8-3.

◎ The Growth Model of Change

CARING THEORY AS A FRAMEWORK

Although care and caring are widely perceived to be important and even possibly central concepts in nursing, "a universal definition or conceptualization of caring does not exist" (Swanson, 1991, p. 161). Morse, Solberg, Neander, Bottorff, and Johnson (1990, p. 2) point out that the literature includes references to care or caring as actions performed (as in to take care of), as well as concern demonstrated (as in caring about). An analysis of the literature reveals at least five perspectives or categories of caring, including caring as a human trait (Benner and Wrubel, Leininger), caring as a moral imperative or ideal (Watson), caring as an interpersonal relationship (Parse), caring as a therapeutic intervention (Orem), and caring as an affect (Morse et al., 1990, p. 3).

Clients perceive as caring "those nursing ministrations that are person-centered, protective, anticipatory, physically comforting, and that go beyond routine care" (Swanson, 1991, p. 161). Kyle (1995) concludes that there is a "marked difference between the patients' perceptions of caring and those of nurses, with the nurses focusing on the psychosocial skills and the patient on those skills which demonstrate professional competency" (p. 509). Caring outcomes may be demonstrated in terms of either subjective experiences or measurable client outcomes.

In recent years, several classifications of the components of caring have been published. Swanson (1991, p. 162) defines caring as "a nurturing way of relating to a valued other toward whom one feels a personal sense of commitment and responsibility." She identified the five caring processes as:

1. Knowing: striving to understand an event as it has meaning in the life of the other
2. Being with: being emotionally present for the other

3. Doing for: doing for the other as he would do for himself if it were possible
4. Enabling: facilitating the other's passage through life transitions and unfamiliar events
5. Maintaining belief: sustaining faith in the other's capacity to get through an event or transition and face a future with meaning

Koldjeski (1990) described five "essences" of caring as:

Interpersonal valuing and involvement
Experiencing-with and being-there
Instilling faith
Concern and love for the other
Actualization

These theoretical components are compared in Table 8-4.

TABLE 8-4

A Comparison of Components of Caring

Swanson	Koldjeski
Knowing	Interpersonal involvement
Being with	Experiencing with
	Concern and love
Doing for	Nursing actions
Enabling	Actualization
Maintaining belief	Instillment of faith

The following section describes nursing models of caring. Orem's model fits within the change as stability paradigm; Watson's model is an example of the change as growth paradigm.

Dorothea Orem's Self-Care Deficit Model
In this model, the purpose of nursing is to help people meet their self-care needs.

TERMS
   Self-care (dependent care): activities that a person performs for self (when able) that contribute to health
   Self-care deficit: a relationship between actions a person should take for healthy functioning and the capability for action
   Self-care requisites: needs that are universal or associated with development or deviation from health
   Self-care demand: therapeutic actions to meet needs
   Agency: capability to engage in self-care

The essence of Orem's model is a three-part nursing theory that "focuses on persons in relations. The theory of self-care focuses on the self, the I; the theory of self-care deficit focuses on you and me; and the theory of nursing systems focuses on we, persons in community" (Orem, 1990, p. 49). Orem's general theory, the self-care deficit theory, integrates the theory of self-care, the theory of self-care deficit, and the theory of nursing systems (Orem, 1995).

Self-care is the "voluntary regulation of one's own human functioning and development that is necessary for individuals to maintain life, health, and well-being" (Orem, 1995, p. 95). Self-care activities are learned as the person matures and are affected by the cultural beliefs, habits, and customs of the family and society. A person's age, developmental state, or state of health can affect the ability to perform self-care activities. For example, a parent or guardian must maintain continuous therapeutic care for a child.

Nursing is concerned with the person's need for self-care action to "sustain life and health, recover from disease or injury, and cope with their effects" (Orem, 1980, p. 6). In Orem's view, nursing care may be offered to "individual and multiperson units," but only persons have self-care requisites. The nurse cares for, assists, or does something for the client to achieve the health results that the client desires (Orem, 1980, p. 126).

Orem (1985, p. 179) implies that health is "a state of a person that is characterized by soundness or wholeness of developed human structures and of bodily and mental functioning." Well-being, which is used "in the sense of individuals' perceived condition of existence" (Orem, 1985, p. 179), is associated with health.

Orem refers to the physical, psychological, interpersonal, and social aspects of health, but indicates that they are inseparable in the person: "Health describes the state of wholeness or integrity of human beings" (Orem, 1995, p. 96). "If there is acceptance of the real unity of individual human beings, there should be no difficulty in recognizing structural and functional differentiation within the unity" (Orem, 1980, p. 180). Orem views individuals as moving "toward maturation and achievement of the individual's human potential" (Orem, 1985, p. 180).

Orem suggests that some people may have self-care requisites (needs) associated with development or with deviation from health. All people have the following universal self-care requisites (Orem, 1980, p. 42):

1. Maintenance of sufficient air, water, and food intake
2. Provision of care associated with elimination processes and excrements
3. Maintenance of a balance between activity and rest and between solitude and social interaction
4. Prevention of hazards to life, functioning, and well-being
5. Promotion of human functioning and development within social groups in accord with potential, known limitations, and the desire to be normal

Identified self-care requisites require actions known as "therapeutic self-care demands." Therapeutic self-care demands can be determined by:

1. Identifying all existing or possible self-care requisites.
2. Identifying methods for meeting self-care requisites, keeping in mind basic conditioning factors (eg, age, developmental state, health state, and pattern of living) that "condition the values of patients' self-care agency and therapeutic self-care demands, as well as the means that are valid for meeting self-care requisites and in regulating self-care agency at particular times" (Orem, 1985, p. 78).
3. Designing, implementing, and evaluating a plan of action. Orem terms this use of nursing process determining a system of nursing.

The theory of nursing systems involves "an interpersonal unity in a particular time–space localization. This unity is formed by nurses, persons who have entered into an agreement to accept and participate in nursing, and the relatives or persons who are responsible for the individuals who require nursing" (Orem, 1990, p. 54). Thus, candidates for nursing care are clients who have insufficient current or projected capability for providing self-care. "It is the need for compensatory action (to overcome an inability or limited ability to engage in care) or for action to help in the development or regulation of self-care abilities that is the basis for a nursing relationship" (Orem, 1980, p. 58).

Orem's model emphasizes a role for the nurse when the client is unable to provide for his or her own self-care requisites. Nursing interventions may be aimed at maintaining health, preventing illness, or restoring health, and they may involve actions for or with the client. The model, which is compatible with the traditional medical model, has been widely used in practice and education and recently has been the basis for research. Major concepts as defined in Orem's model are summarized in Table 8-5.

TABLE 8-5	
Major Concepts as Defined in Orem's Model	
Person	Inseparable physical, psychological, interpersonal, and social aspects
Health	Constancy of internal and external conditions which permits self-care needs to be met
Illness	Deviation from normal structure or function resulting in self-care deficits
Environment	Factors external to the person
Nursing	Actions to overcome or prevent the development of self-care limitations or provide therapeutic self-care for a person who is unable to do so

Jean Watson's Human Science and Human Care Model

In this model, the purpose of nursing is to help persons gain greater harmony within the mind, body, and soul.

TERMS
Phenomenal field: the totality of past, present, and future influences on the person
Carative factors: interventions that demonstrate caring as a moral ideal of nursing

Watson's model represents phenomenologic, existential, and spiritual orientations, blended with Eastern philosophy. The model developed from her conception of "transpersonal caring" as "a moral ideal of nursing with a concern for preservation of humanity, dignity, and freedom of self" (Watson, 1985, p. 74). Watson wants nursing "to concern itself more with meaning, relationships, context, and patterns" (Watson, 1985, p. 2).

"Human life . . . is defined as (spiritual–mental–physical) being-in-the-world which is continuous in time and space" (Watson, 1985, p. 47). Although the soul, mind, and body are explicitly identified as spheres of the human being, they are viewed as integrated and inseparable.

Health is related to "unity and harmony within the mind, body, and soul," and illness is "subjective turmoil or disharmony within a person's inner self or soul at some level or disharmony within the spheres of the person, for example, in the mind, body, and soul, either consciously or unconsciously" (Watson, 1985, p. 48). A distinction is made between the self as perceived and as experienced, with the degree of congruence between these perceptions being related to health.

The human being is viewed as open to the environment, within which interrelationships occur with other humans and nature. Watson uses the concept of a phenomenal field to describe "the totality of human experience" (Watson, 1985, p. 54). The human being, with a unique life history, "imaged future," and "presenting moment," interacts with others in the environment to create an event, "a focal point in space and time from which experience and perception are taking place" (Watson, 1985, p. 59). An event, as a "moment of coming together," provides an actual caring occasion for human care through nursing. "The actual caring occasion, or caring moment, involves action and choice by both the nurse and the other" (Watson, 1996, p. 157).

Nursing

consists of transpersonal human-to-human attempts to protect, enhance, and preserve humanity by helping a person find meaning in illness, suffering, pain, and existence; to help another gain self-knowledge, control, and self-healing wherein a sense of inner harmony is restored regardless of the external circumstances (Watson, 1985, p. 54).

Caring is "a moral ideal, rather than an interpersonal technique" (Watson, 1985, p. 58), which can be demonstrated through the carative factors (nursing interventions) that "allow for contact between the subjective world of the experiencing persons" (Watson, 1985, p. 58). The following carative factors are all presupposed by a knowledge base and clinical competence (Watson, 1989, pp. 227–228):

1. Formation of a humanistic–altruistic system of values
2. Nurturing of faith and hope
3. Cultivation of sensitivity to one's self and others
4. Development of a helping-trusting, human caring relationship
5. Promotion and acceptance of the expression of positive and negative feelings
6. Use of creative problem-solving caring processes
7. Promotion of transpersonal teaching-learning
8. Provision for a supportive, protective, or corrective mental, physical, sociocultural, and spiritual environment
9. Assistance with gratification of human needs
10. Allowance for existential–phenomenologic–spiritual forces

During the human care process (nursing), both the nurse and the client are in a process of "being and becoming." "The agent of change . . . is viewed as the individual patient, but the nurse can be a coparticipant in change" (Watson, 1985, p. 74). Each person has human freedom, choice, and responsibility, with the moral ideal being the "protection, enhancement, and preservation of human dignity . . . . Human caring involves values, a will and a commitment to care, knowledge, caring actions, and consequences" (Watson, 1985, p. 29). "Emphasis is on helping other(s), through advanced nursing caring-healing modalities, to gain more self-knowledge, self-control, and even self-healing potential" (Watson, 1996, p. 148).

This model provides one framework for the study of caring in nursing. The focus on the moral ideals of human care relationships has the potential for significant impact on nursing process. The major concepts as defined in Watson's model are summarized in Table 8-6.

TABLE 8-6

Major Concepts as Defined in Watson's Model

Person	Integrated spiritual–mental–physical being in the world
Environment	An open system continuous with the person in time and space
Health	Unity and harmony within the mind, body, and soul
Illness	Disharmony within mind, body, and soul
Nursing	Transpersonal human care and caring transactions that promote restoration of a sense of inner harmony

COMPLEXITY THEORY AS A FRAMEWORK

Complexity theory assumes that there is an external reality that is changing continuously. Change is not assumed to be regular or predictable. Therefore, the theory emphasizes change over time, long-term unpredictability, and openness to the environment with mutual simultaneous interactions . . . . The complexity perspective seeks to understand patterns of phenomena as wholes within their contexts (Maliski & Holditch-Davis, 1995, p. 25).

This theory replaces the metaphors of separation and interaction (reductionistic) with the metaphor of participation (holistic) (Porter, 1995). The whole cannot be known from the sum of the parts.
Assumptions of complexity theory include:

Nonlinear change over time
Long-term unpredictability
Openness to the environment
Mutual simultaneous interactions
Continual fluctuations reveal patterns.
Patterns are variable at critical points.

Because the theory assumes mutual change of human being and environment, which provides potential for restructuring in new patterns, linear cause and effect is difficult to infer. The theory suggests that multiple, dynamic, mutual relationships rather than enduring "causes" influence change. Thus, change of an individual, because it is related to initial conditions, is not generalizable. In addition, because one cannot observe without changing what is observed, complete objectivity in research methodology is not possible.

The models discussed in the following sections, developed by Peplau, Rogers, Parse, Newman, and Leddy, all emphasize becoming of the human being in terms of potential for change.

Hildegard Peplau's Interpersonal Relations Model

In this model, the purpose of nursing is to foster personality development in the direction of maturity.

TERMS
Tension: discomfort resulting from needs and leading to behavior to meet the needs and reduce discomfort
Therapeutic relationship: interpersonal communication between a client and a nurse to help solve the client's health problems

The essence of Peplau's model, which is a process-organized model, is the human relationship between "an individual who is sick, or in need of health services, and a nurse especially educated to recognize and to respond to the need for help" (Peplau, 1952, pp. 5–6). "The interpersonal process is the central component of the model and describes the method by which the nurse facilitates useful transformations of the patient's energy or anxiety" (Reed, 1996, p. 62). This model, first published in 1952, "initiates a move from an intrapsychic emphasis within psychiatric mental health nursing, and a dominant focus on physical care within general nursing, to an interpersonal focus in both" (Reed & Johnston, 1989, p. 51).

Peplau views the person as "an organism that lives in an unstable equilibrium (ie, physiologic, psychological, and social fluidity) and life is the process of striving in the direction of stable equilibrium; ie, a fixed pattern

Rogers's model is a conceptual system built on an assumption of the person as a unified energy field that is continuously exchanging matter and energy with an environmental energy field. Rogers proposes that "man is a unified whole possessing his own integrity and manifesting characteristics that are more than and different from the sum of his parts" (Rogers, 1970, p. 47). Physical, biologic, psychological, social, cultural, and spiritual attributes are merged into behavior that reflects the total person as an indivisible whole. Rogers believes that it is not possible to describe humans by combining attributes of each of the parts. Only as the parts lose their particular identity is it possible to describe the person.

The person is an organized energy field that has a unique pattern. The continuous exchange of matter and energy between this energy field and the environmental energy field results in continuous patterning of both the person and the environment (Rogers, 1970, p. 53). This results in increasing complexity and innovativeness of the person. Rogers believes that this life process "evolves irreversibly and unidirectionally along the space–time continuum" (Rogers, 1970, p. 59). She conceptualizes this unidirectionality as a spiral, with self-regulation "directed toward achieving increasing complexity of organization—not toward achieving equilibrium and stability" (Rogers, 1970, p. 64). The person is also characterized by "the capacity for abstraction and imagery, language and thought, sensation and emotion" (Rogers, 1970, p. 73).

Rogers believes that health serves as an "index of field patterning" (Malinski, 1986, p. 27). Health and illness are not separate states, good or bad, nor in a linear relationship. "Ease and disease are dichotomous notions that cannot be used to account for the dynamic complexity and uncertain fulfillment of man's unfolding" (Rogers, 1970, p. 42). Observable characteristics (signs) and symptoms are therefore all "manifestations of patterning (that) emerge out of the human/environmental field mutual process and are continuously innovative" (Rogers, 1990, p. 8).

Nursing intervention is aimed toward patterning of humans and the environment to achieve maximum health potential (Rogers, 1970, pp. 86, 127). "People must be informed and active participants in the search for health. Intervention should be directed toward assisting individuals to mobilize their resources, consciously and unconsciously, so that the man–environment relationship may be strengthened and the integrity of the individual heightened" (Rogers, 1970, p. 134). "Maintenance and promotion of health, prevention of disease, nursing diagnosis, intervention, and rehabilitation encompass the scope of nursing's goals" (Rogers, 1970, p. 86).

Rogers (1980, p. 333) has described three principles that explain the life process in humans and predict evolution of the life process: integrality, helicy, and resonancy. The *principle of integrality* emphasizes that the human energy field and the environmental energy field are continuous and must be perceived simultaneously. The relationship is one of constant interaction and mutual simultaneous change. In other words, "they are reciprocal systems in which molding and being molded are taking place at the same time" (Rogers, 1970, p. 97).

The *principle of helicy* predicts that change occurs as a "continuous innovative, unpredictable, increasing diversity of human and environmental field patterns" (Rogers, 1990, p. 8). The human field becomes increasingly diverse with time. As the person ages, behavior is not repeated, but may recur at ever more complex levels. The principle of resonancy indicates that change in pattern and organization toward increased complexity of the field occurs by way of waves, "manifesting continuous change from lower-frequency, longer wave patterns to higher-frequency, shorter wave patterns" (Rogers, 1980, p. 333).

Rogers believes that an understanding of the mechanisms that affect the life process in humans makes it possible for the nurse to purposefully intervene to affect repatterning of a client in a desired direction. In the process, the nurse is also changed. She sees the future as "one of growing diversity, of accelerating evolution, and of nonrepeating rhythmicities" (Rogers, 1992, p. 33). Rogers's emphasis on holism and on the simultaneous and continuous interaction between humans and the environment are concepts that have been widely accepted in nursing and have been incorporated into subsequently developed models. Several theories have been derived from the model, and a number of research studies have been published. Major concepts as defined in Rogers's model are summarized in Table 8-8.

TABLE 8-8	
Major Concepts as Defined in Rogers's Model	
Person	A unified and patterned energy field
Health	An indication of the complexity and innovativeness of patterning of the energy field that is the person
Environment	An energy field continuously interacting with the energy field that is the person
Nursing	Repatterning of person and environment to achieve maximum health potential of the person

Rosemarie Parse's Human Becoming Model

In this model, the purpose of nursing is to improve the quality of life of both client and nurse.

TERMS

Coconstitution: development of patterning through person–environment interaction

Coexistence: dynamic mutual processes between the person and the environment

Situated freedom: freedom of choice in a situation

Parse's model incorporates a combination of Rogers's principles and building blocks "with the tenets of human subjectivity and intentionality and the concepts of coconstitution, coexistence, and situated freedom from existential phenomenological thought" (Parse, 1987, p. 161). The emphasis is on the meaning and values that influence a person's active choices of behavior. "The person constructs his or her own meaning" (Parse, 1996, p. 57).

The person is defined as "an open being, more than and different from the sum of parts in mutual simultaneous interchange with the environment who chooses from options and bears responsibility for choices" (Parse, 1987, p. 160). As a person interacts with the environment, patterns of relating are established that provide insight into his or her patterning and values at that moment. Health is viewed as a "nonlinear entity," a constantly changing process of becoming that incorporates values. Because it is not a state, health cannot be contrasted with disease. Nursing aims to affect the "quality of life as perceived by the person and the family" (Parse, 1987, p. 167).

Parse defines nine concepts in her model (Parse, 1987, pp. 164–165):

1. *Imaging*: "picturing or making real of events, ideas, and people"
2. *Valuing*: "living of cherished beliefs"
3. *Languaging*: "speaking and moving . . . the way one represents the structure of personal reality"
4. *Connecting–separating*: "the rhythmical process of distancing and relating"
5. *Powering*: "the pushing-resisting of inter-human encounters that originates the uniqueness in the process of transforming"
6. *Transforming*: "the changing of change"
7. *Originating*: "generating unique ways of living"
8. *Revealing–concealing*: "rhythmical pattern of relating with others"
9. *Enabling–limiting*: "infinite number of possibilities within choice"

Parse (1987, p. 163) has combined these concepts into three principles. Meaning is structured multidimensionally as humans and the environment together create (cocreate) reality through "the languaging of valuing and imaging." In other words, the meaning of human beliefs and values is developed and demonstrated through words and movement. Rhythmicity of patterns of relating is cocreated through "living the paradoxical unity of revealing–concealing, enabling–limiting, and connecting–separating." In other words, human patterns in relating to others are derived from multiple choices and involve rhythmical processes of moving closer to and away from others. Cotranscendence with possibilities is "powering unique ways of originating in the process of transforming." In other words, it involves the processes of distancing and moving closer in interrelationships that provide the force for change and creativity.

From these concepts and principles, Parse (1987, pp. 168–169) has derived three implications for practice:

1. Illuminating meaning by explicating what is appearing through language
2. Synchronizing rhythms by dwelling with the flow of connecting–separating
3. Mobilizing transcendence by moving toward possibles in transforming

Parse says that, "the way of living the belief system is through true presence" (Parse, 1996, p. 57), "which is a non-routinized, unconditional loving way of being within which the nurse witnesses the blossoming of others" (p. 57). Practicing within this model, the nurse would provide an empathic sounding board for clients and families to express and therefore uncover the meaning of thoughts and feelings, values, and changing views. In the process of expression through language and movement, and in "dwelling with" the rhythm of the client and family, new possibilities for change in the quality of life would become apparent. "The new insights shift the rhythm and all participants move beyond the moment toward what is not-yet. This is mobilizing transcendence" (Parse, 1989, p. 257). In this model, the nurse interacts with clients rather than doing things to or for them (Philips, 1987, p. 182).

Parse has also developed a research methodology to test relationships suggested by the model. The methodology uses "dialogical engagement," a researcher–participant encounter, to uncover the meaning of the lived experience being studied (Parse, 1989, p. 256).

Parse's model emphasizes the importance of the meaning that underlies behavior and provides a structure for the identification and clarification of "manifestations of whole people as they interrelate with the environment" (Phillips, 1987, p. 188). The model is being used in practice and is the basis for an increasing body of research. The major concepts as defined in Parse's model are listed in Table 8-9.

TABLE 8-9	
Major Concepts as Defined in Parse's Model	
Person	A patterned, open being, more than and different from the sum of its parts
Environment	That which is in mutual and simultaneous interchange with the person
Health	Continuously changing process of becoming
Nursing	An interactional process that facilitates the becoming of the participants

Margaret Newman's Model of Health as Expanding Consciousness

In this model, the purpose of nursing is to promote a higher level of consciousness in both client and nurse.

TERMS
Consciousness: capacity of the system (person) to interact with its environment; the informational capacity of the system

Newman's model incorporates Rogers's concept of a unitary person as a center of energy in constant interaction with the environment. Persons are characterized by patterning that is constantly changing. According to Newman, "the focus of nursing is the pattern of the whole, health as pattern of the evolving whole, with caring as a moral imperative" (Newman, 1994, p. xix).

"The total pattern of person–environment can be viewed as a network of consciousness" (1986, p. 33) that is expanding toward higher levels; "the patterns of interaction of person–environment constitute health . . . . Health is the expansion of consciousness" (1986, pp. 3, 18); and "health and the evolving pattern of consciousness are the same" (1990, p. 38). "Consciousness is defined as the information of the system: the capacity of the system to interact with the environment" (Newman, 1994, p. 33).

Health is viewed as a process that encompasses both disease and "nondisease." Instead of the familiar linear relationship between health as good and disease (or illness) as bad, Newman conceptualizes disease as a meaningful component of the whole and a possible facilitator of health. "Sickness can provide a kind of shock that reorganizes the relationships of the person's pattern in a more harmonious way" (Newman, 1994, p. 11). As the person interacts with the environment, "the fluctuating patterns of harmony–disharmony can be regarded as peaks and troughs of the rhythmic life process" (Newman, 1986, p. 21).

Newman posits four major ways in which person–environment patterning is manifested: movement, time, space, and consciousness. Consciousness is expressed in patterns of rhythmic movement toward higher levels that can be described in time and space. Manifestations of these patterns include exchanging, communicating, relating, valuing, choosing, moving, perceiving, feeling, and knowing (Newman, 1986, p. 74). The task for nursing intervention is to recognize patterning and relate to it in an "authentic" (genuine, sincere) way.

> The new paradigm is relational. The professional enters into a partnership with the client with the mutual goal of participating in an authentic relationship, trusting that in the process of its evolving, both will grow and become healthier in the sense of higher levels of consciousness (Newman, 1986, p. 68).

Nursing facilitates the process of evolving to higher levels of consciousness by "rhythmic connecting of the nurse with the client in an authentic way for the purpose of illuminating the pattern and discovering the new rules of a higher level of organization" (Newman, 1990, p. 40).

Newman's model contributes to the development of a body of knowledge about manifestations of healthy patterning of unitary human beings. Newman has described a methodology for using practice as the basis for research within the model, and a few research studies based on the model have been reported in the literature. Table 8-10 lists major concepts as defined in Newman's model.

TABLE 8-10	
Major Concepts as Defined in Newman's Model	
Person	An energy center
Health	Expansion of consciousness
Illness	Part of patterning of the whole person–environment interaction
Environment	An energy field in continuous interaction and patterning with the person
Nursing	Facilitating repatterning of the patient to higher levels of consciousness

Susan Leddy's Human Energy Model

In this model, the purpose of nursing is to facilitate harmonious pattern of the energy fields of both client and nurse.

TERMS
 Energy field: a dynamic web of energy interactions
 Consciousness: expressed through meaning, awareness, and choice
 Energy: conveys and does the work of information
 Pattern: a web of relationships

Leddy's model has been influenced by Rogers's science of unitary human beings, Eastern philosophy, and quantum physics and complexity theories. This model views energy as the essence of the universe.

The human being (*person*) is viewed as a *unitary* energy field that is *open* to and continuously interacting with an environmental energy field. "The human being . . . can only be understood as a whole. Sensitivity to complementary facets and vantage points for observation provides a view of the whole from different perspectives" (Leddy, 1997). *Self-organization* distinguishes the human energy field from the environmental field with which it is inseparably intermingled. "Self-organization is a synthesis of continuity and change, that provides identity while the human evolves toward a sense of integrity, meaning and purpose in living" (Leddy, 1997). The human being is also characterized by *consciousness*, which enables awareness, the construction of self-identity and meaning, and the ability to influence change through choice.

The *environment* is viewed as *dynamic*, changing through continuous transformation of energy with matter and information. These transformations occur as a web of *connectedness* in relationships. "Connections may be with self, the environment, including other humans, and/or an 'ultimate other'" (Leddy, 1997). Change is only partially unpredictable and is also influenced by inherent *order* in the universe. Change is influenced by history, pattern, and choice.

Health is the *pattern* of the whole. This pattern is rhythmic, varying in quality and intensity over *time*. Health is characterized by a changing pattern of harmony/dissonance.

Knowledge-based consciousness in a goal-directed relationship with the client is the basis for *nursing*. "A nurse–client relationship is a commitment characterized by intentionality, authenticity, trust, respect, and genuine sense of connection. The nurse is a knowledgeable, concerned facilitator. The client is responsible for choices that influence health and healing" (Leddy, 1997). The facilitation of harmonious health patterning is accomplished through health pattern appraisal and subsequent energetic interventions (see theory of energetic patterning below).

Leddy has derived three descriptive theories from the model: the theory of healthiness, the theory of participation, and the theory of nursing intervention. In the theory of healthiness, *healthiness* is defined as having perceived purpose and the power to achieve goals.

The Leddy healthiness scale (LHS) (1996) includes items that measure meaningfulness, connections, ends, capability, control, choice, challenge, capacity, and confidence. In studies with the LHS to date (Leddy, 1996, Leddy & Fawcett, 1997) healthiness has been found to be moderately and negatively related to fatigue and symptom experience in women with breast cancer, and moderately and positively related to mental health, health status, and satisfaction with life in a sample of healthy people.

In the theory of participation, *participation* is defined as the experience of continuous human–environment mutual process. The person–environment participation scale (PEPS) (1995) measures expansiveness and ease of participation. In studies with the PEPS to date, participation has been found to be moderately and positively correlated with healthiness, sense of coherence (Antonovsky, 1987), and power (Barrett, 1990), and moderately and negatively correlated with fatigue and symptom experience in healthy people.

The theory of nursing intervention proposes that nursing interventions to facilitate harmonious pattern of both client and nurse are accomplished through energetic patterning. The five domains of energetic patterning are *channeling*, to reestablish free flow of energy; *conveying*, to foster redirection of energy away from areas of excess to depleted areas; *converting*, to augment energy resources; *conserving*, to reduce energy depletion; and *clearing*, to facilitate the releasing of energy tied to old patterns. A number of types of interventions are consistent with this theory, including nutrition, exercise, touch modalities, bodywork, light therapy, music, imagery, relaxation, and stress reduction.

This conceptual model offers a unique and modern perspective for nursing; however, because it is a new model, its usefulness for practice and research remains to be demonstrated. Major concepts as defined in Leddy's model are summarized in Table 8-11.

TABLE 8-11

Major Concepts as Defined in Leddy's Model

Person	A self-organized, unitary, energy field
Environment	An energy field open to the human being
Health	Pattern of the whole
Nursing	Knowledge-based patterning with a goal-directed relationship

Research Related to Models of Nursing

Research based on conceptual models of nursing is in an early stage of development. Currently, three kinds of research related to models of nursing are being conducted: testing the relationships predicted by the model; using the model as a framework for descriptive analysis; and attempting to modify nursing care through use of a model.

For example, Leddy and Fawcett (1997) interpreted the results of a study to explain relationships among theoretical variables (participation, change, energy, and healthiness) derived from the human energy model, as being supportive of the model. In another example, Hart (1995), in a study of pregnant women, derived research variables from Orem's general theory and tested the relationships between the variables. The results were interpreted as supporting Orem's model.

Models have also been used as a framework for descriptive analysis. For example, Frederickson (1993) used Roy's model as a framework to describe the concept of anxiety. Lowry and Anderson (1993) used Neuman's model to derive research variables to study ventilator dependency. In this pilot study they did not test relationships between the variables.

A few studies attempt to modify nursing care through use of a model. For example, Woods (1994) used a group support intervention based on King's model as an intervention with elderly clients. The results were interpreted as being supportive of the model. Biley (1996) discussed the use of a therapeutic touch intervention based on Rogers's model as an effective intervention with clients experiencing phantom pain and sensations.

The issue of the usefulness of nursing models has been raised. A model does provide a useful system for classification of data during the nursing process. A model also proposes theoretical relationships that can be tested through research. But are the differences in terms among models simply a semantic shell game?

Does the model used to organize data make any real difference in the nursing care given the client? What difference does it make if the cause of a problem is labeled a "noxious influence" affecting a behavioral subsystem, a "self-care deficit" leading to a "self-care demand," or a "focal stimulus" that is a stressor? How is the care given any different if its purpose is labeled to "limit self-care deficits," "reduce stressors," or "foster coping"?

Although nursing science is in an early stage of development, there is general agreement on categories of concepts (person, environment, health, and nursing) that are central to nursing knowledge. There has been a great deal of discussion about whether there should be one model for nursing, but the popularity of a growing number of models within different paradigms and frameworks indicates that there is still disagreement about how nursing should be described and how its goals can best be achieved.

However, progress is being made, and there are considerable implications for practice and for further theory development in (1) the centering of all models on nursing practice rather than on medicine; (2) the focus on multiple components of health rather than on pathology; and (3) the consideration of the whole person rather than of fragmented body systems.

◎ Conclusion

All the nursing models discussed in this chapter are based on the metaparadigm concepts of person, environment, health, and nursing. Philosophical differences between the change as stability paradigm and the change as growth paradigm are pronounced. In comparison, there are more differences of emphasis than substance among the models within each paradigm.

A comparison of concepts in selected theories is presented in Table 8-12. The major differences and similarities among models can be seen by comparing Table 8-13 with Table 8-14.

TABLE 8-12

Comparison of Concepts in Selected Theories

Theory	Human	Human–Environment Interaction	Health	Examples of Nursing Implication
Systems	Multiple interacting subsystems that form the human system	Simultaneous change in both systems	Tendency toward increased complexity	Nurse system and client system are mutually affected
Stress and Adaptation	Multiple subsystems that share an internal environment	Humans cope and compensate for environmental change	Constancy of the internal environment within normal parameters	Support coping mechanisms of client
Complexity	Unitary whole	Mutual simultaneous interaction; nonlinear	Pattern of the whole	Stimulate repatterning

TABLE 8-13

Similarities and Differences of Conceptualization in Nursing Models Within the Change as Stability Paradigm

Model	Person		Health	Environment	Nursing	
	Goal	Composition	Health	Environment	Nature	Purpose
King	Functioning in social roles	Open system	Dynamic state of well-being	Internal and external stressors	Goal-oriented interaction	Attainment, mainte-nance, or restoration of health
Orem	Constancy	Whole with physical, psychological, in-terpersonal, social aspects	Meeting self-care needs	External forces	Systems that address self-care requi-sites	Help people to meet self-care needs
Roy	Equilibrium	System with biopsychosocial components	Adaptation	External conditions	Manipulation of stimuli to foster coping	Promotion of adaptation
Neuman	Balance	Composite of physiologic, psychological, sociocultural, developmental variables	Equilibrium	Internal and external stressors	Stress-reducing ac-tivities	Promotion of equilibrium

THOUGHT QUESTIONS

1 Does the human strive toward stability and balance or toward variety and continuous change?

2 Does human behavior reflect an indivisible entity or a composite of various components?

3 What are the roles of innovation and change in the determination of health? Are they dis-ruptive or necessary?

4 Does the person affect the environment or is the person only affected by the environment?

5 Are interactions between the person and the environment cause and effect (linear) or continuous and simultaneous (multidimensional)?

6 Does nursing foster becoming or being (future or present)?

7 Is nursing done with, for, or to the person? Does nursing foster or take responsibility for a person's health?

TABLE 8-14

Similarities and Differences of Conceptualization in Nursing Models Within the Change as Growth Paradigm

	Person				Nursing	
Model	Goal	Composition	Health	Environment	Nature	Purpose
Peplau	Equilibrium	System with physiologic, psychological, and social components	Foreward movement of the personality	Significant others	Therapeutic interpersonal process	Helping people to meet needs and develop
Watson	Sense of inner harmony	Integrated and inseparable spiritual, mental, and physical spheres	Unity and harmony	Energy field external to the person	Transpersonal caring	Promoting harmony
Rogers	Increased complexity of pattern	Indivisible energy field	Increasing innovativeness of patterning	Contiguous, continuously interacting energy field	Promotion of repatterning	Facilitating health potential
Newman	Expansion of consciousness	Center of energy	Patterns of person—environment interaction expanding toward higher levels	Energy field in continuous interaction with the person	Repatterning partnership	Promoting higher level of consciousness
Parse	Process of becoming	Open being	Process of becoming	Energy field in continuous interaction with the person	Interpersonal processes	Improving quality of life
Leddy	Harmony, integrity, meaning, and purpose	Unitary energy field	Pattern of the whole	Energy field in continuous interaction with the person	Goal-directed relationship	Facilitation of harmonious health patterning

REFERENCES

Andrews, H. A., & Roy, C. (1986). *Essentials of the Roy adaptation model.* East Norwalk, CT: Appleton & Lange.

Antonovsky, A. (1987). *The sense of coherence and the mystery of health.* San Francisco: Jossey-Bass.

Auger, J. R. (1976). *Behavioral systems and nursing.* Englewood Cliffs, NJ: Prentice-Hall.

Barone, S. H., & Roy, C. (1996). The Roy adaptation model in research: Rehabilitation nursing. In P. H. Walker & B. Neuman (Eds.). *Blueprint for use of nursing models: Education, research, practice, and administration* (pp. 64–75). New York: National League for Nursing.

Barrett, E. A. M. (1990). A measure of power as knowing participation in change. In O. L. Strickland & C. F. Waltz (Eds.). *Measurement of nursing outcomes* (pp. 159–180). New York: Springer.

Beeber, L., Anderson, C. A., & Sills, G. M. (1990, Spring). Peplau's theory in practice. *Nursing Science Quarterly, 3*, 6–8.

Biley, F. C. (1996). Rogerian science, phantoms, and therapeutic touch: Exploring potentials. *Nursing Science Quarterly 9*, 165–169.

Cannon, W. B. (1932). *The wisdom of the body.* rev. ed. New York: Norton.

Chin, R. (1976). The utility of system models and developmental models for practitioners. In W. G. Bennis, K. D. Benne, R. Chin, & K. E. Corey (Eds.). *The planning of change* (pp. 90–102). New York: Holt, Rinehart, & Winston.

Chinn, P. L., & Kramer, M. K. (1995). *Theory and nursing: A systematic approach* (4th ed.). St. Louis: Mosby-Year Book.

Fawcett, J. (1989). *Analysis and evaluation of conceptual models* (2nd ed.). Philadelphia: Davis.

Fawcett, J. (1995). *Analysis and evaluation of conceptual models* (3rd ed.). Philadelphia: Davis.

Forchuk, C. (1991, Summer). Peplau's theory: Concepts and their relations. *Nursing Science Quarterly, 4*, 54–60.

Forchuk, C. (1995). Hildegard E. Peplau: Interpersonal nursing theory. In C. M. McQuiston & A. A. Webb (Eds.). *Foundations of nursing theory* (pp. 457–514). Thousand Oaks, CA: Sage.

Frederickson, K. (1993). Using a nursing model to manage symptoms: Anxiety and the Roy adaptation model. *Holistic Nursing Practice, 7*, 36–43.

Galbreath, J. G. (1990). Sister Callista Roy. In J. B. George (Ed.). *Nursing theories: The base for professional nursing practice* (3rd ed., pp. 231–258). East Norwalk, CT: Appleton & Lange.

Hart, M. A. (1995). Orem's self-care deficit theory: Research with pregnant women. *Nursing Science Quarterly 8*, 120–126.

Huch, M. H. (1987). A critique of the Roy adaptation model. In R. R. Parse (Ed.). *Nursing science: Major paradigms, theories, and critiques* (pp. 47–66). Philadelphia: Saunders.

King, I. M. (1981). *A theory for nursing: Systems, concepts, process.* New York: Wiley.

King, I. M. (1987). King's theory of goal attainment. In R. R. Parse (Ed.). *Nursing science: Major paradigms, theories, and critiques* (pp. 107–113). Philadelphia: Saunders.

King, I. M. (1989). King's general systems framework and theory. In J. P. Riehl-Sisca (Ed.). *Conceptual models for nursing practice* (pp. 149–158). East Norwalk, CT: Appleton & Lange.

King, I. M. (1995). A systems framework for nursing. In M. A. Frey & C. L. Sieloff (Eds.). *Advancing King's systems framework and theory of nursing* (pp. 12–20). Thousand Oaks, CA: Sage.

King, I. M. (1996). The theory of goal attainment in research and practice. *Nursing Science Quarterly, 9*, 61–66.

Koldjeski, D. (1990). Toward a theory of professional nursing caring: A unifying perspective. In M. Leininger & J. Watson (Eds.). *The caring imperative in education* (pp. 45–57). New York: National League for Nursing.

Kyle, T. V. (1995). The concept of caring: A review of the literature. *Journal of Advanced Nursing, 21*, 506–514.

Leddy, S. K. (1995). Measuring mutual process: Development and psychometric testing of the person–environment participation scale. *Visions: The Journal of Rogerian Nursing Science, 3*, 20–31.

Leddy, S. K. (1996). Development and psychometric testing of the Leddy healthiness scale. *Research in Nursing and Health, 19*, 431–440.

Leddy, S. K. (1997). *The human energy model.* Manuscript in preparation.

Leddy, S. K., & Fawcett, J. (1997). Testing the theory of healthiness: Conceptual and methodological issues. In M. Madrid (Ed.). *Patterns of Rogerian knowing* (pp. 75–86). New York: National League for Nursing.

Lowry, L. W., & Anderson, B. (1993). Neuman's framework and ventilator dependency: A pilot study. *Nursing Science Quarterly, 6,* 195–200.

Magan, S. J. (1987). A critique of King's theory. In R. R. Parse (Ed.). *Nursing science: Major paradigms, theories and critiques* (pp. 115–133). Philadelphia: Saunders.

Malinski, V. M. (1986). *Explorations on Martha Rogers's science of unitary human beings.* East Norwalk, CT: Appleton-Century-Crofts.

Maliski, S. L., & Holditch-Davis, D. (1995). Linking biology and biography: Complex nonlinear dynamical systems as a framework for nursing inquiry. *Complexity and Chaos in Nursing, 2,* 25–35.

Monat A., & Lazarus, R. (Eds.). (1977). *Stress and coping: An anthology.* New York: Columbia University Press.

Morse, J. M., Solberg, S. M., Neander, W. L., Bottorff, J. L., & Johnson, J. L. (1990). Concepts of caring and caring as a concept. *Advances in Nursing Science, 13,* 1–14.

Neuman, B. (1982). *The Neuman systems model: Application to nursing education and practice.* East Norwalk, CT: Appleton-Century-Crofts.

Neuman, B. (1989). *The Neuman systems model* (2nd ed.). East Norwalk, CT: Appleton & Lange.

Neuman, B. (1995). *The Neuman systems model* (3rd ed.). East Norwalk, CT: Appleton & Lange.

Neuman, B. (1996). *The Neuman systems model in research and practice. Nursing Science Quarterly, 9,* 67–70.

Newman, M. A. (1986). *Health as expanding consciousness.* St. Louis: Mosby.

Newman, M. A. (1990). Newman's theory of health as praxis. *Nursing Science Quarterly, 3,* 37–41.

Newman, M. A. (1994). *Health as expanding consciousness* (2nd ed.). St Louis: Mosby.

Orem. D. E. (1980). *Nursing: Concepts of practice* (2nd ed.). New York: McGraw-Hill.

Orem, D. E. (1985). *Nursing: Concepts of practice* (3rd ed.). New York: McGraw-Hill.

Orem, D. E. (1990). A nursing practice theory in three parts, 1956–1989. In M. E. Parker (Ed.). *Nursing theories in practice* (pp. 47–60). New York: National League for Nursing.

Orem, D. E. (1995). *Nursing: Concepts of practice* (5th ed.). St. Louis: Mosby.

Parse, R. R. (1987). *Nursing science: Major paradigms, theories, and critiques.* Philadelphia: Saunders.

Parse, R. R. (1989). Man-living-health: A theory of nursing. In J. P. Riehl-Sisca (Ed.). *Conceptual models for nursing practice* (pp. 253–257). East Norwalk, CT: Appleton & Lange.

Parse, R. R. (1996). The human becoming theory: Challenges in practice and research. *Nursing Science Quarterly, 9,* 55–60.

Peplau, H. E. (1952). *Interpersonal relations in nursing.* New York: G. P. Putnam's Sons.

Peplau, H. E. (1988). The art and science of nursing: Similarities, differences and relations. *Nursing Science Quarterly, 1,* 8–15.

Phillips, J. R. (1987). A critique of Parse's man-living-health theory. In R. R. Parse (Ed.). *Nursing science: Major paradigms, theories, and critiques* (pp. 181–202). Philadelphia: Saunders.

Porter, E. J. (1995). Non-equilibrium systems theory: Some applications for gerontological nursing practice. *Journal of Gerontological Nursing, 21,* 24–31, 1995

Reed, P. G. (1996). Peplau's interpersonal relations model. In J. J. Fitzpatrick & A. L. Whall (Eds.). *Conceptual models of nursing: Analysis and application* (3rd ed., pp. 60–70). Stamford, CT: Appleton & Lange.

Reed, P. G., & Johnston, R. L. (1989). Peplau's nursing model: The interpersonal process. In J. J. Fitzpatrick & A. L. Whall (Eds.). *Conceptual models of nursing: Analysis and application* (2nd ed., pp. 49–67). East Norwalk, CT: Appleton & Lange.

Riehl, J. P., & Roy, C. (1980). *Conceptual models for nursing practice.* New York: Appleton-Century-Crofts.

Rogers, M. E. (1970). *An introduction to the theoretical basis of nursing.* Philadelphia: Davis.

Rogers, M. E. (1980). Nursing: A science of unitary man. In J. P. Riehl & C. Roy (Eds.). *Conceptual models for nursing practice* (pp. 329–337). New York: Appleton-Century-Crofts.

Rogers, M. E. (1990). Nursing: Science of unitary irreducible human beings: Update 1990. In E. A. M. Barrett (Ed.). *Visions of Rogers's based nursing* (pp. 5–11). New York: National League for Nursing.

Rogers, M. E. (1992). Nursing science and the space age. *Nursing Science Quarterly, 5,* 27–34.

Roy, C. (1987). Roy's adaptation model. In R. R. Parse (Ed.). *Nursing science: Major paradigms, theories, and critiques* (pp. 35–45). Philadelphia: Saunders.

Roy, C. (1988). An explication of the philosophical assumptions of the Roy adaptation model. *Nursing Science Quarterly, 1,* 26–34.

Roy, C. (1997). Future of the Roy model: Challenge to redefine adaptation. *Nursing Science Quarterly, 10,* 42–48.

Roy, C., & Roberts, S. L. (1981). *Theory construction in nursing: An adaptation model.* Englewood Cliffs, NJ: Prentice-Hall.

Sills, G. M., & Hall, J. E. (1977). A general systems perspective for nursing. In J. E. Hall & B. R. Weaver (Eds.). *Distributive nursing practice: A systems approach to community health.* Philadelphia: Lippincott.

Swanson, K. M. (1991). Empirical development of a middle range theory of caring. *Nursing Research, 40,* 161–166.

Torres, G. (1986). *Theoretical foundations of nursing.* East Norwalk, CT: Appleton & Lange.

Torres, G. (1990). The place of concepts and theories within nursing. In J. B. George (Ed.). *Nursing theories: The base for professional nursing practice* (3rd ed.). East Norwalk, CT: Appleton & Lange.

Watson, J. (1985). *Nursing: Human science and human care.* East Norwalk, CT: Appleton-Century-Crofts.

Watson, J. (1989). Watson's philosophy and theory of human caring in nursing. In J. P. Riehl-Sisca (Ed.). *Conceptual models for nursing practice* (pp. 219–235). East Norwalk, CT: Appleton & Lange.

Watson, J. (1996). Watson's theory of transpersonal caring. In P. H. Walker & B. Neuman (Eds.). *Blueprint for use of nursing models: Education, research, practice and administration* (pp. 141–162). New York: National League for Nursing.

Woods, E. C. (1994). King's theory in practice with elders. *Nursing Science Quarterly, 7,* 65–69.

Processes of Professional Nursing

LEARNING OUTCOMES

By the end of this chapter, the student will be able to:

1 Describe the strengths and weaknesses of the nursing process.

2 Describe content within the steps of the nursing process consistent with a variety of nursing conceptual models.

3 Differentiate among the stages of the novice to expert model of clinical practice.

4 Differentiate between linear and integrated cognitive nursing processes.

5 Describe interpersonal processes consistent with a variety of nursing conceptual models.

6 Discuss psychomotor processes for patterning of health.

Beliefs about nursing shape the way nurses practice. Consider the nature of nursing when it is based on a model of dependence on medical practice. Much of nursing, as taught and practiced, is standardized according to medical diagnoses and supports medical intervention. The physician does the assessment needed for the medical diagnosis, and this planning is the basis for the medical orders. The focus of nursing is on supporting the medical regimen to cure the client's disease. In this model, the so-called nursing knowledge is actually borrowed from medicine and includes detailed knowledge of pathophysiology, symptoms of disease, and standard medical intervention, as well as a single "best" way to perform treatments and procedures.

In contrast, consider the nature of nursing when it is based on a model of autonomous professional practice. In an autonomous nursing model, the focus is on supporting the client to improve well-being status and potential. Nursing knowledge includes detailed understanding of (1) the client as a whole person; (2) health and the factors that promote health; (3) the environment and the mutual and ongoing interaction between environment and humans; and (4) the purpose and functions of nursing. Nurses do their own assessments of clients, gathering information about each client's well-being status, including

1. Strengths as well as weaknesses
2. Whole response to health concerns
3. Analysis of the circumstances associated with the well-being status
4. Knowledge related to health and well-being
5. Beliefs and values about health
6. Lifestyle
7. Health-related goals
8. Support systems

Because the nurse views the client as a whole person and views nursing and professional nurses as collaborative with other health care professions and providers, the nurse will also have knowledge about the regimens of the other providers, such as physicians, pharmacists, physical therapists, and others. Understanding other regimens helps the nurse more fully appreciate the whole client, who is continually interacting with the whole environment. Understanding the impact of nursing, medical, and other regimens on the client helps the nurse to assume mutual and equal responsibility for the health team's effectiveness in assisting the client to achieve the health goals.

The knowledge projected by the model of nursing accepted by the practitioner is the basis for all nursing processes. Skill in the integrated use of cognitive, interpersonal, and psychomotor processes in client care is basic to the practice of professional nursing. The emphasis in this chapter is on the relationship between nursing processes and the practice of professional nursing according to the nursing models discussed in Chapter 8.

Cognitive Nursing Processes

THE NURSING PROCESS FOR PROBLEM SOLVING

Effective clinical decision-making skill is essential for professional nursing practice. Kataoka-Yahiro and Saylor (1994) suggested that the nursing process, as a method for problem-solving and decision-making, is a discipline-specific version of critical thinking. The steps in the nursing process have also been compared with the scientific method and with steps in problem-solving, as presented in Table 9-1.

The nursing process has been the method used in basic nursing education to teach novice learners how to solve problems. According to Dreyfus and Dreyfus (1996, p. 37):

> normally the instruction process begins with the instructor decomposing the task environment into context-free features which the beginner can recognize without benefit of experience. The beginner is then given rules for determining actions on the basis of these features . . . . Through instruction, the novice acquires rules for drawing conclusions or for determining actions, based upon facts.

The nursing process "provides a systematic guide or method to assist students and novices develop a style of thinking that leads to appropriate clinical judgments" (Christensen & Kenney, 1995, pp. 8–9). The nursing process provides a logical and rational way for the nurse to solve problems and make decisions so that the care given is appropriate and effective. Table 9-2 lists applications of critical thinking skills to phases of the nursing process. However, although the process is a scientific one, it is conducted by human beings who can carry it out in a sensitive and caring manner. Thus, the nursing process is both scientific and humane, just as nursing is perceived as both a science and an art.

TABLE 9-1

Comparison of Steps in Problem-Solving and the Scientific Method with the Nursing Process

Problem-Solving	Scientific Method	Nursing Process
Encountering problem	Recognizing problem	Assessment
Collecting data	Collecting data	
Identifying exact nature of problem	Forming hypothesis	Nursing diagnosis
Determining plan of action	Selecting plan for testing hypothesis	Planning
Carrying out plan	Testing of hypothesis	Implementation
Evaluating plan in new situation	Interpreting results	Evaluation
	Evaluating hypothesis	

From Potter, P. A., & Perry, A. G. (1995). *Basic nursing: Theory and practice* (3rd ed., p. 116). St. Louis: Mosby-Year Book. Used with permission of the publisher.)

TABLE 9-2

Application of Critical Thinking Skills to Components of the Nursing Process

Components and Definitions	Critical Thinking Skills and Activities
Assessment An ongoing process of data collection to determine the client's strengths and health concerns	Collect relevant client data by observation, examination, interview and history, and reviewing the records Distinguish relevant data from irrelevant Distinguish important data from unimportant Validate data with others
Diagnosis The analysis/synthesis of data to identify patterns and compare with norms and models A clear, concise statement of the client's health status and concerns appropriate for nursing intervention	Organize and categorize data into patterns Identify data gaps Recognize patterns and relationships in data Compare patterns with norms and theories Examine own assumptions regarding client's situation Make inferences and judgments of client's health concerns Define the health concern and validate with the client and health team members Describe actual and potential concerns and the etiology of each diagnosis Propose alternative explanations of concerns
Planning Determination of how to assist the client in resolving concerns related to restoration, maintenance, or promotion of health	Identify priority of client's concerns Determine client's desired health outcomes Select appropriate nursing interventions by generalizing principles and theories Transfer knowledge from other sciences Design plan of care with scientific rationale
Implementation The carrying out the plan of care by the client and nurse	Apply knowledge to perform interventions Compare baseline data with changing status Test hypotheses of nursing interventions Update and revise the care plan Collaborate with health team members
Evaluation A systematic, continuous process of comparing the client's response with the desired health outcomes	Compare client's responses with desired health outcomes Use criterion-based tools to evaluate Determine the client's level of progress Revise the plan of care

From Christensen, P. J., & Kenney, J. W. (1995). *Nursing process: Application of conceptual models* (4th ed., p. 8). St. Louis: Mosby-Year Book. Used with permission of publisher.)

Operationally, nursing process is the systematic:

1. Assessment of the client's health status
2. Specification of the client's strengths and problems
3. Determination of the nursing diagnosis
4. Development of a plan to maximize the client's strengths and re-solve the problems or reduce the concerns associated with the problems
5. Use of the nurse–client relationship characterized by empathy, gen-uineness, and respect to implement the plan
6. Engagement in an ongoing evaluation process to measure the effec-tiveness of the process

Invariably, the nursing process is presented as a series of four or five phases, with a number of steps within each phase. The net effect is a pro-cedure that appears linear (or at best overlapping or circular) and cumber-some. However, all parts of the process are interrelated and influence the whole. The parts or phases of the nursing process occur sequentially, but they are not linear. Planning may lead to intervention, or evaluation dur-ing planning may result in more assessment. Figure 9-1 depicts the nurs-ing process viewed from an interactional perspective.

The Assessment Phase

Collection of data about the client's health status is systematic and contin-uous. The data are accessible, communicated, and recorded. Before the nurse can begin collecting data, a degree of trust between the nurse and the client must be established. The nurse should initiate a relationship with the client and begin the definition of the roles each will play in the client's care. In this way, a positive environment for mutuality in the process can be established.

Data collection should be an organized process. The nurse must decide which data are desirable to collect in the particular situation and deter-mine what sources and methods are appropriate to obtain these data. The data collected in each situation should be appropriate and necessary for planning nursing intervention. These data should supplement rather than duplicate data collected by other health professionals (eg, history) and

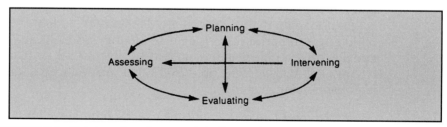

FIGURE 9-1 An interactional approach to the nursing process.

should focus on information needed for nursing care. As data are collected, they are reviewed to determine additional needed data and to begin the process of organizing the data for planning purposes.

Data will be needed about who the client is, why the client is being considered for care, and what factors are influencing the present health status. Necessary data include the client's name, age, gender, marital status, occupation, education, economic status, existing knowledge about health–illness status, and family (and significant others) attitudes toward health care. Information is needed, as well, about the client's personal habits, communication styles, cultural influences, growth and development status, learning capacity, supports and resources, previous experience with the health care system, medical diagnosis and regimen, coping patterns, and desired direction of change. Other needed data are related to the conceptual model being used to organize care, as suggested in Table 9-3. The elements have many similarities, but the emphasis varies.

As data are collected, they must be validated with the client and other sources. If discrepancies are noted, they should be clarified, and those data should not be used as the basis for inferences or judgments. Evaluation of the data should consider accuracy and whether all relevant factors have been included. As data collection continues, the organization and analysis of patterns within the data proceed concurrently, which may identify additional data collection needs.

The Diagnostic Phase
Carpenito (1992, p. 5) defines nursing diagnosis as

> a statement that describes the human response (health state or actual/potential altered interaction pattern) of an individual or group which the nurse can legally identify and for which the nurse can order the definitive interventions to maintain the health state or to reduce, eliminate, or prevent alterations.

Nursing diagnoses are derived from health status data. Using all the data collected in the assessment phase of the nurse–client relationship, the nurse organizes the data into clusters and interprets what those clusters reveal about the client. "Nursing diagnosis expresses [the nurse's] professional judgment of the patient's clinical status, responses to treatment, and nursing care needs" (Sparks & Taylor, 1991, p. 11). The analysis and synthesis of data require objectivity, deliberation, judgment, and discrimination. It is important that the nurse identify strengths as well as obvious and potential problems, but not create problems if they do not exist.

Yura and Walsh (1988, pp. 126–129) have developed a classification for possible nursing diagnoses:

1. No problem exists, and the client's state of wellness is affirmed. A plan to maintain wellness is developed with the client, which the

TABLE 9-3

Implications for Data Collection in Selected Nursing Models Organized by Theoretical Frameworks

Nursing Models	Implications for Data Collection
Systems Theory	
King	Perceptions of self, level of growth and development, level of stress, abilities to function in usual role, decision-making abilities, and abilities to communicate
Neuman	Stressors, indications of disruption of the lines of defense, resistance factors
Stress/Adaptation	
Roy	Adaptation level (related to three classes of stimuli), coping in relation to modes of adaptation, position on the health–illness continuum
Caring	
Orem	Therapeutic self-care demand, presence of self-care deficits, ability of clients to meet self-care requisites
Watson	Phenomenal field (self within life space and motivational factors for health), values, needs for information, problem-solving abilities, developmental conflicts, losses, feelings about the human predicament
Complexity	
Peplau	Physiologic and personality needs, illness symptoms, relationships with significant others, influences on establishment and maintenance of the nurse–client relationship
Rogers	Characteristics of patterning, health potential, rhythms of life, simultaneous states of the individual and environment
Parse	Thoughts and feelings about the situation, the synchronizing rhythms in human relationships, personal meanings, ways of being alike and different, and values
Newman	Person—environment interactions, patterns of energy exchange, client's responses to symptoms, transforming potential, client's feelings and what he does because of those feelings, patterns of life

client then implements. Periodic reassessment of wellness will be made, and the client will be present for these at given intervals. The client will seek reassessment sooner if a problem is suspected.

2. No problem exists, but there is a potential problem that may be offset by giving the client information on prevention and planning for a future interview. It may be necessary to refer the client to another health care member.

3. A problem exists but is being handled successfully by the client or the family, or both. Plans for periodic reassessment will be formulated, but the client will return for these at nonscheduled times whenever the client thinks it is necessary.

4. A problem exists that the client needs help in handling. Providing this assistance will either resolve the problem or make it easier for the client, family, neighbors, or some combination to handle it. Implementation continues until evaluation indicates that the

problem has been resolved or has decreased, or reassessment deems a change in plans is necessary.

5. A problem exists that the client cannot handle at this time, and its nature prevents family and neighbors from helping to resolve it. Health care intervention is needed. Specific members of the health care team, such as the physician, nurse, and dentist, may be assigned to help the client. With health care intervention, the problem can be specifically diagnosed, treated, and resolved (eg, dental caries).

6. A problem exists that must be studied further and diagnosed to resolve it or keep it within manageable proportions. Ambulatory or inpatient health and nursing services may be needed (eg, elevated blood sugar, obstruction).

7. A problem exists that is not incapacitating to the client at present, but its resolution requires intervention that would render the client dependent for a specific period or indefinitely. Inpatient care is generally necessary (eg, surgery).

8. A problem exists that places heavy demands on the client's ability to cope with it and that the family cannot resolve. Immediate and continued intervention by members of the health care team, on an inpatient basis, is required (eg, myocardial infarction, bleeding peptic ulcer).

9. A problem is imposed unexpectedly on the client or the family because of an accident, injury, or natural disaster, or is self-imposed (eg, attempted suicide). The problem may or may not be a threat to life.

10. Problems exist that are long-term and permanent. The client is able to cope with some but not all problems, and other persons may have to intervene to cope with the problem and provide care on a continuing basis (eg, congenital disability).

The three components to a working nursing diagnostic statement are (1) the nursing diagnosis; (2) the etiologic factor(s)—the "related to" phrase; and (3) the supporting signs and symptoms—the defining characteristics phrase (Ackley & Ladwig, 1995, p. 3). All diagnostic categories are associated with a cluster of signs and symptoms that permit discrimination among health problems. A goal is the standardization and publication of nursing diagnostic clusters of signs and symptoms. These are the cues or indications that a particular health problem exists. The signs and symptoms determine the diagnosis and, as changes occur, can be used to monitor progress and evaluate the effectiveness of the nursing care plan.

Although nursing diagnoses are developed by the nurse, they are based on data that have been validated with the client. The nurse and client then need to review the diagnoses to identify the goals (objectives) that will determine what outcomes are to be expected as the result of implementing planned care.

Nursing diagnoses have been classified in several ways:

Human response patterns of exchanging, communicating, relating, valuing, choosing, moving, perceiving, knowing, and feeling (North American Nursing Diagnosis Association, 1995–1996)

Functional health patterns of health perception–health management, nutritional–metabolic, elimination, activity–exercise, sleep–rest, cognitive–perceptual, self-perception–self-concept, role-relationship, sexuality–reproductive, coping–stress tolerance, value–belief (Gordon, 1995).

Some nursing leaders suggest that we need to redefine the essential elements of a nursing diagnosis and to eliminate the use of lists of possible diagnoses as a guide to practice, due to the:

Problem-oriented focus of such diagnoses

Seemingly unilateral response of the client when such diagnoses are used

Etiology aspect of diagnosis that appears to focus on either the past or the future rather than on the always-evolving present

Although the commonly accepted definitions of nursing diagnoses tend to be problem oriented only, it has been argued that the potential health concern aspect of diagnosis provides the opportunity to use nursing diagnosis as a guide even when practicing from a nursing model that focuses on client strengths.

The Planning Phase
The nursing care plan

> includes precise data about a specific client. These data are organized in a systematic, concise manner that facilitates overall nursing and health goals. It clearly communicates the nature of the client's problems. It contains all information about the client, the actual and potential nursing diagnoses and the priorities assigned to each, problems and complications to be prevented, and expected outcomes with prescribed nursing actions (Yura & Walsh, 1988, pp. 147–148).

The purposes of the nursing care plan are to:

1. Give direction, guidance, and meaning to nursing care
2. Provide a means of communicating, synchronizing, and organizing activities of the nursing team
3. Provide for continuity of care

The plan of nursing care includes the priorities and the prescribed nursing approaches or measures to achieve the goals derived from the nursing diagnoses. The nurse and client must agree on the overall goal from within the categories of health restoration, maintenance, or promotion or quality of life. Specific objectives then can be broken down by time frame into long-range, intermediate-range, and short-term behaviors to be expected. It is important that the objectives be both as realistic as possible and clearly stated because they will be the basis for evaluating the effectiveness of the plan of care. Broad guidelines for goal-setting in selected nursing models are presented in Table 9-4.

The objectives are determined by the client, in consultation with the nurse, considering the client's capabilities, limitations, and desired lifestyle. A client's preferences may be difficult for a nurse to accept, particularly if they differ from what would be the nurse's own choices or what the nurse thinks is best for the client. But the nurse cannot plan objectives in isolation from the client nor impose his or her own will on the client. Using change strategies (see Chap. 17), the nurse can attempt to influence goal-setting. However, once the objectives have been identified, the nurse's role must be to support their accomplishment.

After the objectives for care have been selected, priorities must be set among them. When survival is threatened, physical needs must take precedence. Cost, available personnel and resources, and time factors may also influence priorities. For example, for a student with a broken leg, weight loss may be considered an important goal, but because of the time needed to accomplish substantial weight loss, it may be assigned a lower priority than learning how to use crutches needed for mobility now. The theories or model being used to organize care can also influence determination of priorities. For example, use of Maslow's theory would assign

TABLE 9-4

Broad Guidelines for Goal Setting in Selected Nursing Models Organized by Theoretical Frameworks

Nursing Models	Broad Guidelines for Goal Setting
Systems Theory	
King	Achievement of goals and solution of problems related to personal, interpersonal, and social systems
Newman	Maintenance or restoration of dynamic equilibrium or the normal line of defense
Stress/Adaptation	
Roy	Promotion of adaptation from successful coping
Caring	
Orem	Restoration of external and internal constancy
Watson	Meeting human needs and solving problems in a caring interpersonal relationship
Complexity	
Peplau	Physiologic or psychological equilibrium, met needs, capabilities demonstrated (learning)
Rogers	Increasing complexity and innovativeness of patterning, facilitating health through evolutionary change
Parse	Illuminating meaning, synchronizing rhythms, and mobilizing transcendence
Newman	Transformation of patterns of life and facilitation of evolving consciousness

higher priority to physiologic, safety, and security needs, and lower priority to love, self-esteem, and self-actualization needs. In addition, as always, the client must be closely involved in the decisions.

Once the priorities among objectives have been determined, alternative options for care can be generated and their probability for success predicted. The possible solutions or approaches are heavily influenced by availability of resources and by factors in the client's lifestyle and cultural background. For example, weight loss could be achieved by 2 weeks' residence at a clinic, a diet requiring weighing portions of food, an exercise program, and so forth. However, financial constraints may make the clinic nonfeasible, and time and lifestyle constraints may influence the desirability of the exercise or food-weighing approaches.

This process of choosing approaches from among a number of alternatives is frequently neglected in the rush to take action. As a result, the first solution thought of may be the one implemented, with limited assessment of its likelihood of success or its appropriateness in the particular situation. This tendency to avoid brainstorming is also fostered by a belief that there is only one best way to accomplish a particular goal.

A conscious effort may have to be made to avoid choosing a prescribed "cookbook recipe," and instead for the nurse and client together to select the alternative that has the best likelihood of success for this unique client. This approach can then be translated into specific actions, the desired frequency of the actions, who will be assigned to carry them out (eg, nurse, client, other health team members), and the timetable for expected achievements.

The writing of the nursing care plan by students is often a rigorous exercise in complexity and volume, which results in avoidance and dread of the procedure. However, once the intellectual process has been completed, the actual writing of the plan can be accomplished fairly quickly. The care plan should include the (1) nursing diagnosis; (2) objectives associated with the diagnosis in order of priority; and (3) blueprint for accomplishing the objectives, including actions, assigned resources, and timetable.

The Intervention Phase

Nursing actions provide for client participation in health promotion, maintenance, and restoration and assist clients to maximize their health capabilities. The actions performed by the nurse are those previously determined to have the highest likelihood of success in meeting the objectives sought by the client. In addition, nursing actions support the medical regimen of care. Accomplishing these actions requires diverse skills, possibly including teaching, learning, leadership, management, group process, psychomotor ability, and, in all cases, communication.

All interactions with the client should be goal-directed and purposeful. As the actions are carried out, the nurse continues to collaborate with the client and significant others, and continues to involve the client in the care. Interventions are carried out with sensitivity to the client's feelings and are based on the client's individuality. The conceptual model being used to organize care has possible implications for intervention strategies, as suggested in Table 9-5.

The results of actions and the client's reactions to them should be recorded so that the progress can be shared by all involved in the client's care. The nurse needs to remain flexible so that actions can be modified as needed. As data are accumulated, they are evaluated in relation to the behaviors sought and to the previously set timetable. This assessment may indicate continuation of the plan, modification of the actions or the timetable, or possibly the need to reconsider the importance of the previously defined objective. Thus, the process of intervention is integrally involved with concurrent evaluation of its effectiveness.

The Evaluation Phase

The client's progress or lack of progress toward goal achievement is determined by the client and the nurse. This determination directs reassessment, reordering of priorities, new goal-setting, and revision of the nursing care plan. Evaluation should be continuous and ongoing

---

TABLE 9-5

Implications for Nursing Interventions in Selected Nursing Models Organized by Theoretical Frameworks

Nursing Models	Implications for Nursing Interventions
Systems Theory King	Emphasis is on exploration of the situation, shared information, mutually set goals, and explored means to resolve problems, achieve goals, and move forward.
Newman	Emphasis is on primary, secondary, or tertiary prevention to reduce stressors or strengthen the lines of defense.
Stress/Adaptation Roy	Emphasis is on increasing, decreasing, or maintaining focal, contextual, or residual stimuli.
Caring Orem	Emphasis is on self-care actions for or with the client if he is unable to perform them for himself.
Watson	Emphasis is on caring that reflects interpersonal teaching–learning, mutual formulation of the problem, joint appraisals, shared need for problem-solving, joint planning, provision of cognitive information, and evaluation of helpfulness for learning and coping.
Complexity Peplau	Emphasis is on the therapeutic relationship between the client and the nurse.
Rogers	Emphasis is on mobilization of the client's resources and repatterning of the human–environment interaction.
Parse	Emphasis is on guidance to relate the meaning of the client's situation, to share thoughts and feelings with one another, and to change the meaning of the situation by making it more explicit.
Newman	Emphasis is on the process of growth in which the nurse focuses on the client's evolving capacities, diversity, and complexity in the process of expanding consciousness.

throughout the nursing process. At this phase, however, the purpose of the evaluation is to compare changes in client behavior or health status with the desired behaviors or indicators defined in the objectives. Yura and Walsh (1988, pp. 168–169, enumeration added) have suggested that the outcome of evaluation may be any one or a combination of the following:

1. The client responded as expected and the problem is resolved. No further nursing action is needed. A plan to maintain the client's state of optimal wellness is formulated jointly by the nurse and the client. . . . A future appointment may be made to reaffirm the client's problem-free status.
2. Behavioral manifestations of the client's situation indicate that the problem has not been resolved; evidence demonstrates that short-term results, but not intermediate long-range expectations, have been achieved. . . . Reevaluation is to continue.
3. Behavioral manifestations of the client are similar to those evidenced during the assessment phase. Little or no evidence is available that the problem has been resolved. . . . Reassessment with replanning is needed.
4. Behavioral manifestations indicate new problems resulting from unmet or poorly met human needs. Assessing, planning, and implementing a plan of action to resolve these problems (nursing diagnoses) are in order. Planning action to resolve the new problem must be coordinated with the planning for the previously diagnosed problems. Evaluation will follow implementation.

It is difficult to develop valid and reliable tools to objectively measure progress toward some goals. It may be helpful to consider whether there are appropriate tools to measure progress toward goals when the goals are established. For example, weight loss and blood pressure reduction are easily validated. However, it is difficult to objectively assess improved self-concept or valuing of a more healthful lifestyle. Assumptions must be made about the meaning of observed behavior and whether it contributes to the specified goal.

Because the nursing process is systematic, logical, and goal-directed, it is assumed that adherence to the process will result in accomplishment of the desired goals. When evaluation of progress indicates that the problem is not resolved, it is necessary to consider possible reasons, which may involve the client, the nurse, the client's significant others, or health care team members.

Depending on the outcome of evaluation, the nurse and client may need to modify the goals or interventions, continue the planned strategies with a modified timetable, or, if the goals have been met and no new ones have emerged, terminate the relationship. Both the client and the nurse may have difficulty terminating the relationship. Clients may be unsure of their ability to maintain the changes in health behavior or well-being status on their own. The nurse may be ambivalent about not being needed any longer. Awareness and an open sharing of these feelings can lead to satisfaction in having accomplished the desired goals and acceptance of the need to end the relationship.

Despite the extensive attention given to nursing process, many nurses continue to intervene using standardized procedures based on medical diagnoses. "Thus, the nursing process would appear not to be an accurate description of how nursing is actually performed" (Lundh, Soder, & Waerness, 1988, p. 37). In the following section, two brief examples will illustrate that nursing care can be based on modifications of the nursing process within nursing conceptual models.

Conceptual Models Emphasizing the Nursing Process
THE ROY ADAPTATION MODEL

In the Roy adaptation model, the goal of nursing is to promote adaptation. The nurse manipulates stimuli to move the client in the desired direction of change toward adaptation. The process of nursing is described as a six-step problem-solving method (Andrews & Roy, 1991):

> First level assessment
>> Examine client behaviors in the adaptation modes.
>> Make a judgment about whether behaviors in the four modes are adaptive or ineffective.
> Second level assessment
>> Analyze stimuli that influence ineffective behaviors.
>> Determine priorities.
> State problem areas as nursing diagnoses.
> Determine specific goals.
> Determine interventions.
> Evaluate as behavior changes, and modify as needed.

THE NEUMAN SYSTEMS MODEL

In the Neuman systems model, the purpose of nursing "is to assist clients to retain, attain, or maintain optimal system stability" (Neuman, 1995, p. 69). "The major concern for nursing is in keeping the client stable through accuracy both in assessing the effects and possible effects of environmental stressors" (Neuman, 1995, p. 33). A three-step modification of the nursing process is proposed:

> Determine a nursing diagnosis.
> Establish nursing goals.
> Determine nursing outcomes—interventions take the form of primary, secondary, and tertiary prevention.

The American Nurses Association (ANA) "Standards of Clinical Practice" (ANA 1991) are related to application of the nursing process.

- Assessment: Client health data are collected
- Diagnosis: Diagnoses are determined and expected outcomes are individualized to the client
- Planning: A plan of care that prescribes interventions to attain expected outcomes is developed
- Implementation: Interventions identified in the plan of care are implemented
- Evaluation: The client's progress toward attainment of outcomes is evaluated

Research has demonstrated that nurses hold a relatively positive attitude toward the nursing process (Martin et al., 1994).

However, although there are several assumed benefits of the nursing process, a number of concerns have also been expressed.

Benefits and Criticisms of the Nursing Process

A number of benefits of the nursing process for problem-solving have been suggested:

Provides an orderly and systematic method for planning and providing care
Enhances efficiency by standardizing nursing practice
Facilitates documentation
Provides a unity of language
Is economical
Stresses the independent functions of nurses
Increases quality of care through the use of deliberate actions

However, in many practice settings, the perception is that the nursing process is too time-consuming to be practical. In addition, with an emphasis on "nurse-centered power," (Varcoe, 1996), the essential rights and responsibilities of clients and their families and collaboration with other health care providers are lacking. A number of other concerns with the nursing process have been identified (Henderson, 1987; Lindsey, 1996; Rew, 1996; Varcoe, 1996), including:

- A linear, rational problem-solving process is not consistent with the real world of clinical practice
- It focuses on problems, not strengths and potential
- Elaborate and time-consuming nursing jargon is used
- Rules take precedence over interaction
- It is antithetical to holism
- Diagnoses label patients
- Intuition is minimized or not allowed
- Appropriateness for expert practice is questionable

The formula-like structure of the nursing process has been found to be a useful way to teach rules to novice learners. However, many nurses treat the nursing process as if it were the only process in nursing practice. Research has demonstrated that the nursing process is inadequate "when sensory data are changing rapidly or are ambiguous, uncertain, or conflicting" (Rew, 1996). Interestingly, a relationship between critical thinking ability and professional competence has not been demonstrated (Maynard, 1996). In addition, Benner, Tanner, and Chesla (1996) found that clinically proficient and expert nurses use intuitive cognitive processes (rather than rule-based thinking) in their clinical judgments. These processes are discussed in the next section.

INTEGRATED MODELS FOR CLINICAL JUDGMENT

In the preceding section, the nursing process was presented as "an objective, empirically based form of analysis with emphasis on the development of sound arguments" (Pless & Clayton, 1993, p. 426). However, it has been suggested that "the clinical judgment of experienced nurses resembles much more (the) engaged, practical reasoning . . . than the disengaged, scientific, or theoretical reasoning . . . represented in the nursing process" (Benner et al., 1996, p. 1).

The Novice-to-Expert Practice Model

The novice-to-expert practice model is based on inductive studies of clinical practice settings (Benner et al., 1996). The model proposes that

> experienced nurses reach an understanding of a person's experience with an illness, and hence their response to it, not through abstract labeling such as nursing diagnoses, but rather through knowing the particular patient . . . and through advanced clinical knowledge, which is gained through experience with many persons in similar situations. This experientially gained clinical knowledge sensitizes the nurse to possible issues and concerns in particular situations (Benner et al., p. 1).

Based on the five-stage model of skill acquisition in clinical practice of Dreyfus and Dreyfus (1996), this model is individualized rather than rule based, and emphasizes the integration of nonconscious, nonanalytical aspects of judgment, experience, and reflection on rational critical thinking.

THE NOVICE STAGE

In the novice stage, which occurs during the educational process, tasks are presented as context-free. Examples include a client assignment to make an "occupied bed" or chart fluid intake and output. The instructor provides rules for determining actions related to these abstract tasks. In the above example, the novice nurse learns to "always" put up the opposite side rail when making an occupied bed. As a result of this teaching approach, the novice nurse tries to learn as many rules as possible for drawing conclusions or for determining actions.

THE ADVANCED BEGINNER STAGE

Dreyfus and Dreyfus (1996) propose that "performance improves to a marginally acceptable level only after the novice has considerable experience coping with real situations" (p. 38). Over time, there is beginning ability to intuitively recognize meaningful "situational" elements that are not definable objectively. Because many new elements (and more rules) are now recognized as relevant, tasks appear to become more difficult. Benner and coworkers (1996) describe the following clinical behaviors of advanced beginner nurses:

They are open, yet apprehensive and anxious about task accomplishment; may feel overwhelmed
Practice is viewed as a set of tasks to be accomplished
Concern is to organize, prioritize, and complete tasks
They have a fragmented or only partial grasp of situations
They view practice as a test of personal capabilities
They base practice on standardized procedures or orders that are external to the immediate situation
They depend on the expertise of others
They question their capacity to contribute

THE COMPETENT STAGE

In the competent stage, the nurse has a limited sense of what is important in the clinical situation. A hierarchy, such as a plan, facilitates decision-making. The nurse becomes emotionally involved in making choices, which makes it more difficult to base care exclusively on detached rules. Benner and colleagues (1996) describe the following clinical behaviors of competent nurses:

Have improved organizational ability and technical skills
Have increased understanding and are able to anticipate in familiar situations
Focus care on managing the patient's condition
Are disillusioned with gaps in their own ability and in the fallibility of others

THE PROFICIENT STAGE

By the proficient stage, the nurse has achieved situational discrimination accompanied by associated responses. There is a growing intuitive appreciation of what is important in a situation. As a result, thinking about alternatives is easier and less stressful, but decisions are still based on detached rules. Benner and coworkers (1996) describe the following clinical behaviors of proficient nurses:

Able to recognize patterns (qualitatively different from preceding stages)
Have increased perceptual acuity and responsiveness to the situation
Identify similarities and differences in situations

Develop engaged reasoning in transitions
Are emotionally attuned to do what needs to be done
Recognize changing relevance
Have achieved differentiated skills of involvement with patients and
   families

THE EXPERT STAGE

Expert nurses normally do not solve problems. They use subtle and refined discrimination. Reasoning involves deliberative rationality with a
background of intuition, in which critical thinking involves detached, rea-
soned observation of intuitive behavior. In novel situations, the expert
uses theory or seeks advice from other experts. Benner and colleagues
(1996) describe the following clinical behaviors of expert nurses:

Increased links between seeing issues and ways of responding
Use engaged, practical reasoning
See big picture and can anticipate the unexpected
Know the patient
Have moral agency

The validity of the novice-to-expert model in describing actual clinical
practice has been supported by research (Benner et al., 1996; Tabak, Bar-
Tal, & Cohen-Mansfield, 1996). Studies have shown that although

> the prevailing conception of clinical judgment in nursing is the diagnosis–
> treatment model, which relies on explicit identification of patient's deficits
> and deliberation on and selection of treatment options, with experience, nurses
> become more involved, rather than more detached; they grasp the meaning of
> the situation directly, rather than through analytic thinking (Benner et al.,
> 1996, p. 311).

INTUITION

Studies of expert clinical practice have identified intuition, knowing the
patient, and reflection as important characteristics. Intuitive awareness
has been described as "another way of knowing wherein facts or truths are
known or felt directly rather than arrived at through a linear process of rational analysis" (Rew, 1996, p. 149), or as "an instantaneous, direct grasping of reality" (Mishlove, 1994, p. 32). In a study that supported the
novice-to-expert model, Polge (1995) found that "as the level of nursing
proficiency increases from advanced beginner to expert, there is a significant increase in the use of intuitive critical thinking to make clinical nursing judgments" (p. 8). At least a minimum amount of time and concrete
learning experiences in practice are required before nurses can pass to a
higher level of proficiency.

Young (1987) has proposed that intuition is multidimensional. The
functional dimension, which operationalizes intuition, is comprised of
cues and judgment, in which actions do not have a logical link with data.
The personal dimension, a form of personal knowing, may include:

Direct patient contact
Self-receptivity
Experience
Energy
Self-confidence

REFLECTION

Reflection is a process of thinking about concerns associated with an experience. "The aim of one's deliberations is to make sense or meaning out of the experience and to incorporate this experience into one's view of the self and the world" (Baker, 1996, p. 19). Reflection develops the affective domain of learning and allows nurses to relate to the aspects of their experience that are the most profound at the time. As a result, reflection has the potential to provide for personal growth.

Reflective learning has been associated with the following aspects:

Triggering of a sense of inner discomfort
Identification or clarification of the concern in relation to the individual
Openness to new information
Resolution (an "aha") with the feeling of having changed or learned something that is personally significant
Change in oneself
Deciding whether to act on the outcome of the process

KNOWING THE PATIENT

Tanner, Benner, Chesla, and Gordon (1993) argue that when nurses are constrained from knowing their clients by "organizational arrangements and economic constraints of practice . . . then the very ground for safe and astute nursing care is undermined . . . and nursing is reduced to a technology" (p. 279). Knowing the client involves knowing the client as a person and knowing the client's typical pattern of responses.

Jenny and Logan (1992) view knowing the client as a process for acquiring and using individualized clinical knowledge. They have identified actions involved in knowing the client:

1. Perceiving/envisioning—"the active transformation of observations of patients' behavior into a direct, non-mediated perception of what was significant in it" (p. 256)
2. Communicating
3. Self-presentation—"the nurses' conscious efforts to gain the patients' trust by displaying professional knowledge, self-confidence, dependability and concern" (p. 256)
4. Showing concern—"the demonstration of a caring attitude to the patient and responding to their concerns" (p. 256)

In contrast, Radwin (1995) identifies familiarity and intimacy as the properties of knowing the patient. Time, the nurse's experience, and other nurses' input are described as conditions. Four strategies for knowing the client include:

1. Empathizing—"the nurse imagines what her feelings and perceptions might be if she were in the patient's situation" (p. 367). This strategy is used when time periods are short and familiarity is low.
2. Matching a pattern—the nurse matches knowledge about the patient being cared for with "a pattern or configuration comprising the experiences, behaviors, feelings, and/or perceptions of previously cared for patients in similar situations" (p. 367).
3. Developing a bigger picture—"the nurse combines understanding of the patient within and outside the acute care setting to produce a broader perspective" (p. 367).
4. Balancing preferences with difficulties—"the nurse has an understanding of patient experiences, behaviors, feelings, and/or perceptions . . . and preferences" (p. 368).

Intuition and reflection are approaches to practice that integrate experience with cognition. Knowing the client integrates experience and cognition and also adds the dimension of interpersonal processes.

Although cognitive processes receive the bulk of attention when nursing process is discussed, interpersonal processes are also essential. The next section discusses interpersonal processes as guided by selected nursing conceptual models/theories.

Interpersonal Processes

Nursing occurs within a relationship between the client and the nurse. However, many nursing conceptual models and theories differ in their descriptions of interpersonal processes, as illustrated by the following brief examples.

KING'S THEORY OF GOAL ATTAINMENT

In King's theory (King, 1995), the goal of nursing is to help individuals maintain their health so they can function in their roles. Nursing is a process of action, reaction, and interaction that results in goal attainment. Although the the process proposed by this theory is classified according to the steps in the nursing process, the emphasis is on interpersonal processes within the steps:

Assessment: Incorporates perception, communication, and interaction of nurse and client

Planning: Includes decision-making about goals and agreement on means to attain goals

Implementation: Transactions are made
Evaluation: Was the goal attained?

PEPLAU'S INTERPERSONAL RELATIONS MODEL

In Peplau's model (Reed, 1996), nursing is a therapeutic, interpersonal process. It is an educative instrument, a maturing force, that aims to promote forward movement of the personality. The interpersonal process is the method by which the nurse facilitates useful transformations of the client's energy or anxiety. The interpersonal process is based on a participatory relationship between the nurse and the client in which the nurse governs the purpose and the process in the relationship, and the client controls the content. The process consists of four phases:

Orientation: Clients become aware of the availability of and trust in the nurse's abilities
Identification: Nurse facilitates expression of feelings without rejection
Exploitation: The client derives the full value from the relationship
Resolution: The client is gradually freed from an identification with the helping professional. The client's ability to meet his or her own needs is strengthened

PATERSON AND ZDERAD'S HUMANISTIC THEORY

In this humanistic nursing practice theory, nursing is perceived as an experience lived between human beings. "Nursing is a response to the human situation. One human being needs a kind of help and another gives it" (Paterson & Zderad, 1988, p. 11). The humanistic nursing effort is directed toward increasing the possibilities of making responsible choices. The process, which is labeled the phenomenologic method of nursology, consists of five phases:

Phase I: The nurse knower prepares for coming to know
Phase II: The nurse intuitively knows the "other"
Phase III: The nurse scientifically knows the other
   Analyze
   Consider relationships between components
   Synthesize themes or patterns
   Conceptualize or symbolically interpret a sequential view of this postlived reality
Phase IV: The nurse complementarily synthesizes known others
   Compare similarities and differences
   Synthesize

> Phase V: Succession within the nurse from the many to the paradoxical one—"a conception or abstraction that is inclusive of and beyond the multiplicities and contradictions" (Paterson & Zderad, 1988, p. 74)

Parse's Human Becoming Theory

In Parse's theory, the goal of practice is quality of life from the client's perspective, with the focus on the meaning constructed by the client (Parse, 1996). The nurse is present in a nonroutinized, unconditional, loving way of being with the client. The full attention of the nurse is with the client "as they move beyond the moment." The methodology in this theory consists of three processes:

> Explicating (illuminating meaning)—making clear what is appearing now through languaging
> Dwelling with (synchronizing rhythms)—giving of self over to the flow of the struggle in connecting-separating
> Moving beyond (mobilizing transcendence)—propelling with visioned possibles in transforming

Newman's Theory of Health as Expanding Consciousness

Newman describes nursing as "caring in the human health experience" (Newman, 1994, p. 139). "The responsibility of the nurse is not to make people well, or to prevent their getting sick, but to assist people to recognize the power that is within them to move to higher levels of consciousness" (Newman, 1994, p. xv). The focus of nursing in this theory is the pattern of the whole that is clarified through a praxis (practice) method:

> A partnership with the client is established, with a mutual goal of participating in an authentic relationship.
> Meeting and forming a connection
> Forming shared consciousness
> Moving apart
> Participants tell their stories in their own way.
> Nurse is free to be authentic and fully present. "Awareness of being, rather than doing, is the primary mechanism of helping" (Newman, 1994, p. 104)
> Data are organized in chronological order as a narrative (sequential pattern over time)

In addition to cognitive and interpersonal processes, nursing care also includes psychomotor processes. Skill in the performance of physician-ordered, often invasive, disease or problem-related interventions is a major emphasis in much of nursing clinical practice. The next section, however, discusses noninvasive, patterning interventions that fall within nursing's autonomous scope of practice.

◎ Patterning Processes

ROGERS'S SCIENCE OF UNITARY HUMAN BEINGS

Rogers states that "the purpose of nursing is to promote human health and well being" (Rogers, 1988, p. 100). For Rogers, health is not a separate state, nor is it good or bad, nor in a linear relationship with disease or illness. Instead, health is viewed as "an index of field patterning" (Malinski, 1986, p. 27), and nursing intervention is aimed toward patterning of humans and the environment to achieve maximum health potential (Rogers, 1970).

In Rogerian science, behavior patterns are viewed as manifestations of the human–environment field. Field manifestations may include lifestyle parameters such as:

Nutrition
Work and play
Exercise
Sleep–wake cycles
Safety
Interpersonal networks
Decelerated–accelerated field rhythms

Examples of field rhythm manifestations might include diversity (from greater to lesser), motion (from slower to seeming continuous), time (from slower to timelessness), and creativity (from pragmatic to visionary).

The client is a knowing participant in change in this model. Through being aware, having choices and the freedom to act intentionally, and being involved in creating changes, the client is a mutual participant with the nurse in the patterning process. A healing relationship is characterized by certain principles:

■ The focus is on strengths and skills
■ Nurse and client are involved in creating changes and influencing outcomes
■ Nurse and client are equal partners, but the client has the major responsibility for change decisions
■ A balance of exchange or reciprocity
■ Presence and involvement, or connectedness
■ Flow and harmony

The patterning process has two phases, appraisal and deliberative patterning. The elements of appraisal in phase one include:

Using multiples modes of awareness including recognizing, being aware of, and being sensitive to
Tuning into a person's unique patterns
Appreciating manifestations of the human field in the form of experience, perception, and expressions

> Constructing pattern knowing through synthesis
> Verifying with the client

Phase two involves the mutual deliberative patterning of behavior, which is possible because of the integral connectedness of the person–environment. Although diversity is considered to be a norm, patterning of each individual is unique. Each individual has an intrinsic potential for growth, which can be identified through exploring the meaning of experiences for the individual. The client and nurse are viewed as connected, and the healing milieu is as important as the particular modality selected as a treatment. Because change is viewed as inevitable, the challenge is to reframe problems into opportunities for positive becoming. By tuning in to the client's rhythms, the nurse can help the client to free energy for self-patterning through a number of possible noninvasive interventions such as:

> Imagery
> Relaxation
> Affirmation
> Sound (music)
> Exercise
> Color/light (wave modalities)
> Nutrition (diet, vitamins, minerals, herbs)
> Meaningful presence
> Humor
> Authentic dialogue (guided reminiscence)
> Wellness counseling (health education)
> Therapeutic touch (centering)
> Movement (dance, imposed motion)
> Journal-keeping
> Balance between activity and rest
> Bibliotherapy
> Acupressure
> Bodywork (massage, touch for health)

Conclusion

Cognitive, interpersonal, and patterning nursing processes provide methods by which the nurse sensitively and systematically approaches practice to achieve mutually determined health goals with the client. The use of these processes provides an enriching relationship for both the client and the nurse and a basis for autonomous practice emerging from a professional nursing model.

THOUGHT QUESTIONS

1 When is it desirable to use the nursing process in giving care?

2 How useful is the nursing process for experienced nurses?

3 What are the key differences of interpersonal process as proposed by King, Peplau, Paterson and Zderad, Parse, and Newman.

4 How are nursing processes guided by Rogers's science different from those suggested by any of the other nursing models and theories? Why is that so?

REFERENCES

Ackley, B. J., & Ladwig, G. B. (1995). *Nursing: A guide to diagnosis planning care handbook* (2nd ed.). St. Louis: Mosby-Year Book.

American Nurses Association. (1991). *ANA standards for practice.* Kansas City: Author.

Andrews, H. A., & Roy, S. C. (1991). The nursing process according to the Roy adaptation model. In S. C. Roy & H. A. Andrews (Eds.). *The Roy adaptation model. The definitive statement.* East Norwalk, CT: Appleton & Lange

Baker, C. R. (1996). Reflective learning: A teaching strategy for critical thinking. *Journal of Nursing Education, 35,* 19–22.

Benner, P., Tanner, C. A., & Chesla, C. A. (1996). *Expertise in nursing practice: Caring, clinical judgment, and ethics.* New York: Springer.

Carpenito, L. J. (1992). *Nursing diagnosis: Application to clinical practice* (4th ed.). Philadelphia: Lippincott.

Christensen, P. J., & Kenney, J. W. (1995). *Nursing process: Application of conceptual models* (4th ed.). St. Louis: Mosby-Year Book.

Dreyfus, H. L., & Dreyfus, S. E. (1996). The relationship of theory and practice in the acquisition of skill. In P. Benner, C. A. Tanner, & C. A. Chesla (Eds.). *Expertise in nursing practice: Caring, clinical judgment, and ethics* (pp. 29–47). New York: Springer.

Gordon, M. (1995). *Manual of nursing diagnosis, 1995–1996.* St. Louis: Mosby-Year Book.

Henderson, V. (1987). Nursing process: A critique. *Holistic Nursing Practice, 1,* 7–18.

Jenny, J., & Logan, J. (1992). Knowing the patient: One aspect of clinical knowledge. *Image, 24,* 254–258.

Kataoka-Yahiro, M., & Saylor, C. (1994). A critical thinking model for nursing judgment. *Journal of Nursing Education, 33,* 351–356.

King, I. M. (1995). The theory of goal attainment. In M. A. Frey & C. L. Sieloff (Eds.). *Advancing King's systems framework and theory of nursing* (pp. 23–32). Thousand Oaks, CA: Sage.

Lindsey, E., & Hartrick, G. (1996). Health-promoting nursing practice: The demise of the nursing process? *Journal of Advanced Nursing, 23,* 106–112.

Lundh, U., Soder, M., & Waerness, K. (1988, Spring). Nursing theories: A critical view. *Image, 20,* 36–40.

Malinski, V. M. *Explorations on Martha Rogers' science of unitary human beings.* East Norwalk, CT: Appleton-Century-Crofts.

Martin, P. A., Dugan, J., Freundl, M., Miller, S. E., Phillips, R., & Sharritts, L. (1994). Nurses' attitudes toward nursing process as measured by the Dayton attitude scale. *Journal of Continuing Education for Nurses, 25,* 35–40.

Maynard, C. A. (1996). Relationship of critical thinking ability to professional nursing competence. *Journal of Nursing Education, 35,* 12–18.

Mishlove, J. (1994). Intuition: The source of true knowing. *Noetic Science Review, 29,* 31–36.

Neuman, B. (1995). *The Neuman systems model* (3rd ed.). East Norwalk, CT: Appleton & Lange.

Newman, M. A., (1994). *Health as expanding consciousness* (2nd ed.). New York: National League for Nursing.

North American Nursing Diagnosis Association. (1995). *Nursing diagnoses: Definitions and classification 1995–1996.* Philadelphia: Author

Parse, R. R. (1996). The human becoming theory: Challenges in practice and research. *Nursing Science Quarterly, 9,* 55–-60.

Paterson, J. G., & Zderad, L. T. (1988). *Humanistic nursing.* New York: National League for Nursing.

Pless, B. S., & Clayton, G. M. (1993). Clarifying the concept of critical thinking in nursing. *Journal of Nursing Education, 32,* 425–428.

Polge, J. (1995). Critical thinking: The use of intuition in making clinical nursing judgments. *Journal of the New York State Nurses Association, 26,* 4–9.

Potter, P. A., & Perry, A. G. (1995). *Basic nursing: Theory and practice* (3rd ed.). St. Louis: Mosby-Year Book.

Radwin, L. E. (1995). Knowing the patient: A process model for individualized interventions. *Nursing Research, 44,* 364–370.

Reed, P. G. (1996). Peplau's interpersonal relations model. In J. J. Fitzpatrick & A. L. Whall (Eds.). *Conceptual models of nursing* (pp. 62–69). Stamford, CT: Appleton & Lange.

Rew, L. (1996). *Awareness in healing.* Albany, NY: Delmar.

Rogers, M. E. (1970). An introduction to the theoretical basis of nursing. Philadelphia: Davis.

Rogers, M. E. (1988). Nursing science and art: A prospective. *Nursing Science Quarterly, 1,* 99–102.

Sparks, S. M., & Taylor, C. M. (1991). *Nursing diagnosis reference manual.* Springhouse, PA: Springhouse.

Tabak, N., Bar-Tal, Y., & Cohen-Mansfield, J. (1996). Clinical decision making of experienced and novice nurses. *Western Journal of Nursing Research, 18,* 534–547.

Tanner, C. A., Benner, P., Chesla, C.,& Gordon, D. R. (1993). The phenomenology of knowing the patient. *Image, 25,* 273–280.

Varcoe, C. (1996). Disparagement of the nursing process: The new dogma? *Journal of Advanced Nursing, 23,* 120–125.

Young, C. E. (1987). Intuition and nursing process. *Holistic Nursing Practice, 1,* 52–62.

Yura, H., & Walsh, M. B. (1988). *The nursing process* (5th ed.). East Norwalk, CT: Appleton & Lange.

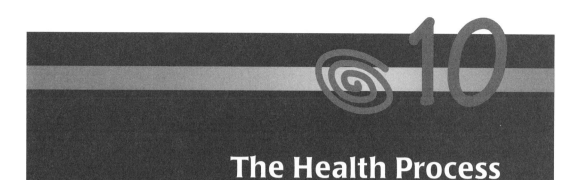

The Health Process

LEARNING OUTCOMES

By the end of this chapter, the student will be able to:

1 Explain how well-being differs from health, and illness from disease.

2 Differentiate between the interaction and integration worldviews of health.

3 Identify what factors cause individual variability in wellness.

4 Describe how health and illness can be explained as a unitary concept.

5 Compare and contrast models for health protection and promotion.

6 Discuss strategies for changing lifestyle behaviors and health patterning.

VIGNETTE

Michael, a staff nurse on a general medical–surgical unit, says: "In the hospital, health is a distant goal. My job is to take care of sick people, and I don't have time to even think about health! I guess it might be important for nurses who work in ambulatory care."

When asked why they went into nursing, many nurses answer "to help people." By this, they usually mean to help sick people get better. Nursing, in the minds of many people, is associated with medicine and hospitals because most nurses have worked for hospitals caring for sick people.

The major purpose of the hospital is to support the medical regimen in treating disease and dysfunction. The public image of what nursing is and what nurses do has been influenced by the medical definition of health as "the absence of disease." The association of nursing with disease and sickness is at the heart of the traditional characterization of the nurse as the physician's handmaiden.

Cure of disease is the major purpose of medicine, but health care delivery aimed predominantly at cure of disease is wasteful of resources and costly. Increasingly, the public is becoming aware of the need to prevent illness and promote wellness. Through roles designed to (1) promote health, (2) capitalize on the healthy outlook of people, and (3) reinforce their strengths, the nursing profession has the potential to make a major impact on our society's philosophy and delivery of health care. Health promotion and patterning are considered to be essential nursing activities in all (including acute care) settings for nursing care.

In this chapter, the interaction and the integration worldviews of health are presented as organizing frameworks for alternate views of the concepts of health, well-being, wellness, disease, illness, and sickness. Later sections of the chapter consider models and nursing interventions for the protection, promotion, and patterning of health.

◎ Worldviews of Health

Basic philosophic assumptions about the nature of reality, including human beings and the human–environment relationship, are referred to as paradigms or worldviews. Worldviews that have been described by nursing scholars include change/persistence (Hall, 1981); totality/simultaneity (Parse, 1987), particulate–deterministic/interactive–integrative/unitary–transformative (Newman, 1992); and reaction/reciprocal interaction/simultaneous action (Fawcett, 1993). Elements of these classifications have been synthesized into the interaction/integration worldview (Leddy, 1996), which is summarized below.

THE INTERACTION WORLDVIEW

In the interaction worldview, the human being is usually conceptualized as a whole comprised of parts. The human being interacts with a physically separate environment. The environment contains stressors that act on a person and to which a person must react. Therefore, there is a belief in linear, predictable, and quantifiable cause-and-effect relationships.

In this worldview, because the goal for the person is to maintain balance, or stability, environmental change is seen as a threat. The threat may involve disease, illness, or sickness, affecting well-being, wellness, and health.

Disease

Disease is a medical term consistent with the interaction worldview. It is a "dysfunction of the body" (Benner, Tanner, & Chesla, 1996, p. 45). The objective of the physician is to classify observable changes in body structure or function (signs) into a recognizable clinical syndrome. A correct label, or diagnosis, implies disease course and duration, communicability, prognosis, and appropriate treatment. Medical intervention is aimed at curing the disease. Part of nursing intervention supports and promotes the medical regimen through, among other things, administering treatments, encouraging rest, and evaluating the effectiveness of interventions.

Historically, diseases were believed to be due to one agent, which, in a sufficient dose, caused certain predictable signs and symptoms. Increasingly, however, a variety of factors related to the person (host), agent, and environment have been viewed as being interrelated in the cause and in effective treatment of disease. All these interactions must be considered in determining a plan for care.

Illness

Illness is a subjective feeling of being unhealthy that may or may not be related to disease. A person may have a disease without feeling ill and may feel ill in the absence of disease. For example, a person may have hypertension (a disease), controlled with medication, diet, and exercise, and may have no symptoms (no illness). Another person may have pain, and thus feel ill, but may not have an identifiable disease. What is important is how the person feels and what he or she does because of those feelings.

Nursing intervention aims to identify a cause for symptoms and to decrease them, if possible, by focusing on the client's responses to the symptoms. In contrast, medical care focuses on efforts to label and treat the symptoms. When a person's illness is accepted by society, and thus given legitimacy, it is considered "sickness."

Sickness

Sickness is a status, a social entity usually associated with disease or illness, although it may occur independently of them (Twaddle, 1977, p. 97). Once the person is defined as sick, various dependent behaviors are condoned that otherwise might be considered unacceptable. The nurse's role is to assist until the person is able to independently reassume responsibility for decision-making.

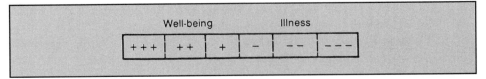

FIGURE 10-1 The well-being continuum. (Modified from Terris, M. [1975]. Approaches to an epidemiology of health. *American Journal of Public Health, 65,* 1039. Used with permission from publisher).

Well-Being

Well-being is a subjective perception of vitality and feeling well that is a component of health within the interaction worldview. It is a variable state that can be described objectively, experienced, and measured. Experienced at the lowest degrees, a person might feel ill. Experienced at the highest levels, a person would perceive maximum satisfaction, understanding, and feelings of contribution. Thus, well-being status can be plotted on a continuum, as shown in Figure 10-1.

Health as Wellness

Health is difficult to define. Health is described in various sources as a value judgment, a subjective state, a relative concept, a spectrum, a cycle, a process, and an abstraction that cannot be measured objectively. In many definitions, physiologic and psychological components of health are dichotomized. Other subconcepts that might be included in definitions of health include environmental and social influences, freedom from pain or disease, optimum capability, ability to adapt, purposeful direction and meaning in life, and sense of well-being.

In the interaction worldview, health indicates the absence of disease and presence of normal functioning in roles or tasks. In this book, health has been defined as a state or condition of integrity of functioning (functional capacity and ability), and perceived well-being (feeling well). As a result, a person is able to:

Function adequately (can be observed objectively)
Adapt adequately to the environment
Feel well (as assessed subjectively)

Wellness, as defined in the literature, is similar to the open-ended and eudaimonistic models of health described below, and in this book will be considered synonymous. Dunn (1977, p. 9) describes wellness as "an integrated method of functioning which is oriented toward maximizing the potential of which the individual is capable, within the environment where he is functioning." Others have characterized wellness–illness as "the human experience of actual or perceived function–dysfunction" (Jensen & Allen, 1994, p. 349). Indications of wellness (health) might include:

A person's capacity to perform to the best of his or her ability
The ability to adjust and adapt to varying situations
A reported feeling of well-being, and
A feeling that "everything is together."

Smith (1981, p. 47) presents four models of health consistent with the interaction worldview that "can be viewed as forming a scale—a progressive expansion of the idea of health": the clinical model, the role performance model, the adaptive model, and the eudaimonistic model.

The *clinical model* is the most narrow view. People are seen as physiologic systems with interrelated functions. Health is identified as the absence of signs and symptoms of disease or disability, as identified by medical science. Thus, health might be defined as a "state of not being sick" (Ardell, 1979, p. 18) or as a "relatively passive state of freedom from illness . . . a condition of relative homeostasis" (Dunn, 1977, p. 7). Much of our present health care delivery system is set up to deal with disease and illness after it occurs, based on this model of health. In the clinical model of health, the opposite end of the continuum from health is disease.

Next on the scale is the idea of health as *role performance*. This model adds social and psychological standards to the concept of health. The critical criterion of health is the person's ability to fulfill roles in society with the maximum (eg, best, highest) expected performance. If a person is unable to perform the expected roles, this inability can mean illness even if the individual appears clinically healthy. For example, "Somatic health is . . . the state of optimum capacity for the elective performance of valued tasks" (Parsons, 1958, p. 168). In the role performance model of health, the opposite end of the continuum from health is sickness.

Incorporating the clinical and role performance models is the *adaptive model*. Health is perceived as a condition in which the person can engage in effective interaction with the physical and social environment. There is an indication of growth and change in this model. For example, McWilliam, Stewart, Brown, Desai, and Coderre define health as "the individual's ability to realize aspirations, satisfy needs, and respond positively to the challenges of the environment" (1996, p. 1). In the adaptive model of health, the opposite end of the continuum from health is illness.

Smith (1981) considers the *eudaimonistic model* to be the most comprehensive conception of health. In this model, health is a condition of actualization or realization of the person's potential. For example, human health is "the actualization of inherent and acquired human potential" (Pender, 1990, p. 116). Health "transcends biological fitness. It is primarily a measure of each person's ability to do what he wants to do and become what he wants to become" (Dubos, 1978, p. 74). In the eudaimonistic model, health is consistent with high-level wellness and at the opposite end of the continuum from disabling illness.

Examples of nursing conceptual models that are consistent with the interaction worldview are King's systems interaction model, Neuman's health care systems model, Roy's adaptation model, and Orem's self-care deficit model (see Chap. 8).

THE INTEGRATION WORLDVIEW

In the integration worldview, the human being is considered to be a unitary, indivisible whole. The human, although distinct, is embedded in and inseparable from environment. Therefore, the human–environment participation is a mutual process of nonlinear changes. Multiple "causes" and "effects" make prediction probabalistic.

In this worldview, the goal for a person is to develop his or her potential toward increased diversity. Change is inevitable and provides an opportunity for growth. Health is viewed as a unitary pattern, with manifestations of health reflecting the whole of the human.

Disease and Illness as Manifestations of Health

In the integration worldview, health is viewed as encompassing both disease and "non-disease" (Newman, 1994). Disease can be considered to be "a manifestation of health . . . a meaningful aspect of health" (Newman, 1994, p. 5) and "a meaningful aspect of the whole" (p. 7). Illness and health are viewed as a single process of ups and downs that are manifestations of varying degrees of organization and disorganization. Disputing that death is the antithesis of health, Newman (1994, pp. 11) says that disease and nondisease are not opposites, but rather are complementary factors of health, a unitary process. Illness, like health, simply represents a pattern of life at a particular moment. The tension characteristic of disease throws one off balance, which promotes growth toward a new level of evolving capacities, diversity, and complexity.

In this nursing definition, disease and nondisease are aspects of the unitary phenomenon of health, as discussed later in the chapter. Both disease and nondisease are viewed as manifestations of person–environment interaction and both represent the underlying pattern of energy exchanges in this interaction. Given this definition, disease can be viewed as an integrating factor: "Disease can help people see themselves and their interactions with others more clearly" (p. 27). Viewing disease this way permits the nurse to focus on the transforming potential of disease rather than on the disabling outcomes of disease.

Health can be conceptualized as an actively continuing process that involves initiative, ability to assume responsibility for health, value judgments, and integration of the total person. It is a goal, a fluid process, rather than an actual state. Thus, health is difficult to quantify for objective evaluation. Nurses try to help clients promote growth toward a potential for health by focusing on strengths as well as acknowledging weaknesses, and by collaborating with clients. A client's goals and feelings are major determinants of nursing intervention.

Nursing models and theories that are consistent with the integration worldview include Rogers's science of unitary human beings, Parse's theory of human becoming, Newman's theory of health as expanding consciousness, and Leddy's human energy model (see Chap. 8). These models and theories describe health as an evolving or emerging process, a forward movement with mutual person–environment patterns.

◎ Health Protection and Promotion

The *Cumulative Index of Nursing and Allied Health Literature* (CINAHL) defines health promotion as "the process of fostering awareness, influencing attitudes and identifying alternatives so that individuals can make informed choices and change their behavior to achieve an optimum level of physical and mental health, and improve their physical and social environment" (CINAHL, 1992, p. 118).

Pender differentiates between disease prevention and health promotion. According to Pender (1996, p. 7):

> the most important difference between health promotion and health protection or illness prevention is in the underlying motivation for the behavior on the part of individuals and aggregates. Health promotion is motivated by the desire to increase well-being and actualize health potential. Health protection is motivated by a desire to actively avoid illness, detect it early, or maintain functioning within the constraints of illness.

Pender (1996) differentiates between health promotion and health protection as follows (p. 8):

1. Health promotion is not illness- or injury-specific; health protection is.
2. Health promotion is "approach" motivated; health protection is "avoidance" motivated.
3. Health promotion seeks to expand positive potential for health; health protection seeks to thwart the occurrence of insults to health and well-being.

GOALS FOR HEALTH PROMOTION AND PROTECTION

The U.S. health care system remains disease-oriented today, despite increased valuing of health promotion and fitness by society.

The major portion of national expenditures for medical care goes for the cure and control of illness; relatively little is spent for prevention and health education. Even efforts toward prevention and health education are illness-oriented. For example, children are taught to brush their teeth to avoid cavities (not because the mouth will feel, look, taste, and smell better) and to dress warmly so they will not catch a cold (rather than so that they will feel better).

In 1990, the U.S. Department of Health and Human Services published *Healthy People 2000*. This report described national objectives for health promotion and disease prevention, including three overarching goals (p. 43):

- Increase the span of healthy life for Americans
- Reduce health disparities among Americans
- Achieve access to preventive services for all Americans

Objectives (each with multiple subobjectives) were proposed in 22 categories:

1. Physical activity
2. Nutrition
3. Tobacco
4. Alcohol and other drugs
5. Family planning
6. Mental health and mental disorders
7. Violent and abusive behavior
8. Educational and community-based programs
9. Unintentional injuries
10. Occupational safety and health
11. Environmental health
12. Food and drug safety
13. Oral health
14. Maternal and infant health
15. Heart disease and stroke
16. Cancer
17. Diabetes and chronic disabling conditions
18. Human immunodeficiency virus (HIV) infections
19. Sexually transmitted diseases
20. Immunization and infectious diseases
21. Clinical prevention services
22. Surveillance and data systems

All of these objectives fit within Pender's description of health protection. The concepts of health protection and promotion are consistent with the interaction worldview. In the next section, models and strategies for changing lifestyle behavior are discussed.

MODELS FOR CHANGING LIFESTYLE BEHAVIOR

Health Belief Model

Why do people behave in certain ways in certain situations? What kinds of nursing intervention would be most effective in modifying a person's behavior to reduce risk of disease? Rosenstock (1966), in his "health belief" model, included the following aspects:

1. Perceived susceptibility—the client's perception of the likelihood of experiencing a particular illness

2. Perceived severity—the client's perception of the severity of the illness and its potential impact on his or her life

3. Benefits of action—the client's assessment of the potential of the health action to reduce susceptibility or severity

4. Perceived threat of disease

5. Costs of action—the client's estimate of financial costs, time and effort, inconvenience, and possible side effects such as pain or discomfort

6. Cues that trigger health-seeking behaviors, such as information in newspapers or on television, internal signals such as symptoms, and interpersonal relationships with the health care provider and significant others

The health belief model is called a "rational model" for well-being behavior. The model assumes that well-being is a common objective for all. Individual differences are explained largely in terms of differing perceptions in interaction with motivation. Kasl and Cobb (1966) extended the basic model by specifying a relatively positive variable, the "perceived importance of health matters," in addition to perceived value and perceived threat. Becker and Malman (1975) expanded the model even further by including positive health motivation. In 1988, Rosenstock, Strecher, and Becker urged incorporation of self-efficacy into the model. In a review of 10 years of studies related to the model, Janz and Becker (1984) concluded that only two of the model components, perceived barriers and perceived susceptibility, explained or predicted preventive behaviors.

Revised Pender Health Promotion Model
The health promotion model (HPM) (Pender, 1996) was developed in the early 1980s and revised in 1987, "as a framework for integrating nursing and behavioral science perspectives on factors influencing health behaviors" (p. 51). Determinants of health-promoting behavior were categorized into cognitive–perceptual factors (individual perceptions); modifying factors; and variables affecting the likelihood of action. Pender describes this model as "competence- or approach-oriented" (p. 52), emphasizing that "fear" and "threat" have not been included as sources of motivation for health behavior.

Based on extensive research, the HPM has recently been revised (Figure 10-2) (Pender, 1996). The revised model proposes that health-promoting behavior is related to direct and indirect influences among the 10 determinants of individual characteristics and experiences (eg, prior related behavior and personal factors); behavior-specific cognitions and affect (eg, perceived benefits of action, perceived barriers to action, perceived self-efficacy, activity-related affect, interpersonal influences, and situational influences); commitment to a plan of action; and immediate competing demands. Pender (1996) considers the behavior-specific cognitions and affect category of variables "to be of major motivational significance . . .

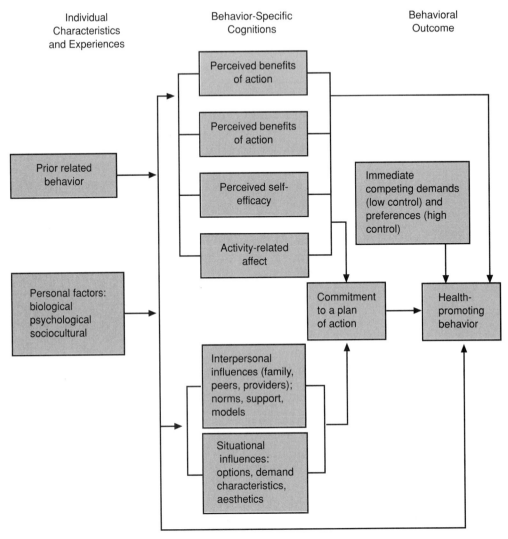

FIGURE 10-2 Revised health promotion model. (From Pender, N. J. [1996]. *Health promotion in nursing practice*, [3rd ed., p. 67]. Stamford, CT: Appleton & Lange. Used with permission of publisher.)

(and) constitute a critical 'core' for intervention, as they are subject to modification through nursing actions" (p. 68).

Prior research has supported the predictive validity of some of the constructs in the HPM, such as perceived benefits of action, perceived barriers to action, perceived self-efficacy, interpersonal influences, and situational influences. The entire revised model now needs to be tested.

The Transtheoretical Model
The transtheoretical model assumes that change requires movement through discrete motivational stages over time, with the active use of different processes of change at different stages. The model has been sup-

ported in studies of a number of lifestyle behaviors including smoking cessation, weight control, sunscreen use, exercise acquisition, mammography screening, and condom use (Prochaska, Velicer et al., 1994).

According to Prochaska, Redding, Harlow, Rossi, and Velicer (1994), the stages of change in this model represent a continuum of motivational readiness for behavior change. The stages include:

Precontemplation—not intending to change
Contemplation—intending to change within 6 months
Preparation—actively planning change
Action—overtly making changes
Maintenance—taking steps to sustain change and resist temptation to relapse

Westberg and Jason (1996, p. 147) describe steps of successful change that are consistent with the stages of the transtheoretical model. The steps are:

1. Acknowledging that something is not right in one's life
2. Deciding that a change is wanted
3. Setting a goal or goals
4. Exploring options for the achievement of goals
5. Deciding on and trying to implement a plan
6. Assessing progress
7. Guarding against backsliding

Also included in the transtheoretical model is the concept of *decisional balance.* It is believed that part of the decision to move toward the action stage of change is based on the relative weight given to the pros and cons of changing behavior to reduce risk. "The pros represent the advantages or positive aspects of changing behavior, and may be thought of as facilitators of change. The cons represent the disadvantages or negative aspects of changing behavior, and may be thought of as barriers to change" (Prochaska, Redding et al., 1994, pp. 478–479).

This model provides a rationale for individualizing interventions based on a client's readiness for change. It remains to be demonstrated whether stage-appropriate interventions are effective not only in encouraging behavior change progress, but also in promoting maintenance of the desired change.

LIFESTYLE BEHAVIOR CHANGE

Lifestyles and Health

Lifestyle has been described as a "general way of living based on the interplay between living conditions in the wide sense and individual patterns of behavior as determined by sociocultural factors and personal characteristics" (World Health Organization, 1986, p. 118). It has been shown that the length of life can be increased by modifying simple lifestyle habits.

Pender suggests that a healthy lifestyle has two complementary parts: health-protecting behavior and health-promoting behavior. *Health-protecting* behavior includes activities such as:

1. Getting adequate sleep (7–8 hours a night)
2. Eating regular meals (not eating between meals); reducing dietary cholesterol and salt intake; and eating a diet with sufficient vitamins, calcium, and fiber
3. Participating in recreational activity (eg, long walks, gardening, swimming)
4. Consuming moderate or no alcohol
5. Never smoking tobacco
6. Maintaining near-average weight
7. Establishing the habit of eating breakfast (Belloc & Breslow, 1972)

In contrast, *health promotion* "is motivated by the desire to increase well-being and actualize human health potential" (Pender, 1996, p. 7). Thus, health-promoting lifestyle activities might promote feelings of vitality, vigor, improved mood and affect, flexibility, relaxation, confidence, and harmony.

Why does a person make healthy lifestyle choices? What factors are important in promoting and sustaining positive changes in lifestyle habits? The answers to these questions are not clear, but some of the variables believed significant include:

Motivation for change
Perceived self-efficacy
Supportive relationships
Knowledge of benefits
Perceived control
Definition of health
Lack of significant barriers
Modifying demographic, interpersonal, and situational variables
Positive reinforcement

People must take the responsibility for their own lifestyle choices. The nurse can help facilitate change in behavior, but only for a sufficiently motivated client. Therefore, the nurse must understand the meaning of health promotion to the client and the client's expectations of outcomes of health promotion interventions. The nurse must shift thinking from use of professional expertise to overcome client weaknesses, to empowering clients to help themselves by building on their strengths.

Health Strengths

A large body of literature associates stress with illness. Stress is assumed to arise when a situation is appraised as threatening or otherwise demanding, and an appropriate coping response is not immediately available (Lazarus & Folkman, 1984). When an event is appraised as stressful, emotionally linked responses occur that result in vulnerability to illness.

Certain characteristics, including social support, self-efficacy, and internal locus of control, seem to decrease the relationship between stress and illness. Two models explain the process by which these characteristics might influence well-being. One model suggests that the person is protected, or buffered, from the potentially pathogenic influence of stressful events. In this case, these characteristics would be related to well-being only (or primarily) for persons under stress (Cohen & Wills, 1985, p. 310). The alternative model suggests that health strengths have a beneficial effect irrespective of whether the person is under stress.

It has been suggested that certain personality characteristics reduce perception of stress or increase resistance to stress and, therefore, may be considered health strengths. In her theory of *hardiness*, Kobasa (1979) assumes that life is always changing and thus is inevitably stressful. However, people who have a sense of commitment (an overall sense of purpose), control (a belief that one can influence the course of events), and challenge (a view of change as opportunity and incentive for personal growth) are thought to be more resistant to stress. In the *sense of coherence* theory, Antonovsky (1987) proposes that confidence in comprehensibility (a cognitive sense that information is consistent, clear, and ordered); manageability (a belief that resources are adequate to meet demands); and meaningfulness (a motivational commitment and engagement), provides generalized resistance resources and promotes health. These two theories are compared in Table 10-1.

Strategies for Lifestyle Behavior Change

The idea of changing health behavior is uncomfortable for many people. Deeply ingrained habits, even harmful ones, can be difficult to change, and most people have difficulty making even minor changes. According to Westberg and Jason (1996, pp. 147—148), people tend to resist change because change of behavior may:

Require giving up pleasure (eg, eating high-fat ice cream)
Be unpleasant (eg, doing certain exercises)
Be overtly painful (eg, discontinuing addictive substances)
Be stressful (eg, facing social situations without alcohol)

TABLE 10-1

Comparison of the Subconcepts of the Sense of Coherence and Hardiness Models

Antonovsky	Kobasa
Sense of coherence	Hardiness
Comprehensibility—cognitive sense	Challenge—change is normative
Manageability—adequate resources	Control—internal locus of control
Meaningfulness—motivation	Commitment—self-involvement

Jeopardize social relationships (eg, engaging in unprotected adolescent sex)

Not seem important anymore (eg, in the case of older individuals)

Require alteration in self-image (eg, in the case of a hard-working executive learning how to play)

As a result, giving up long-standing habits and attitudes is not easy for most people.

Given that health behavior change is difficult for most people, Westberg and Jason (1996, pp. 148–150) suggest that, in order to promote "what it takes" to make meaningful, lasting changes in lifestyle, the individual should:

- Endorse the need for change
- Have "ownership" of the need for change
- Feel that there is more to gain than to lose
- Develop an enhanced sense of self-worth
- Identify realistic goals and workable plans
- Seek gradual change rather than a "quick fix"
- Have patience
- Address starting new behaviors instead of just focusing on what behaviors should be stopped
- Practice new behaviors
- Seek the support of family, friends, colleagues, or health professionals
- Gain positive reinforcement for the desired behavior
- Have a strategy for monitoring progress and making needed changes
- Seek constructive feedback
- Have a mechanism for follow-up to reduce backsliding

Learning how to help people adopt and sustain healthy attitudes and habits is a challenge for health professionals. "There are no miracle drugs available for helping people change long-standing patterns of living. Simply telling people to stop smoking, eat less fat, have safe sex, exercise more, discontinue their abusive practices, or reduce their life stresses seldom works" (Westberg & Jason, 1996, pp. 146). Clients often do not follow the advice of nurses or physicians, particularly when authoritarian "orders" are given. Clients must be actively involved as collaborative partners who assess their own current health and develop and monitor their own long-term health plans. The nurse can best help to promote and sustain change by educating, facilitating, and advising.

According to Prochaska, Redding, and colleagues (1994), some of the most frequently replicated strategies and techniques to help clients modify their behavior include:

Consciousness raising
Self-reevaluation
Environmental reevaluation

Self-liberation
Social liberation
Helping relationships
Stimulus control
Counterconditioning
Reinforcement management

During the contemplation stage of behavior change, *consciousness raising* occurs as the individual seeks information. The nurse can provide potential information resources so that the individual can be actively involved. The client's perceived incentives and barriers to change can be clarified, and the nurse can help explain and interpret often conflicting or unclear information. In addition, the knowledge and interest of family members can be assessed. It may be helpful for the individual to talk with others who have successfully made the contemplated changes.

As movement occurs toward the preparation and action stages of change, the individual engages in *self- and environmental reevaluation*. The individual considers how the current problem behavior (or lack of positive behavior) affects the physical and social environment, and personal standards and values. Questions that might be asked include: Will I like myself better as a (thinner, nonsmoking, less-stressed) person? Is my environment supportive of the proposed changes? Do I believe that I am able to make and continue the changes needed? The assumption is that changes will not occur unless they are congruent with a person's self-concept.

A strategy that can assist with *self- and social liberation* is cognitive restructuring. "Cognitive restructuring focuses on client's thinking, imagery, and attitudes toward the self and self-competencies as they affect the change process" (Pender, 1996, p. 171). The nurse can help clients clarify the messages they give themselves about their health and health-related behaviors. Certain beliefs can be irrational compared with actual reality. Positive affirmations and imagery, repeated several times a day, can help clients to believe that they have the power to think positively and make desired lifestyle changes.

Helping relationships with family members, friends, colleagues or health care professional can be critical in helping to move the individual through the preparation, action, and maintenance stages of change. A self-help group is a strategy that has been found to be very helpful for modeling, support, and reinforcement of desired behavior.

Stimulus control, emphasizing activities that precede the desired behavior, can be helpful during the action and maintenance stages of change. The activities, which must be personally relevant for the individual client, might include a postcard reminder for mammography screening, a personal call from the nurse to encourage continued exercise, or a scheduled group meeting to practice relaxation. To encourage the development of a desirable behavior habit it may be helpful to promote the behavior in the same setting or context and time on a daily basis. For example, the client can be encouraged to exercise in a consistent place, early each morning before other activities intervene.

Counterconditioning to break an undesirable association between a stimulus and a response can be desirable during the later part of the action stage and during the maintenance stage. Undesirable associations can occur that create a negative emotional response to the behavior. For example, many people indicate that exercising can become boring. The nurse can encourage a varied routine, walking outside whenever the weather permits, and at least occasional exercise with a partner to counteract boredom.

Reinforcement management is an effective strategy, especially during the preparation and action stages of change. "It is based on the premise that all behaviors are determined by their consequences. If positive consequences occur, the probability is high that the behavior will occur again. If negative consequences occur, the probability is low for the behavior's being repeated" (Pender, 1996, p. 172). Immediate reinforcement of the desired behavior is important, especially in the early phases of change. Personalized attention and positive verbal feedback are helpful. Eventually, a desirable consequence of the behavior can become an intrinsic reward. For example, a weekly scale reading indicating decreasing weight can be a reward in itself for continuing on a weight reduction diet.

The object of these strategies is to decrease barriers and increase incentives to change of behavior. Barriers to change include lack of:

Knowledge
Skills
Perception of control
Facilities
Materials
Clear goals
Social support
Time
Motivation

Incentives to change behavior include (Leddy, 1997):

Expectation of benefit
Sense of personal responsibility
Enjoyment of the activity
Previous experience
Guilt
Support from family, peers, or professionals

The choice of appropriate strategies to foster incentives and reduce barriers and thereby promote behavior change should be based on an individualized and collaborative assessment by the nurse and the client.

The previous section addressed models and strategies for health promotion consistent with the *interaction* worldview of health. In the final section, models and strategies for health patterning consistent with the *integration* worldview for health are discussed.

Health Patterning

MODELS FOR HEALTH PATTERNING

For centuries, the concept of vital life energy, or chi, has been a part of Eastern religion and culture. For example, the ancient Chinese originated the belief that chi circulates through invisible channels called meridians that can be blocked by stressors or by living excesses. A blockage in energy flow results in energy imbalances and areas of the body with energy deficits, producing symptoms or disease.

Leddy's theory of energetic patterning (see Chap. 8) proposes that consciousness, or focused attention by the nurse, can pattern client–nurse energy by clearing (releasing), converting (transforming), channeling (reestablishing free flow), or conveying energy (redirecting to depleted areas).

The concept of the person as an energy field interacting with an environmental energy field was introduced to nursing by Martha Rogers (see Chap. 8). Rogers conceptualizes that patterning of the human energy field occurs simultaneously and mutually with changes in the environmental energy field. The nurse (part of the environmental energy field) can influence the client's health by redistributing energy and thus repatterning the client's energy field. This focus on enhancing patterning or strength of a client's energy field is the basis for many nursing interventions.

HEALTH PATTERNING MODALITIES

Categories of interventions include:

1. Energy-based body therapies, including acupuncture, reflexology, touch for health, therapeutic touch, and massage
2. Therapeutic exercise, including yoga, Tragerwork, T'ai chi, rolfing, and Feldenkrais method
3. Nutritional therapies, including herbal remedies, supplements, and aromatherapy
4. Relaxation techniques, including meditation, biofeedback, imagery, music color and light therapy, and breathing methods

The literature contains increasing evidence that these kinds of therapies, most of which are noninvasive and involve the client as an active participant in the process, have tangible and highly desirable outcomes for health and healing. It can be expected that nurses will increasingly incorporate patterning methods as an integral part of care in all settings.

◎ Implications of the Nurse's View of Health for Role Performance

"In a positive model of health, emphasis is placed on strengths, resiliencies, resources, potentials, and capabilities rather than on existing pathology" (Pender, 1996, p. 16). We believe that nurses are not dealing with persons who move between states of wellness and illness in a linear fashion; rather, it is more likely that we are dealing with persons who display areas of strength and weakness in their health patterning at any given moment. Because human beings are more alike than different, we suggest that every one of us, under the best of circumstances, can experience a high level of wellness; that every one of us, under the worst of circumstances, can experience a high level of illness; and that, in predominant average circumstances, every one of us simultaneously experiences well-being as a state inclusive of strengths (wellness) and weaknesses (illness).

In trying to improve the quality of health of clients and self, the nurse is obligated to fulfill roles that incorporate promoting health, systematically and strategically planning changes, and using the strengths displayed by the client. Note that we did not say "promotion and maintenance of health." We believe that "maintenance" is an obsolete concept because wellness (health) is an active process, life moves forward, and the client is always evolving. The nurse may promote well-being and may restore perceptions of well-being, but the process of health does not permit the status quo that maintenance implies.

If we view health as a process, and if we believe that nursing focuses on the person's responses, as a whole, to the environment and to a perception of well-being, then nurses have a basis for our professional roles:

When clients are perceiving a sense of harmony, vitality, and ability
When clients can learn most effectively about how they can enhance strengths and gain greater control of their life
When clients are perceiving a lack of harmony, when they feel that their weaknesses are paramount and that they are most vulnerable (generally referred to as illness state)

◎ Conclusion

In our society, responsibility for illness has been delegated to health professionals who have been prepared and are rewarded for delivering care to the sick. Short-term incentives and rewards to maintain health do not exist for the recipient; in addition, the health care system is not organized to reward providers for keeping clients well.

Clients must be encouraged to assume an increased concern and responsibility for their own health potential. Nurses can support, facilitate, and encourage those positive skills, qualities, and plans that will promote health. Interventions can then be devised collaboratively by the client and the nurse, based on goals and a timetable determined by the client.

THOUGHT QUESTIONS

1 Is it possible for a nurse to implement health promotion and health patterning interventions in the hospital setting? How would you respond to Michael in the opening vignette?

2 Which of the worldviews of health (interaction or integration) seems more compatible with your personal philosophy? What about the nurses with whom you work?

3 How might nurses increase the attention paid to health promotion in the health care delivery system?

4 Are you interested in incorporating health patterning modalities into your practice? How can you learn more about these noninvasive strategies?

REFERENCES

Antonovsky, A. (1987). *The sense of coherence and the mystery of health.* San Francisco: Jossey-Bass.

Ardell, D. B. (1979). The nature and implications of high level wellness, or why "normal health" is in a rather sorry state of existence. *Health Values, 3,* 17–24.

Becker, M. N., & Malman, L. A. (1975). Sociobehavioral determinants of compliance with health and medical care recommendations. *Medical Care, 13,* 10–24.

Belloc, N. E., & Breslow, L. (1972, August). Relationship of physical health status and health practices. *Preventive Medicine, 1,* 409–421.

Benner, P., Tanner, C. A., & Chesla, C. A. (1996). *Expertise in nursing practice: Caring, clinical judgment, and ethics.* New York: Springer.

Cohen, S., & Wills, T. A. (1985). Stress, social support, and the buffering hypothesis. *Psychological Bulletin, 98,* 310–357.

Cumulative index to nursing and allied health literature. (1992). Glendale, CA: CINAHL Information Systems.

Dubos, R. (1978, January). Health and creative adaptation. *Human Nature, 1,* 74–82.

Dunn, H. L. (1977, January/February). What high-level wellness means. *Health Values, 1,* 9–16.

Fawcett, J. (1993). *Conceptual models of nursing* (3rd ed.). Philadelphia: Davis.

Hall, B. A. (1981). The change paradigm in nursing: Growth versus persistence. *Advances in Nursing Science, 3,* 1–6.

Janz, N. K., & Becker, M. H. (1984). The health belief model: A decade later. *Health Education Quarterly 11,* 1–47.

Jensen, L. A., & Allen, M. N. (1994). A synthesis of qualitative research on wellness–illness. *Qualitative Health Research 4,* 349–369.

Kobasa, S. C. (1979). Stressful life events, personality and health: An inquiry into hardiness. *Journal of Personality and Social Psychology, 37,* 1–11.

Kasl, S., & Cobb, S. (1966). Health behavior, illness behavior, and sick role behavior. *Archives of Environmental Health, 12,* 246–266.

Lazarus, R. S., & Folkman, J. (1984). *Stress, appraisal, and coping.* New York: Springer.

Leddy, S. K. (1997). Incentives and barriers to exercise in women with breast cancer. *Oncology Nursing Forum, 24.*

Leddy, S. K. (1996). Unifying the interaction and integration worldviews. Unpublished manuscript.

McWilliam, C. L., Stewart, M., Brown, J. B., Desai, K., & Coderre, P. (1996). Creating health with chronic illness. *Advances in Nursing Science, 18,* 1–15.

Newman, M. A. (1992). Prevailing paradigms in nursing. *Nursing Outlook, 40,* 10–13, 32.

Newman, M. A. (1994). *Health as expanding consciousness* (2nd ed.). New York: National League for Nursing.

Parse, R. R. (1987). *Nursing science: Major paradigms, theories, and critiques.* Philadelphia: Saunders.

Parsons, T. (1958). Definitions of health and illness in the light of American values and social structure. In E. G. Jaco (Ed.). *Patients, physicians, and illness* (pp. 120–144). Glencoe, IL: The Free Press.

Pender, N. J. (1990). Expressing health through lifestyle patterns. *Nursing Science Quarterly, 3,* 115–122.

Pender, N. J. (1996). *Health promotion in nursing practice* (3rd ed.). Stamford, CT: Appleton & Lange.

Prochaska, J. O., Redding, C. A., Harlow, L. L., Rossi, J. S., & Velicer, W. F. (1994). The transtheoretical model of change and HIV prevention: A review. *Health Education Quarterly, 21,* 471–486.

Prochaska, J. O., Velicer, W. F., Rossi, J. S., Goldstein, M. G., Marcus, B. H., Rakowski, W., Fiore, C., Harlow, L. L., Redding, C. A., Rosenbloom, D., & Rossi, S.R. (1994). Stages of change and decisional balance for 12 problem behaviors. *Health Psychology, 13,* 39–46.

Rosenstock, I. M. (1966, July). Why people use health services. *Milbank Memorial Fund Quarterly, 44,* 94–127.

Rosenstock, I. M., Strecher, V. J., & Becker, N. H. (1988, Summer). Social learning theory and the health belief model. *Health Education Quarterly, 15,* 175–183.

Smith, J. A. (1981, April). The idea of health: A philosophical inquiry. *Advances in Nursing Science, 3,* 43–50.

Terris, M. (1975). Approaches to an epidemiology of health. *American Journal of Public Health, 65,* 1039.

Twaddle, A. C. (1977). *A sociology of health.* St. Louis: Mosby.

U.S. Department of Health and Human Services. (1990). *Healthy people 2000.* (Public Health Service Publication No. 91-50213). Washington, DC: U.S. Government Printing Office.

Westberg, J., & Jason, H. (1996). Fostering healthy behavior: The process. In S. H. Woolf, S. Jonas, & R. S. Lawrence (Eds.). *Health promotion and disease prevention in clinical practice* (pp. 145–162). Baltimore: Williams & Wilkins.

World Health Organization Health Education Unit (1986). Life-styles and health. *Social Science Medicine, 22,* 117–124.

The Changing Health Care Context

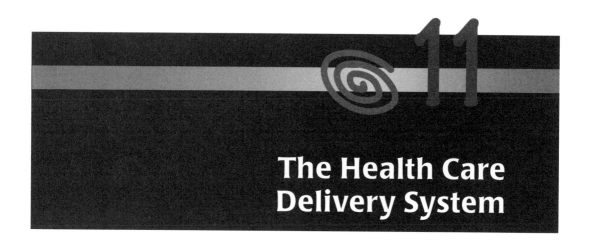

The Health Care Delivery System

HISTORIC DEVELOPMENT
  1850–1900
  1900–1945
  1945–1990s

FORCES INFLUENCING CHANGE IN THE HEALTH CARE DELIVERY SYSTEM
  Demographic Forces
  Epidemiologic Forces
  Economic Forces
  Changing Attitudes
  Changes in the Nursing Labor Force

CHANGES IN THE HEALTH CARE DELIVERY SYSTEM AND THEIR IMPLICATIONS FOR NURSING
  Structure and Organization
  Nursing Care Delivery Models
  Costs of Health Care
  Ethical Considerations

LEARNING OUTCOMES

By the end of this chapter, the student will be able to:

1 Appreciate how the historic development of the health care delivery system led to current issues and concerns.

2 Understand what major forces are influencing change in the system.

3 Understand what the gaps are between needs and services.

4 Understand the implications for nursing of the changes.

5 Appreciate the ethical issues being raised by competing values and goals.

The U.S. health care delivery system is in the process of a radical transformation. In the past, the "system" was a collection of fragmented services provided on a fee-for-service basis by numerous organizations and providers. The care was dominated by physicians and focused on cure of illness. The cost of health care escalated rapidly, given both the lack of control of expenditures and the belief that someone else will pay. However, changes in demography, the economy, and attitudes toward health care, as well as in available labor forces, have resulted in unprecedented changes in the delivery of health care, with significant implications for nursing as a critical component of the system.

◎ Historic Development

1850–1900

Until the middle of the 19th century, most American physicians had less than a high school education, and a minimal apprenticeship with a European-trained physician. Because physicians had few therapeutic tools, the focus was on nursing care through environmental manipulation provided by family members within the home. Education for nursing began only in 1873. Epidemics of acute infectious diseases were the predominant health problems. Most diseases were the result of impure food, contaminated water supplies, inadequate sewage disposal, or the poor condition of urban housing. No organized health programs existed because the predominant ethic of the time said that "each person should care for himself, should be self-sufficient, and, should he become dependent, should take advantage of the various charities . . . established for that specific purpose and be grateful for the charity" (Torrens, 1978, p. 12).

The hospital was an almshouse and pesthouse used almost exclusively by socially marginal, overwhelmingly poor people without roots in the community (Vogel, 1979, pp. 105–106). Because hospitals were supported by the philanthropy of the wealthy, class distinctions were considered to be justified, and hospital patients were stigmatized as dependent and somehow unworthy.

In the mid-to-late 1800s, health care delivery was revolutionized by scientific discoveries. Anesthesia was perfected by 1847 and antisepsis by 1865, leading to the need for centralized facilities to support expensive equipment for surgery. The typhoid bacillus was isolated in 1880 (with vaccination available in 1896), and the cause of diphtheria in 1883, which reduced the epidemic spread of those diseases. By 1860, the thermometer, ophthalmoscope, and laryngoscope were in use, joined by the gastroscope, cystoscope, and sphygmomanometer by 1883. X-rays were discovered in 1895. Conquest of hospital infections and advances in medical diagnostics and therapeutics increasingly led to the referral of middle class and even wealthy clients to hospitals for treatment.

As immigration and industrialization propelled population increases and urbanization, hospitals flourished. By increasing the number of students in the "schools" of nursing, hospitals could inexpensively meet the demand for care. The medical community became aware of the rich learning resource that hospitalized patients provided for nursing students, and regular hospital affiliations as part of a 4-year university medical education slowly became established, following the lead of Johns Hopkins University in 1893. While medicine developed its independent prestige based on a body of continually increasing scientific knowledge, nursing became associated with a medically dependent scope of practice, with an apprenticeship type of education totally dominated by hospitals.

1900–1945

As the private patients of a greatly expanded class of hospital physicians increasingly provided the money that kept hospitals going, "the poor and penniless, whom the institution had originally been meant to serve, became a liability" (Vogel, 1979, p. 115). A growing system of public institutions developed to meet the needs of poor patients; private hospitals were owned and controlled largely by physicians. Industrialization and urbanization led to increased specialization of workers, separation of the home from the workplace, and transformation of the social structure. The nuclear family was separated from extended kin, and the streetcar and the telephone became important communication links, especially for the middle classes. Whereas health care had been home oriented and family centered, it now became a stratified and localized system closely attuned to the city. Trained nurses were employed in the home to give the care once provided by family members.

In 1901, the American Medical Association was restructured, and "doctors sought to assure their financial security and power through their own organization and reform of medical education" (Markowitz & Rosner, 1979, p. 186), as well as by restriction of competition. Foundations added their resources to the centralization of power and decision-making in medicine and medical education. There was an effort to replace the rather haphazard art of medical practice with the new scientific medicine, which increasingly involved hospital treatment. As technology developed, it tended to be concentrated in hospitals. The primary causes of death were pneumonia and tuberculosis, with heart disease, nephritis, and accidents close behind.

Nursing also made efforts to differentiate trained nurses from those with no formal training, through state laws mandating registration and eventually licensure of all seeking to give nursing care. Thus, rigid requirements and an apprenticeship system of education became legally mandated.

The Depression of the 1930s had major impact on the developing health care system. The federal, state, and local governments, which had been primarily concerned with quarantines and relatively ineffective attempts to improve sanitation (Raffel, 1980, p. 241), increasingly assumed responsibility for providing and funding services. In 1935, the Social Security Act included provisions for the indigent and for the infirm elderly.

Accident and life insurance companies, which had originally covered the loss of earned income due to diseases such as typhus, typhoid, scarlet fever, and smallpox, increased their hospital services. In 1939, the first Blue Shield plan for medical and surgical expenses was sponsored by the California Medical Society. The social philosophy that "society should take care of those who, through no fault of their own, could no longer take care of themselves" (Torrens, 1978, pp. 13–14), became accepted, and the system increased in complexity to provide increased services. However, because there was no coordination of growth, expansion was indiscriminate and often led to duplicative services.

Up to the time of the Great Depression, most trained nurses worked in clients' homes, paid directly by the families. Hospitals did not want to pay for nursing care they could obtain for nothing through student labor. However, as private families became unable to pay for nursing, starving nurses agreed to work in hospitals—some solely for room and board. By World War II, most nurses had become employees of hospitals.

1945–1990s

After World War II, the influence of the federal government increased through a growing belief that health care was a right of every individual. For example, the Hill-Burton Act (1946) stimulated hospital construction; creation of the Department of Health, Education, and Welfare in 1953 provided a mechanism to coordinate research and service programs; and Congress amended the Social Security Act (1965–1966) to include Medicare and Medicaid. The federal government assumed major responsibility for providing health care for all elderly and most poor people by the end of the 1960s. Whereas the 1960s had emphasized equity, the 1970s concentrated on access, with tremendous growth in the number of hospitals, hospital employees, ancillary services, and sophisticated technology. But the emphasis on research and technology led to specialization and depersonalization, as well as rapidly escalating expenses.

The increasing cost of health care was also fueled by the developing health insurance industry. "The percentage of Americans covered by some form of health insurance rose from less than 20% prior to World War II to more than 70% by the early 1960s" (Torrens, 1978, p. 13). Health insurance funded the increased costs caused by inflation and by additional optional services, greater number of beneficiaries, and increased use of services, and all costs were essentially unmonitored.

The entire system became increasingly complex with the:

■ Haphazard growth of nursing homes to provide care covered by Medicare and Medicaid

- Expansion of military and veterans' hospitals to care for returning veterans and their families
- Expansion of city and state hospitals
- New construction of research facilities

Further, although infectious illnesses were nearly eradicated due to the introduction of antibiotics in the 1940s,* the fragmented and discontinuous health care delivery system continued to be modeled on acute illness. Thus, although chronic illnesses dominated health care needs, long-term illness—an area in which nursing has a great deal of expertise and potential power—was treated as a series of separate acute episodes.

By the late 1970s, it became impossible to continue to ignore what had become an unacceptable cost for health care, and the emphasis shifted from access to cost. But "attention focused only on parts of the system, particularly hospitals, not on the system as a whole" (Ehlinger, 1982, p. 518). The federal government established new regulations and began to reduce funding of social programs. The changes emphasized efficiency rather than equity or quality and competition rather than access. Prospective payment reimbursement for hospital expenses for Medicare patients (1983) was instituted to significantly reduce the rate of increase in hospital costs. Prospective payment sets a prearranged reimbursement amount (by diagnostic category) that the federal government pays hospitals for the care given to patients covered by Medicare. The hospital receives the prearranged amount regardless of the actual cost of care for an individual patient. This initial change resulted in multiple ripple effects that are dramatically affecting the entire system.

Forces Influencing Change in the Health Care Delivery System

DEMOGRAPHIC FORCES

One of the most significant influences affecting health care delivery is the increasing population of older Americans. As a result of improvements in life expectancy at birth, the age-65-or-over population is expected to grow from 12.7% in 1986 to 17% in 2020, and 30% in 2050 (U.S. Bureau of the Census, 1996, pp. 15, 17). The ratio of people under 65 to those over 65 will shrink from the current ratio of 9:1 to 5:1 by 2030. The Census Bureau projects that the 85-and-older group, mainly "frail elderly," will double from about 3.5 million people currently to about 7 million in 2020, and then double again to 14 million by 2040 (Waite, 1996). Worldwide, the population over age 65 is expected to grow from 10% in 1975 to 18%–20% by 2030 (Bezold, 1982).

The infectious diseases, including AIDS and associated diseases and tuberculosis are major health problems in the 1990s.

Because older persons often have chronic conditions that require treatment and care, their increasing numbers will exert a continuing upward pressure on health care costs. "Half of all oldest-old adults require assistance with everyday activities" (Waite, 1996, p. 222), and recently, nearly half of the average daily census in short-term hospitals consisted of people over age 65.

> Three-quarters of all home health visits are made to elderly people, who comprise nine patients of every ten in nursing homes. If current usage rates were to continue, there would be twice as many physician visits and hospital stays in the year 2020 than at present and almost three times as many elderly residents in nursing homes than the current 1.3 million (U.S. Department of Health and Human Services [USDHHS], 1990, p. IIIB-3).

Skilled nursing care for the critically ill and the handicapped and disabled will be in high demand, but demand for general duty nursing in hospitals is predicted to be low. These anticipated shifts in the locations for care offer both significant opportunities and possible threats for nursing.

Other demographic influences include changes in geographic distribution and composition. Areas of the northeasthern United States are losing population, while urban midsized cities in the South and Southwest are experiencing rapid growth in the need for health care delivery services for the very young, as well as for the elderly. The "baby boom" generation, born between 1946 and 1964, is now settling into middle age and creating a baby boom "echo." "As one of the best educated generations of Americans, they will be more prevention-oriented, but the care they seek will push demands in the health sector for the next fifty years" (Pew Health Professions Commission, 1991, p. 32).

As a result of the increased pregnancy rate in teenagers with poor health habits, the continuing needs of low-birth weight infants have assumed major importance. In addition, immigration and population growth among ethnic minorities such as Hispanics, African Americans, and Asians present significant challenges for the provision of culturally acceptable health care. By 2025 the Hispanic and African American populations will together represent 32% of the U.S. population (U.S. Bureau of the Census, 1996, p. 14). They are currently underserved by the delivery system and underrepresented in all the health professions.

EPIDEMIOLOGIC FORCES

Age-Related Factors

The increasing numbers of older adults will fuel need for "acute care hospitalization for diseases of the heart, malignant neoplasms, and chronic incurable diseases with multisystem failures and functional decline" (USDHHS, 1990, p. IIIB-3). Chronic disorders such as diabetes and osteoarthritis, cognitive impairment, and the increased fragility of advancing age are of major concern. Mental health and dental needs will also increase. Nursing home and home health programs are an especially high priority. Health promotion, illness prevention, and rehabilitative services are needed to enhance the quality of life for the elderly. Older adult caregivers (primarily women) of their oldest-old parents will need support and assistance. The increasing need for coordination and continuity of care provides an opportunity for managed care by professional nurses.

Infant mortality continues to be of major concern, although there is evidence that primary care directed at high-risk mothers can be effective. Good prenatal care can prevent prematurity and low-birth weight infants. Health promotion efforts aimed at influencing high-risk behaviors among adolescents are especially needed.

The Impact of AIDS

Acquired immunodeficiency syndrome (AIDS) is now a world pandemic. It is estimated that 21.8 million adults and 830,000 children worldwide are living with human immunodeficiency virus (HIV) or AIDS (NIAID, 1997). By the year 2000, an estimated 40 million people worldwide will be HIV-infected, 90% of them in developing counties. It has been estimated that 650,000 to 900,000 U.S. residents were living with HIV infection in 1992, and, as of mid-1996, an estimated 223,000 people in the United States were living with AIDS (NIAID, 1997). AIDS is now the leading cause of death in the United States among people aged 25 to 44 (NIAID, 1997). A number of therapies have been developed, but no cure is known. There will be an increasing need for acute and community care, education, and counseling. Nurses are the largest group of health professionals caring for HIV-infected people.

Drug and Alcohol Abuse

Abuse of alcohol and other drugs is a causative factor in various severe health and social problems, including:

Traffic accidents (implicated in 50%)
Transmission of HIV through contaminated needles
Lost wages and productivity (an estimated 5% of the U.S. gross national product)
Increased pregnancy and infant mortality among teenagers
Increased "crack" and "ice" babies
Increased homelessness, disability, poverty, and crime

The inner-city poor are at particularly high risk for drug and alcohol abuse. Community health nurses, in particular, provide essential services for prevention, detection, referral for treatment, and education.

Environmental Factors

Our industrial age is associated with numerous environmental problems that have an impact on health, including:

- Air pollution
- The "greenhouse effect"
- Acid rain
- Deforestation
- Increased ultraviolet radiation (eg, holes in the ozone layer)
- Toxic and nuclear wastes
- Lead-based paints and asbestos
- Radon gas

ECONOMIC FORCES

In this century health care costs have constituted an increasing percentage of the U.S. gross national product (GNP), from 3.5% in 1929 to 13.7% in 1994. Inflation in health care costs has also increased at a rate higher than that of general inflation. In the past 10 years, the inflation rate in health care costs has been more than twice the overall inflation rate.

Physician Fees

A number of factors have influenced health care costs. "In all but one year of the 1980s, growth in spending for physician services outpaced growth in total health spending" (Levit et al., 1991, p. 120). High physician fees were encouraged by lack of competitive pressures and by insurance reimbursement practices that allowed physicians to determine both fees and the level of insurer reimbursement. However, the physician surplus, along with prospective payment, caps on Medicare reimbursement for physicians, and changes in the structure of medical practice, have begun to moderate increases in physicians' fees.

Despite resistance by organized medicine, in 1996, 43 states allowed advanced practice RNs access to third-party reimbursement, with legislation in progress in three additional states (Pearson, 1997). Care given by nurse practitioners results in demonstrably lower costs and higher benefits. Nurse practitioners are reimbursed by Medicaid in most states at 60% to 100% of the physician rate. In July 1997, direct Medicare reimbursement for nurse practitioners and clinical nurse specialists was approved by Congress at 85% of the physician payment rate (Sharp, 1997).

Hospital Costs

Hospital costs have been a major component of rising health care costs. Several factors have influenced hospital costs. The development and intense use of advanced technology was encouraged both by federal monies for medical research and by almost automatic insurance reimbursement. In the past, insurers unquestioningly paid costs, and consumers had limited out-of-pocket costs for health care. As a result, no group perceived responsibility for rising costs.

Specialization of knowledge promoted growth of medical specialties supported by a complex network of nonphysician health care workers. In the past, physicians and third-party reimbursers urged consumers to expect extensive use of hospital resources for diagnosis as well as treatment. Many hospitalizations were unnecessary; costs also were increased by multiple unnecessary laboratory tests, by procedures to avoid the threat of lawsuit, and by excessive lengths of stay (Califano, 1988). Although these practices have been changing, the costs of hospital care have continued to increase.

New technologies, such as magnetic resonance imaging (MRI), genetic engineering, the artificial heart, monoclonal antibodies for the treatment of cancer, and organ transplantation, create pressures on health care costs, just as hip replacement, chronic dialysis, coronary bypass grafts, and computed tomography CT scans did in earlier years.

Federal costs for Medicare and Medicaid comprise a significant proportion of the burden of health care costs—at least 20.7% of the health services and supplies in 1994 (U.S. Bureau of the Census, 1996, p. 114). "The Medicare market, with its enormous size and explosive growth potential, is the most important future market for managed care" (Etheredge, Jones, & Lewin, 1996, p. 96). Efforts to contain increases in health care costs will need to influence changes in every aspect of the health care delivery system, including the psychology of the consumer.

CHANGING ATTITUDES

Over the last two decades, the American public has become increasingly aware of and interested in promoting health. People are more aware of the relationship between lifestyle and incidence of stress-related diseases, chemical and drug dependencies, and predisposition to other diseases. To prevent illness and promote health, many people have focused attention on moderating stressful aspects of their lifestyles: developing habits of good nutrition and adequate exercise, rest, and relaxation; and controlling the use of abusive substances such as tobacco, alcohol, and other drugs.

People are seeking increased responsibility for personal health and self-care, requiring increased health education. As consumers have requested and received information, they have begun to question the adage that "the doctor (or nurse) knows best." Evidence suggests a shift in attitudes toward personal involvement in choices affecting health status. As informed consumers become more involved in health-related decision-making, they may increase the emphasis on expressive values, research on noninvasive (and cost-effective) preventive and therapeutic interventions, and the demand for mutuality rather than paternalism by health care professionals. This movement has created a real opportunity for nursing to:

- Disseminate information and promote an educated public
- Strengthen the profession's influence on health promotion
- Foster alliances with consumers and collaborative relationships with physicians
- Become accepted as a primary care provider for long-term care

CHANGES IN THE NURSING LABOR FORCE

Trends in Staffing

Recent years saw two major "shortages" of nurses, from 1979–1980 and from 1986–1988. The shortage in the 1980s was due to increased demand for RNs by hospitals. In the early 1980s, nurses' salaries were reasonable compared with less versatile providers. The ratio of nurses to patients in hospitals rose by 29.4% between 1984 and 1994 (Aiken, Sochalski, & Anderson, 1996). As demand and the subsequent perception of "shortage" grew, hospitals finally responded with substantial increases in RN salaries. As a result, nurses became more expensive compared with licensed practical nurses (LPNs) and aides. By 1991, there was a 1.7% decline in full-time-equivalent RN openings and a record increase in the employment of "nurse extenders" (AJN News, 1991).

There is a perception of widespread reductions in the hospital RN work force in the mid-1990s (and an increase in unlicensed assistive personnel [UAP]) that has not been reflected yet in regional and national data (Aiken et al., 1996). However, a national survey of RNs (Shindul-Rothschild, Berry, & Long-Middleton, 1996) documented a number of perceived trends, including:

Part-time or temporary RNs being substituted for full-time RNs
UAP being substituted for RNs
Increase in "deskilling"—the substitution of temporary RNs or unskilled aides or technicians for full-time RNs
Nurses taking care of more patients
Increase in cross-training of nurses to take on more responsibilities
Less time to care for patients (speed-up)
Continuity of care decreasing
Unexpected readmissions increasing, especially in emergency and psychiatric and mental health
Better patient outcomes in hospitals than in subacute care settings
Increase in consumer discontent about health care

Declining Enrollments

In 1994, overall enrollments in basic RN programs decreased for the first time in 6 years (*Nursing Data Review*, 1996). This decrease is continuing, with 1996 enrollment in entry-level bachelor's programs falling 6.2% from the previous year. Thus, supply is decreasing in response to a number of factors, including:

1. Decrease in the population of people aged 18 to 24
2. Shift in interest from a career in nursing, compounded by the number of career choices available to women (who comprise 97% of nurses)
3. Compression of salary and promotion increases throughout a nursing career

4. Image problems, including an emphasis on hard technical work, low entry salaries and limited career financial potential, limited return for increased education, an "employee image," and low status
5. Increased labor intensity of acute illness, coupled with attention given to understaffing
6. Widespread fear of contracting AIDS
7. Perceived lack of hospital jobs coupled with lack of awareness of community-based employment

Job Satisfaction

Job satisfaction is also an issue, as nurses express dissatisfaction with basic working conditions, such as scheduling, adequate numbers of staff, and the correct mix of nursing and support personnel, and with professional issues, including control over nursing practice, adequate autonomy for client care, respect from others (especially physicians and administrators), and opportunities for growth and promotion.

With an emphasis on cost rather than quality, there has been an increase in the use of nursing registries, which facilitate part-time, flexible shifts, and higher hourly wages with no benefits. Because registry nurses are not regular employees of a hospital, they may have limited influence on working conditions and quality of patient care, and they may be assigned wherever they are needed. The ability to obtain "outside" nurses as needed gives the employer increased control over numbers, allowing reduction of full-time staff or the requirement of "on-call" time. Hospitals also have been hiring unlicensed workers who depend on the hospital for employment.

Not surprisingly, the number of nurses stating that they are going to leave the profession is increasing (Shindul-Rothschild et al., 1996). Given the existence of deterrents to increasing supply, the lack of substantial long-term reform in hospital working conditions and governance, and increasing nonhospital demand for RNs, it is likely that there will soon be another cycle of imbalance between supply and demand.

The Physician Surplus

Nursing supply and demand is affected by the supply of physicians. Since 1960, the number of physicians in the United States has climbed four times as fast as the population—from 142 to 274 physicians per 100,000 people (*Hospitals & Health Networks*, 1997). There is a growing oversupply in urban areas and specialties, and a shortage in family practice and in rural and poverty areas, although there are indications that medical student choice of family practice has begun to increase (Ruhnke, 1997). The increasing competition generated by oversupply is already creating significant changes in the organization and reimbursement of health care delivery. Physicians are increasingly working on a salary or capitation (fixed payment per person) basis, rather than the traditional fee-for-service basis.

The surplus of available physicians will have a significant impact on nursing practice, as well as on other aspects of the health care delivery system. As competition among physicians has increased, the organized medical community has increased its opposition to expanded role functions by nurses. Physicians have become more active in prevention, elderly ambulatory care, and community settings that previously were less appealing, thereby threatening nonhospital jobs and the status of many nurses. Physicians already are showing increased interest in health promotion activities and in relocation to rural and underserved areas that previously had been served by nurse practitioners.

Although structural changes already underway in the system will reduce the influence of physicians in the hospital industry, physicians will have financial incentives to exert professional power to limit the growth of third-party reimbursement competition by nurses.

Changes in the Health Care Delivery System and Their Implications for Nursing

STRUCTURE AND ORGANIZATION

The health care delivery system provides primary care for health promotion and prevention of illness, secondary care for treatment toward the cure of illness, and tertiary care for technologically complex diagnostic, treatment, and rehabilitative services. Although hospitals have been the dominant provider of care, alternative structures have been developed recently.

Alternative Delivery Systems

Alternative delivery systems, particularly for ambulatory secondary care, have developed over the past few years, primarily to provide care at a lower cost than is possible through hospitalization. Some examples of alternative ambulatory care systems include diagnostic, minor emergency, and surgery centers; birthing centers; substance abuse facilities; and rehabilitation sites. Additionally, home health agencies and hospices provide continuity of nursing care to the home setting. Hospitals are increasing outpatient services in an effort to balance the loss of inpatient revenue.

Group Practices by Physicians

Alternative delivery systems are being supplemented by a dramatic movement toward group practice by physicians. In 1980, it was estimated that 30% of physicians were in group practice and 50% of licensed active physicians were on full-time salaries (Roemer, 1982). By 1996, more than 50% of physicians had joined group practices (Frenkel, 1996). The greatest growth in physician group practice is expected to be in either individual practice associations (IPAs) or preferred provider organizations (PPOs), associated with a health maintenance organization (HMO) or primary case management model (PCMM).

A PPO or IPA enables a group of providers to negotiate fee schedules with hospitals and third-party reimbursers to reduce out-of-pocket expenses and receive rapid payment for claims. However, increasingly the financial risk has been shifted from health plans to physicians. "Physicians are rewarded for practicing efficiently, or denying care, depending on one's ideological interpretation" (Gabel, 1997, p. 140). The advantage to the system is the incentive toward decreasing the use of resources and thereby decreasing costs.

The HMO was designed to emphasize preventive care and consumer education to reduce the cost of treatment (including hospitalization) for illness. The traditional group- or staff-model HMO is a vertically integrated organization which operates its own physical facilities in different geographic locations, and whose salaried physicians work solely for the HMO. However, by the end of 1994, only 31% of HMOs were of this type. "Increasingly, HMOs are 'virtual organizations' or 'organizations without walls,' built on contractual relationships with community providers . . . . Today, most HMOs do not view themselves as HMOs but as managed care organizations that offer an array of managed care plans" (Gabel, 1997, p. 136).

The Hospital Industry

Hospital industry occupancy is expected to continue to decline, and capacity will contract by about 200,000 RN hospital jobs as a result of closings and permanent destaffing of floors and wings of hospitals. Although occupancy rates have been decreasing, the severity of illness of clients who are hospitalized has been increasing (Brewer, 1997).

Another change in the hospital industry involves the movement toward large corporations. Multiunit organizations "set out to provide what they sell in an efficient and effective manner" (Brown & McCool, 1990, p. 88) by providing economies of scale, no unnecessary duplication, channeling of referrals, and organizational stability. The linking of similar kinds of services or institutions located in different geographic areas is called "horizontal integration." In contrast, "vertical integration" involves relationships between and control of an array of different services—for example, hospitals, nursing homes, and ambulatory care services, drug and equipment suppliers, insurance services, and health care providers such as physicians and nurses.

The centralization of control in large corporations, both horizontally and vertically integrated, is promoted as economical. "Today, approximately 25 managed care organizations account for an estimated two-thirds of national membership" (Gabel, 1997, p. 138). However, the emphasis on the bottom line of cost efficiency is associated with risks of reduced access and decreased influence of nurses on a quality environment for care. "Managed care is managed care, not health maintenance and not necessarily consumer-friendly" (Brown & McCool, 1990, p. 92).

Criticisms of managed care are growing. Editorials in both the *New England Journal of Medicine* (Ginzberg & Ostow, 1997) and the *American Journal of Public Health* (Silver, 1997) have indicated that:

- "A cost containment focus can only achieve that objective at the expense of appropriate care"
- "Managed care neither saves money nor improves quality"
- "Public concern, discontent, and distrust have grown as enrollees have become increasingly aware of the more egregious profit-oriented practices of their managed-care plans"
- The rapid expansion of enrollment in managed care has not prevented a quadrupling of overall health care outlays between 1980 and 1995

However, continued increases in managed care enrollment are probable, given the shift of Medicare and Medicaid beneficiaries, voluntarily or under government compulsion, into managed care (Ginzberg, 1997). Given that "the primary factor driving down hospital utilization is managed care" (Shindul-Rothschild et al., 1996, p. 26), hospital downsizing and restructuring is expected to continue. As a result, the Bureau of Labor Statistics has estimated that "by 2005 the percentage of nurses employed in hospitals will decrease to 57.4% from 63.8%" (Shindul-Rothschild et al., 1996, p. 29). In addition, "it's unlikely that every RN job lost in the hospital sector will be replaced" (Shindul-Rothschild et al., 1996, p. 35).

Pluralistic Choices

The changes occurring in the structure and organization of the health care delivery system are associated with increased competition among providers, which gives the consumer pluralistic choices for health care. The philosophy of a competitive marketplace is firmly entrenched in the American system, and competition is expected to lead to higher quality of service at lower cost. But it also leads to confusion among consumers, increased potential for fragmentation, and lack of clear access to care.

Nurses can help bridge the gap between consumers and the delivery system, promoting both continuity of care and education to foster appropriate use of services. A major way that the system reduces health care costs is to limit the needs and desires for medical care. However, reduction of cost must not be allowed to jeopardize access to needed care. Millions of adults, insured and uninsured, have reported problems in getting needed medical care (Donelan et al., 1996). Nurses need to advocate for consumer protection. In addition, nursing has a major role in helping consumers fulfill their personal responsibility for health promotion, to reduce the need for treatment of illness.

NURSING CARE DELIVERY MODELS*

Historical Patterns of Nursing Care

The management of patient care has always fallen within the purview of nurses. The care of patients was accomplished in a variety of ways depending on nurse–patient ratios and the patient care environment. Functional nursing, team and district nursing, and primary nursing are examples of historical patterns of nursing care (Ellis & Hartley, 1995).

Functional nursing was considered efficient for use in acute care when a limited nursing staff was assigned to care for a large number of patients on a nursing unit for one shift. Nursing responsibilities were task oriented and assigned to staff according to levels of training and licensure. Efficient care was considered more important than continuity of care (Ellis & Hartley, 1995).

The following example describes a functional nursing pattern. An RN is assigned to administer intravenous and parenteral medications and complete the charting for all patients on the unit. An LPN is assigned to administer oral medications and perform treatments, such as dressing changes. A nurse aide is responsible for vital signs and hygiene measures for all patients.

Team nursing was a staffing pattern that also divided patient care duties for one shift but focused on patient needs. A team of nursing staff would provide care for a limited number of patients on an acute care nursing unit. There were sufficient teams to care for all patients. Each team cared for approximately the same number of patients with a similar patient acuity. Team nursing responsibilities were assigned according to level of training and licensure, where the RN was usually the team leader (Ellis & Hartley, 1995). The entire nursing team was familiar with the patient's progress and condition. However, overlapping responsibility was a limitation of this approach.

Team nursing responsibilities might be distributed to staff in the following manner. A team, consisting of an RN, LPN, and nurse aide, was assigned to care for 9 patients in close proximity to each other. All team members worked together, but with specific duties. The RN team leader "took off" orders, documented, and hung intravenous medications for all 9 patients, and delegated the patient care duties to the LPN and nurse aide. The LPN administered oral and parenteral medications and performed treatments. The nurse aide was responsible for patient hygiene measures and dietary assistance (Ellis & Hartley, 1995).

District nursing is a variation of team nursing. The chief difference was the physical layout of the nursing unit, divided into defined areas called districts. The district nurse, an RN, was coassigned with other nursing staff to care for patients in the specified district regardless of patient acu-

Section author: Carol Sando, R.N., D.NSc.

ity level. One district might be very busy during the shift while other districts might be moderately so.

Primary nursing was a patient care approach that used only RNs. On primary care nursing units, an RN was the principal nursing care provider for a limited number of patients over a 24-hour period. The primary nurse developed and implemented the entire care plan for the patient and delegated responsibilities to nurses on other shifts. Often the admitting nurse was the primary nurse. A primary nurse working day shift may also have had nursing care responsibilities for other patients delegated by their admitting nurses on other shifts (Ellis & Hartley, 1995).

Primary nursing was an expensive venture, but more cost-effective if operated efficiently. It was successful in a variety of health care settings. The RN was the most knowledgeable among nursing team members, hence, most costly to employ. Yet job satisfaction due to direct patient care was high for this type of nursing pattern, and desired patient outcomes were achieved more often than not (Ellis & Hartley, 1995).

Redesigned Patient Care

The current pattern of nursing care in acute care settings may disregard the patient care staff's level of educational training. Cross-training or redesigned staffing patterns are taking hold as a cost-effective method of meeting patient needs during a limited length of stay. In contrast to nurses, staff assigned to the patient may have no formal training.

For example, in addition to originally assigned duties, housekeeping staff may also be responsible for feeding and bathing patients. Unit clerks may be "trained" by staff developers to obtain electrocardiographs or to initiate oxygen therapy or perform respiratory treatments. Previously labeled nurse aides may go by a new title, "patient care technicians," and be trained to draw blood samples for laboratory tests.

The use of UAP is one method of containing costs for health care providers. These individuals are paid at a lower rate than licensed health care personnel. Task-oriented patient care is accomplished at a lower cost to the health care institution.

As hospitals and health care agencies merge as for-profit organizations, the "bottom line" becomes survival in a competitive market. Cost-effective health care is the objective for these corporations. However, the quality of health care provided by UAP is subject to ongoing criticism by consumers and health care professionals.

Case Management

Case management, a relatively new patient care model in health care, is defined as a system of patient care delivery that focuses on the achievement of outcomes within effective time frames and with appropriate use of resources (McElroy & Campbell, 1992). The *CareMap*, a problem list with expected outcomes, provides the framework for planning patient care, in conjunction with the *critical path*. The critical path is "a time line that depicts key incidents that must occur in a predictable and timely fashion to achieve an appropriate length of stay" (McElroy & Campbell, 1992, p. 750). A *variance* is anything that occurs to alter the patient's progress through the normal critical path.

Case management is a long-term approach that considers both the objectives of cost containment through the avoidance of variances to the critical path, and continuity of care, by encompassing the entire length of stay, regardless of the multiple areas in which the patient receives care.

Recidivism and the use of the emergency department for treatment of symptoms of chronic disease are not cost-effective, nor do they reflect continuity of care. Patient populations, such as the frail elderly; patients with AIDS, transplants, or multisystem failure; and low-birth-weight babies, may benefit from the services of a nurse case manager. Ineffective and costly medical care can be avoided when the case manager assesses the patient's home environment, client and family teaching requirements, the need for long-term treatments and procedures, or the benefit of a skilled nursing facility before discharge to home (Concept Media, 1995; Pollack, 1996).

In the acute care setting, the nurse case manager is a coordinator of care that is timely and necessary. Communication with the patient, family, and physician before admission to the hospital can serve many purposes. Among these are an orientation to the hospital; explanations of the case manager's role, expected length of stay, routine hospital events, preprocedure teaching, and the plan of care; and assessments of the patient's needs and coping abilities. Identification of patient needs includes insurance for durable medical equipment, the patient's ability to use stairs at home after discharge, and family or support persons available to assist the patient. The outcome of the preadmission encounter with the case manager is that the patient feels more in control because of a greater understanding and involvement in care (Concept Media, 1995; Ellis & Hartley, 1995).

The case manager in the acute care setting integrates nursing processes with management processes to achieve patient outcomes in a fiscally responsible manner (McElroy & Campbell, 1992). Patient assessments involve the collection of clinical data, such as health history information, physical examination findings, and functional and mental capabilities. Other factors affecting the patient's well-being are also evaluated. Among these are the patient's needs after discharge, abuse of alcohol or drugs, referrals after discharge (ie, physical therapy or diabetic education), and verification of insurance coverage for hospitalization, prescription medicine, long-term care, and durable medical equipment (Concept Media, 1995; Ellis & Hartley, 1995).

A cost-effective plan of care is also assessed. The case manager determines the patient's understanding of the plan of care. The patient's strengths and limitations are considered relative to the projected length of stay. Previous admission charts are reviewed for patterns. The medical record for the current admission is reviewed for redundancy between admission orders and preadmission procedures (Concept Media, 1995; Ellis & Hartley, 1995).

Planning short-term and long-term goals requires the participation of the patient and the multidisciplinary health care team. The patient's strengths and limitations determine time frames for goal achievement. The plan of care is updated with the collaboration of those involved (Concept Media, 1995).

Implementation of the plan of care requires vigilance and time management. The client's progress is compared daily to the goals of the plan of care. The case manager assertively coordinates procedures and referrals. Team meetings are scheduled to identify the possibility of early discharge to home or the unexpected need for a skilled nursing facility after discharge from the hospital. The case manager acts as the patient's advocate in obtaining benefits and services from health care payers (Concept Media, 1995).

Evaluation of the patient's progress is compared to the length of stay. This comparison may identify new goals or require goal revision. Deviations from expected outcomes may be observed, identifying trends in the hospital's delivery or performance of services. Any delays or repeated procedures compromise efficient and optimum care. The case manager monitors the patient's progress in terms of recovery, cost, and efficiency of the facility (Concept Media, 1995; Ellis & Hartley, 1995).

When the patient's care is overseen by the case manager, it is less fragmented and more comprehensive. The case manager employed by a health care organization comprised of various settings may follow the patient over time, to multiple clinical sites. The patient and family perceive the case manager as an advocate, knowledgeable about the care involved. Their confidence is increased and a sharing of the responsibilities of care is the desired result (Concept Media, 1995; Ellis & Hartley, 1995).

In summary, the case manager has three primary roles that are multifaceted and require critical analytical thinking. As a clinician, the case manager communicates effectively with a multidisciplinary health care team. As a manager, the patient's care is coordinated among professionals and consultants. The case manager also has a financial role, one that ensures economic care but does not compromise quality for cost containment.

Table 11-1 compares nursing care delivery models.

COSTS OF HEALTH CARE

Insurance

In the 1950s and 1960s, criticism of the cost of health care to the individual, and the resulting low level of access to care, stimulated the rapid growth of employer-provided and privately purchased health insurance; the initiation of federal government Medicare insurance for the elderly and disabled; and state government Medicaid insurance for the poor.

TABLE 11-1

Comparison of Healthcare Delivery Systems

	Case Method	Functional	Team Nursing	Primary	Case Management
Origin date; reason designed	1800s; patients were home	1940s; shortage of nurses	1950s; move away from tasks	1960s; nurses move toward independence	1980s; DRGs and budget awareness
Clinical decision-making	Done per shift	Done per shift	Shift based	Continuous, 24 h/d	Case managers, continuous 24 h/d
Responsibility and authority	Autonomous for a small group of patients	Autonomous for large group of patients	Large group of patients	Small group of patients; very personal; great autonomy	Includes coordination with other departments
Work allocation	Total care to assigned patients	Specific task for all patients	Some tasks, assigned per skill patients require	Total care of own patients	Case manager can be the coordinator or provide total patient care
Professional nursing satisfaction	Yes	No	Yes	Yes	High for the case managers and the nursing staff
Major advantage	Patient receives continuous care for 8 h by one nurse	Cost-effective for a large number of patients	Cost-effective, work in small groups to provide care	Satisfied patient and nurses	Cost-effective care coordinated to achieve patient outcomes
Major disadvantage	No continuity of care	Task-oriented fragmented care	Do not always have leaders to coordinate the team	Not cost-effective to have all RN staff	Costly to implement correctly

*Adapted from Manthey, M. (1991). Delivery systems and practice role models. *Nursing Management, 22*(1), 28–30.
From Wise, P. S. Y. (1995). *Leading and managing in nursing* (p. 430). St. Louis: Mosby-Year Book.

However, the current health insurance system, developed largely as a passive risk-sharing system, has contributed to overwhelming inflationary pressure on the costs of health care. In addition, in 1994 there were more than 40 million uninsured Americans, including many full-time employees and their dependents; another 29 million were underinsured (Donelan et al., 1996). The moral concern about access to care has contributed to major proposals for national health insurance.

In 1991, "Nursing's Agenda for Health Care Reform" was released by the American Nurses Association (ANA, 1991). This plan, supported and lobbied for by most nursing organizations, emphasized:

- A core of essential services available to everyone, financed by integration of public and private funding
- A shift from a predominant emphasis on illness toward wellness and care
- Direct access to "a full range of qualified providers"
- Provisions for long-term care and vulnerable populations (including pregnant women and children)
- Managed care, case management, and incentives for cost efficiencies
- A restructured system that enhances consumer access and fosters consumer responsibility

Many major health reform bills have been introduced in Congress, and there is growing consensus on the need to deal with the problem of those who lack medical insurance problem and to develop a strategy to fill the gaps left by current public programs such as Medicaid (Etheredge, 1991). However, the cost-containment environment of the 1990s, a lack of congressional commitment to health care reform, and public disagreement over the best design of any national health care plan, indicate that passage of comprehensive reform is unlikely. More likely are incremental changes within the framework of the existing pluralistic system.

In the past, the medical model of episodic care for acute illness dominated insurance reimbursement philosophy. The system allowed free choice of provider (physician and hospital) regardless of cost; reimbursement based on cost-plus charges; fee-for-services; and subsidies favoring inpatient hospital care. Individual physician judgment determined treatment, with automatic reimbursement and limited out-of-pocket costs to the client. This approach favored use of elaborate technologies even in questionable cases, extensive use of laboratory testing, and excessive hospitalization. Consumers developed unrealistic expectations of the system and were not restrained from using services excessively.

This system has undergone radical change in the 1990s. Corporations are now the largest purchasers of private health insurance. In an effort to contain costs, companies have:

- Limited consumer choice of providers through HMOs or PPOs
- Increased cost sharing by shifting more cost to the consumer through larger premiums, deductibles, and out-of-pocket charges

- ▪ Required authorization for hospitalization and second opinions for medical treatments
- ▪ Substituted ambulatory and home care reimbursement for hospitalization
- ▪ Encouraged reduced use of services

As a result of expenditures that double almost every 5 years, the federal government has instituted prospective payment procedures for hospital and physician Medicare costs based on diagnostic categories of care or diagnosis-related groups (DRGs). There is increased emphasis on physician documentation of "outcomes" that warrant the intervention provided. Increasing attention has been given to the morality of rationing services as a cost-containment mechanism. A major concern is the typically American valuing of unrestricted choice, progress, and profit. But, as Callahan puts it, "what we do need to do is to restrain our demands for unlimited medical progress, maximal choice, perfect health, and profits and income. This is not the same as rationing good health care" (Callahan, 1990, p. 1813).

Pressures for change in insurance policies have potential opportunities for nursing. Nurses are a competitive alternative choice as both gatekeepers and care providers, decreasing costs and improving quality of care. Nurses also are appropriate providers to educate consumers in reducing unnecessary use of services and practice healthful living to improve the quality of life and prevent illness. It is hoped that nurses, as responsible client advocates, will actively participate in the process of creating change in the delivery system.

Competition

Increased competition as a cost-containment mechanism provides an opportunity for nurse practitioners to expand primary and secondary health care services with direct reimbursement from the client and from third-party insurers. For effective competition, consumers must be actively involved in choosing alternatives, and qualified providers must have free entry into the system.

"Not only are (nurses') direct costs lower than those of physician providers, but (also) the cost of ancillary services is greatly reduced when nurses are the primary carers" (Fagin, 1982, p. 59). Numerous studies (Bissinger, Allred, Arford, & Bellig, 1997; Fagin & Jacobsen, 1985; Hylka & Beschle, 1995) have documented the cost effectiveness of nursing care.

Clearly, expanding the scope of services reimbursed for, or substituting nurses for other providers, leads to head-on competition with physicians. It is thus understandable that expanding competition by nurses has been strenuously resisted by organized medicine. Although substituting nursing care for physician care reduces costs, the concern is that providing third-party reimbursement to nurses will ultimately increase system costs as additional health care providers such as pharmacists and social workers also seek direct reimbursement.

Quality of Care

Cost effectiveness provides a source of potential power when viewed in relation to the impact of nursing care on the quality of care provided to the consumer. "The quality of medical care services provided by nurse practitioners is at least comparable to the quality of services provided by physicians. Furthermore, in some cases, nurse practitioners following protocols have shown performance superior to physicians in symptom relief, diagnostic accuracy, and patient satisfaction" (LeRoy, 1982, p. 299).

From 70% to 90% of primary care services could safely be delegated to nurses by physicians (Andrews, 1986). Nurses contribute to reduced morbidity, reduced mortality, and improved quality of life (Fagin, 1982, p. 59). Nurse practitioners do a better job than physicians in areas such as continuity of care and emphasis on prevention, amount of advice offered and amount of time spent listening to clients, and communication skills and support (Andrews, 1986, p. 53). Holistic and individualized nursing care can provide a highly desirable alternative to medicine's "intrusive, disease-oriented model" (Andrews, 1986, p. 56).

Although it is difficult to quantify quality of care, it is critical that nursings make increased efforts to document effectiveness by determining what nursing activities and interventions produce beneficial outcomes under which conditions. As efforts to contain costs increase, quality of care and other ethical issues become increasingly urgent. Nurses must be able both to communicate their unique contributions to quality health care and to exert moral leadership as advocates for access and consumer choice in the system.

ETHICAL CONSIDERATIONS

Nursing "is responsible for ensuring that its members act in the public interest" (ANA, 1995, p. 17). Therefore, it is imperative that nurses take an active leadership role in discussing and resolving a number of philosophic issues and ethical concerns that affect the delivery of health care.

Ethical Concerns

Ethical concerns have been raised by an increasing life span, the development of health care technology, and the increasing cost of delivering care. Curtin (1996, p. 19) states that "the critical ethical problem in health care today is that ability to pay determines the availability and quality of care."

Because it is not possible to meet all goals of accessibility, equity, and quality given available resources, difficult choices must be made among competing values and multiple desirable alternatives. One basic issue is the relative valuing of predictability and containment of the costs of health care, versus the access to health care for all persons.

Ethical questions raised by these choices include:

- How willing are some people to assume the costs to make the system affordable, acceptable, and available to all?

- How much is health care a basic right?
- If there are limits on access to health care, who should have priority?
- What is an acceptable level of health care?
- Should technology be available to all regardless of cost or should it be rationed?
- What should be the criteria for rationing?
- Who should determine the criteria?
- How much choice should be determined by ability to pay?
- What (and when) is death?
- How much is the prolongation of life worth?
- Does reducing costs reduce the quality of care?
- What rights do clients have?
- Is cure of all disease possible?
- Is it desirable at any cost?

"Treating health care primarily as a business and a commodity to be sold like cars is an impoverished notion of health care in relation to the concept of health care as a human service created by society to meet the needs of vulnerable people who are ill or at risk of becoming ill" (Aroskar, 1995, p. 65). It is critical that the voice of the nursing profession be added to that of the public in discussions of the philosophic considerations and values that will shape the decisions concerning the size, shape, and direction of the American health care system.

Philosophic Issues

Until now, philosophical considerations of the role of the health care delivery system have been affected by the domination of the medical model of curing disease. "One can continue to engage in risky lifestyle behaviors, while medicine provides 'magic bullets' to prevent diseases that it cannot treat. I have called this trend the medicalization of prevention" (Micozzi, 1996, p. 5).

> Medical care in America requires a better balance between prevention and treatment, promotion of function and cure, and educational as compared to technical approaches to care . . . . Most of the great advances in health status arise from basic improvements in economic status, education, nutrition, lifestyles and the environment (Mechanic, 1986, pp. 23, 30)

Nursing can advocate for increased emphasis on:

- Promotion of health and prevention of illness
- Maintenance of function in the elderly and chronically ill
- Reduction of stress
- Attention to quality of education, nutrition, and other aspects of the environment

In the past, physicians have assumed a paternalistic attitude toward health care decision-making by consumers: the doctor knows best. With cost pressures, government has become intimately involved in almost every aspect of planning and provision of services. However, nurses can help consumers to understand that availability of more services does not necessarily mean better health or better care. Nurses can advocate for more egalitarian relationships between providers and clients and an increased role of the consumer in:

1. Setting the values of the system
2. Having an enlarged knowledge base to increase self-reliance, self-determination, and autonomy in health care choices
3. Assuming increased personal responsibility for health promotion through risk reduction in lifestyle

The role of the provider is to provide sensitive, competent care reflecting respect for each client's autonomy. Nursing's potential contribution has been limited by:

Lack of an adequate educational base of the majority of its practitioners

Inability of nursing leadership to mobilize collective professional action

Historic lack of involvement and influence in political decision-making

However, the changes that have occurred in the system provide an ideal opportunity for nursing to secure influence and power for the profession, thereby assuming a major role in shaping the future direction of health care delivery.

◎ Conclusion

As a result of significant demographic, economic, attitudinal, and available manpower forces, the health care delivery system is in the process of structural change and reorganization, raising multiple ethical considerations. The nursing profession has the opportunity to influence the direction of change to ensure the improvement of health and health care.

THOUGHT QUESTIONS

1 What are the issues concerning the increasing domination of managed care strategies in the health care delivery system?

2 When you think about nursing practice in the future, are you more concerned about threats or excited about opportunities? What are the implications of the changing system for you?

3 What are the strengths and limitations of the major nursing care delivery models in use today? What can you do to improve care within the model used in your practice setting?

REFERENCES

Aiken, L. H., Sochalski, J., & Anderson, G. F. (1996). Downsizing the hospital nursing workforce. *Health Affairs, 15,* 88–92.

American Journal of Nursing News (1991). Nursing extenders now found in 97% of hospitals, 91:88.

American Nurses Association. (1991, June). Nursing's agenda for health reform. *The American Nurse Supplement.*

American Nurses Association. (1995). *A social policy statement.* Kansas City: Author.

Andrews, L. B. (1986, January/February). Health care providers: The future marketplace and regulations. *Journal of Professional Nursing, 2,* 51–63.

Aroskar, M. A. (1995). Managed care and nursing values: A reflection. *Journal of Nursing Law, 2,* 63–70.

Bezold, C. (1982, August). Health care in the U.S. Four alternative futures. *Futurist, 16,* 14–18.

Bissinger, R. L., Allred, C. A., Arford, P. H., & Bellig, L. L. (1997). A cost-effectiveness analysis of neonatal nurse practitioners. *Nursing Economics, 15,* 92–99.

Brewer, C. S. (1997). Through the looking glass: The labor market for registered nurses in the 21st Century. Nursing and Health Care Perspectives, 260–269.

Brown, M., & McCool, B. P. (1990). Health care systems: Predictions for the future. *Health Care Management Review, 15,* 87–94.

Califano, J. A., Jr. (1988, March 20). The health-care chaos. *New York Times Magazine,* pp. 44, 46, 56–57.

Callahan, D. (1990). Is rationing inevitable? *New England Journal of Medicine, 322,* 1809–1813.

Concept Media (Producer), & Walters, T. (Director). (1995). Hospital-based case management [videocassette]. Irvine, CA: Producer.

Curtin, L. L. (1996). The ethics of managed care—Part I: Proposing a new ethos. *Nursing Management, 27,* 18–19.

Donelan, K., Beelendon, R. J., Hill, C. A., Hoffman, C., Rowland, D., Frankel, M., & Altman, D. (1996). Whatever happened to the health insurance crisis in the United States? *Journal of the American Medical Association, 276,* 1346–1350.

Ehlinger, E. P. (1982). Implications of the competition model. Nurse Outlook, 30, 518–521.

Ellis, J., & Hartley, C. (1995). *Nursing in today's world.* Philadelphia: Lippincott.

Etheredge, L. (1991, Spring). Negotiating national health insurance. *Journal of Health Politics and Law 16,* 157–167.

Etheredge, L., Jones, S. B., & Lewin, L. (1996). What is driving health system change? *Health Affairs, 15,* 93–104.

Fagin, C. M. (1982). Nursing's pivotal role in American health care. In L. H. Aiken (Ed.). *Nursing in the 1980s: Crises, opportunities, challenges* (pp. 459–473). Philadelphia: Lippincott.

Fagin, C. M., & Jacobsen, B. S. (1985). Cost-effectiveness analysis in nursing research. In H. H. Werley & J. J. Fitzpatrick (Eds.). *Annual review of nursing research* (Vol. 3, pp. 215–238). New York: Springer.

Frenkel, M. (1996). Caveats for physicians in the financing of practice networks. *Journal of Health Care Financing, 22,* 49–51.

Gabel, J. (1997). Ten ways HMOs have changed during the 1990s. *Health Affairs, 16,* 134–145.

Ginzberg, E., & Ostow, M. (1997). Managed care—A look back and a look ahead. *New England Journal of Medicine, 336,* 1018–1020.

Hospitals & Health Networks. (1997). *71,* 12.

Hylka, S. C., & Beschle, J. C. (1995). Nurse practitioners, cost savings, and improved care in the department of surgery. *Nursing Economics, 13,* 349–354.

LeRoy, L. (1982). The cost-effectiveness of nurse practitioners. In L. H. Aiken (Ed.). *Nursing in the 1980s: Crises, opportunities, challenges.* Philadelphia: Lippincott.

Levit, K. R., Lazenby, H. C., Letsch, S. W., & Cowan, C. A. (1991, Spring). National health care spending 1989. *Health Affairs, 10,* 117–130.

Markowitz, G. E., & Rosner, D. (1979). Doctors in crisis. Medical education and medical reform during the progressive era, 1895–1915. In S. Reverby & D. Rosner D (Eds.). *Health care in America. Essays in social history* (pp. 185–205). Philadelphia: Temple University Press.

McElroy, M. J., & Campbell, S. (1992). Case management with the nurse manager in the role of case manager in an interventional cardiology unit. *AACN Clinical Issues, 3,* 749–760.

Mechanic, D. (1986). *From advocacy to allocation.* New York: Free Press.

Micozzi, M. S. (1996). *Fundamentals of complementary and alternative medicine.* New York: Churchill Livingstone.

NIAID. (1987). *Fact sheet: HIV/AIDS statistics.* Bethesda, MD: National Institutes of Health.

Nursing Data Review. (1996). New York: National League for Nursing.

Pearson, L. J. (1997). Annual update of how each state stands on legislative issues affecting advanced nursing practice. *The Nurse Practitioner, 22,* 18–86.

Pew Health Professions Commission. (1991). *Health America. Practitioners for 2005: An agenda for action for U.S. health professional schools.* Durham, NC: Author.

Pollack, A. M. (1996). Analysis of U.S. health-care. Unpublished manuscript, Widener University, School of Business Administration, Chester, PA.

Raffel, M. W. (1993). *The U.S. health care system. Origins and functions.* New York: Wiley.

Roemer, M. I. (1982). *An introduction to the U.S. health care system.* New York: Springer.

Ruhnke, G. W. (1997). Physician supply and the shifting paradigm of medical student choice. *Journal of the American Medical Association, 277,* 70–71.

Sharp, N. J. (1997). Internet electronic mail message.

Shindul-Rothschild, J., Berry, D., & Long-Middleton, E. (1996). Where have all the nurses gone? *American Journal of Nursing, 96,* 25–39.

Silver, G. (1997). Editorial: The road from managed care. *American Journal of Public Health, 87,* 8–9.

Torrens, P. R. (1978). The American health care system. Issues and problems. St. Louis: CV Mosby.

U.S. Bureau of the Census. (1996). *Statistical abstract of the US: 1996* (116th ed.). Washington, DC: Author.

U.S. Department of Health and Human Services. (1990, March). *Seventh report to the President and Congress on the status of health personnel in the United States.* Springfield, VA: U.S. Department of Commerce National Technical Information Service.

Vogel, M. J. (1979). The transformation of the American hospital, 1859–1920. In S. Reverby & D. Rosner (Eds.). *Health care in America. Essays in social history* (pp. 105–116). Philadelphia: Temple University Press.

Waite, L. J. (1996). The demographic face of America's elderly. *Inquiry, 33,* 220–224.

Wise, P. S. Y. (1995). *Leading and managing in nursing.* St. Louis: Mosby-Year Book.

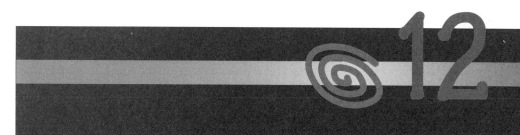

The Professional Nurse's Role in Public Policy

LEARNING OBJECTIVES

By the end of this chapter, the student will be able to:

1 Define public policy, politics, lobbyist, and political action committee.

2 Differentiate between the roles of lobbyists and political action committees.

3 List strategies used to lobby elected officials.

4 Distinguish direct lobbying from indirect lobbying techniques.

5 Discuss key elements of effectively written letters to elected officials.

6 Outline a plan for a personal visit with an elected official.

7 Discuss ways for nurses to become involved in politics and public policy development.

Chapter author: Lucy Hood, R.N., D.NSc.

VIGNETTE

As a result of budget cuts, school districts in a midwestern state no longer have to provide RNs for health screening, medication administration, and health teaching for their students. State law specifies that a licensed practical nurse (LPN) may outline health promotion classes and health programs for a school district. Since enactment of the budgetary cut, the following child and adolescent health problems have risen: obesity, ethanol abuse, drug abuse, sexually transmitted diseases, teenage pregnancy, and immunization noncompliance.

While acting as client advocates and change agents, a group of nurses approaches a member of the state legislature to see if she would propose legislation mandating "A nurse in every school." The legislator declines, stating that it would be political suicide to propose such a measure because of declining state revenues earmarked for state health services and education.

What can these nurses do to promote their legislative goal?

Working to lower the speed limit on a busy stretch of highway; petitioning city legislators to limit traffic in a residential neighborhood; writing or visiting an elected official to persuade him or her to support limited use of unlicensed assistive personnel (UAP) in acute health care institutions; organizing a group of nurses to develop a legislative agenda; visiting formally or informally with an elected official; protesting legislation aimed at limiting health care access for the poor; lobbying for a bill aimed at increasing governmental funding for breast cancer research, nursing education, or nurse run health centers. . . these are a few examples of how professional nurses can influence governmental and institutional policies. Governmental and institutional policies greatly affect nursing practice and health care delivery in the United States.

This chapter provides an overview of public policies, various levels of governmental influence on the development and implementation of public policies, and the roles assumed by professional nurses concerning public policies. It offers strategies for professional nurses to use while influencing public policy development, implementation, and revision. Finally, it presents examples of nurses who have influenced public policy development and strategies for nurses to learn the art and science of political action.

The Nurse's Role in Influencing Public Policy

THE NURSE'S ROLE AS A RESPONSIBLE CITIZEN

The United States Constitution ensures the right of American citizens to have a voice in the government. Americans have the freedom to ask questions, offer suggestions, and debate effects of public policies (deVries & Vanderbilt, 1992).

A *policy* is an established course of action determined to achieve a desired outcome. Governments and institutions create policies to achieve their missions. However, policy development and implementation are not limited to governments and institutions. Any health care providing agency, professional organization, nonprofit organization, or family may make policies for members to follow. When health care policies are developed and revised, nurses bring special expertise to issues. This expertise brings a holistic approach that helps to protect the health and safety of the public.

KEY DEFINITIONS

Politics plays a key role in policy development. *Merriam Webster's Collegiate Dictionary* (1994) defines *politics* as "the art or science concerned with guiding or influencing governmental policy" and "the art or science of winning and holding control over a government" (p. 901). When the specified course of action is to develop or revise a policy, persons use political activities to influence policy development and implementation.

Some policies may evolve into law. *Laws* are a set of established rules that create a system of privileges and process for persons to solve problems with minimal force. Laws outline and govern relationships of individuals to other individuals, organizations, and their government. In addition, laws outline and govern the relationships of the government to its citizens. In democratic societies, citizens use political action to influence the legislative process required for law enactment.

Once laws become established, polices must be developed to ensure consistency in procedures to uniformly enforce the laws. *Policies* are formalized procedures that are followed by persons responsible for delivering governmental or institutional services (Stanhope, 1996). In most cases, the government acts as the ultimate authority within society for policy enforcement (except in cases of rebellions or coups). Most laws are public policies. However, not all public policies are laws.

GOVERNMENTAL ROLE IN PUBLIC POLICY DEVELOPMENT

The federal and most state governments are organized using three branches: the legislative, executive, and judicial. The *legislative branch* develops and approves legislation for executive branch consideration. The *executive branch* approves legislative acts and administers and regulates governmental policies. Once laws are passed, the government must develop policies to enact them. The *judicial branch* interprets laws and meaning of approved policies.

Legal bases for legislative action in health care are found in Article I, Section 8 of the United States Constitution, which states that the government bears the responsibility to provide for the general welfare of its citizens, regulate interstate commerce, fund the military, and provide funds for governmental operations. Each state bears the responsibility to enforce national policies while protecting the safety, health, and welfare of its citizens. State and national governments award grants for funding programs that enhance citizen safety, health, and welfare. Local governments implement national programs and develop laws, regulations, and policies to ensure public health.

THE NURSE'S ROLE IN PUBLIC POLICY-MAKING

Because laws govern professional nursing practice, nurses have a stake in public policy legislation and enforcement. Legislators pass laws and provide funding for health care programs, access, professional education, and research. Nurses might react to proposed legislation by writing their elected officials to influence their action during the legislative process. Some nurses engage in proactive political action by proposing legislation, persuading an elected official in the legislature to introduce a bill, devising public relation campaigns around their proposal, lobbying to get the bill passed by both houses of Congress, and influencing the head of the executive branch to sign it.

Nurses participate in national, state, and local legislative efforts. A national or statewide effort to pass legislation requires the participation of many for success. However, once legislation becomes law, some nurses continue to work with state or federal agencies responsible for devising the regulations to implement the law.

Nursing's Legislative Agenda

The American Nurses Association (ANA) develops an annual legislative agenda. A legislative agenda needs goals to direct the process. Legislative goals are developed and approved by the ANA board. Once approved, the organization publicizes it agenda. Its membership bears the responsibility to support the agenda while the ANA staff advances it. State nurse associations (SNAs) and the ANA hire professional lobbyists to promote legislation that favorably affects the practice of professional nursing (deVries & Vanderbilt, 1992). The current legislative agenda approved by the ANA outlines the following legislative and regulatory goals:

1. Maintain control of nursing practice
2. Influence health care policy development and reform
3. Advocate on the behalf of health care consumers
4. Initiate workplace reforms (deVries & Vanderbilt, 1992)

The first step to publicize a legislative agenda is the development of position papers on the legislative goals. A position paper is a one-page paper that specifies a goal. A position paper forces clear, concise communication of the rationale behind the agenda based on solid facts and persuasive arguments.

During preparation of the position paper, some effort should be spent exploring the opposition's viewpoints on the issue. Time spent here prepares the organization to anticipate arguments that will be used when confronted by the opposition. Supportive data including documents, articles, and statistics may be attached.

Printing the paper on an organizational letterhead adds to its credibility. Elements of the position paper include the background, position, rationale, group name, and contact person (name, address, and telephone number) (deVries & Vanderbilt, 1992).

The Art of Lobbying

The world of politics moves quickly. Sometimes a piece of legislation changes in less than an hour. To stay abreast of proposed legislation and its changes, nursing organizations hire lobbyists. The ANA has lobbyists for federal legislation. Most SNAs hire a lobbyist for state legislation. Lobbyists visit with elected officials in hopes of influencing action on a piece of pending legislation. In addition, lobbyists are responsible for keeping their organizational membership informed of proposed changes to a piece of legislation. At the local level, nurses attend city council and other community organizational meetings.

Besides hiring lobbyists, the ANA and SNAs offer the Nurses Strategic Action Team (N-STAT) a coordinated effort to ensure that nurses' voices are heard at the federal and state governmental levels. When presenting information on a legislative or local issue, nurses and lobbyists must do their homework to develop expertise on the impending issue.

Before briefing an elected official on an issue, it is mandatory to develop expertise on it. Having facts and statistics related to an issue provides a solid foundation for the art of persuasion. Effective use of statistics involves:

1. Putting the numbers in human terms
2. Reporting the statistics in simple terms while avoiding the use of percentages
3. Including practical and statistical significance when reporting numbers
4. Using national, state, and local statistics (legislators concern themselves with the local impact of an issue)
5. Citing the source of information (deVries & Vanderbilt, 1992)

Besides statistics, personal stories may be used effectively to influence elected officials. Effective use of personal stories involves:

1. Using a personal story about a citizen who resides in the elected official's district
2. Telling the true story in clear, concise, declarative, strong, and simple terms
3. Requesting a specific action by the legislator
4. Emphasizing the importance of the issue (deVries & Vanderbilt, 1992)

A clear, concise, precise, and persuasive presentation is mandatory to provide information to elected officials because they deal with many issues that multiply daily.

Before effective lobbying can occur, nurses must be aware of current changes in proposed legislation. Staying abreast of constant changes in issues surrounding a piece of legislation is an important, never-ending challenge. Table 12-1 provides a list of helpful resources that can be used by nurses to stay abreast of current legislative activity. Many of these resources can be found in a public or academic library.

Besides printed materials, the Library of Congress has an electronic information site (http://thomas.loc.gov/) to link citizens to legislative literature. This Internet site has the following information available for downloading, printing, or studying: pending legislation, committee hearing transcripts, electronic mail addresses of senators and representatives, and the *Federal Register* (Skaggs, 1997).

The Federal Legislative Path

Because of the complex process set forth by the authors of the Constitution, the path of legislation provides ample opportunity for citizen input. A bill must be introduced by a member of the House of Representatives or the Senate before it can be considered. Once a bill is introduced, it goes to a committee where it may be referred (passed to another committee), become the topic of a hearing, marked up (rewritten and amended), or reported out (sent to the House or Senate for floor action).

The chair of the committee considering the bill decides on its action. This person possesses much power because he or she may delay presentation of the bill to the committee (deVries & Vanderbilt, 1992). During this phase of the legislative process, nurses may brief the committee chair to attempt to influence scheduling of the bill for committee discussion or to be sent to the floor for action.

Once a bill has been approved by the full committee, it is placed on a legislative calendar. Only the Senate has filibuster privileges, where one or more senators may speak indefinitely about anything until 60 senators vote to end the discussion.

Once a bill is passed by either chamber, it goes to the other chamber and is subjected to the entire legislative process again. After the bill is approved by the second chamber, it is submitted to a conference committee that consists of members from both chambers. The conference committee negotiates differences between the two bill versions, adopts the conference bill, then submits (reports) the bill to both chambers for adoption or rejection. If the conference bill is adopted by both chambers, it becomes an Act of Congress.

Each Congressional Act (also known as an enrolled bill) is referred to the president (or governor in state legislatures), who signs or vetoes it. If the bill is signed, it becomes law. If the bill is vetoed, the House and Senate may override the veto by a two-thirds majority vote and the bill become public law. If the veto is sustained, the bill dies (deVries & Vanderbilt, 1992).

During the legislative process, nurses must communicate with their legislators to ensure that no bill adversely affects health care recipients and professional nursing practice.

The United States Constitution provides the president 10 days (excluding Sundays) to act on an enrolled bill. The president has four possible options. The bill may be approved; approved by inaction (ie, the president takes no action within 10 days, an option used when it is considered unnecessary or politically unwise to sign a bill or if there are questions about its constitutionality); pocket veto (used at the end of the legislative session when Congress adjourns before the 10-day expiration date); or veto (the president refuses to sign the bill, with a message stating his or her objections to it) (deVries & Vanderbilt, 1992). When the enrolled bill is submitted for executive approval, nurses should call, fax, or write the president or governor to voice support for the desired action.

Lobbying Strategies

Lobbying techniques are classified into two types: direct and indirect. *Direct lobbying* involves personal contact with elected officials. *Indirect lobbying* involves influencing public opinion on a particular issue. Table 12-2 outlines direct and indirect lobbying strategies.

Before implementing lobbying strategies, a nurse should outline a working plan that includes a chronological record of accomplishments. By keeping records of reactions and responses from elected officials, the nurse may use this information in future interactions. Appointment of a spokesperson helps maintain a consistent lobbying approach and enhances public recognition of a particular issue viewpoint.

Constituent pressure is perhaps the most effective weapon for the lobbyist. Mobilization of a group of individuals for collective action involves educating nurses, other health team members, and the general public. Letter-writing campaigns are effective when a bill is pending in Congress or in a state legislative body. A well written letter received from a constituent may appear in the *Congressional Record*. Because the elected official relies on voter support for reelection, each letter and personal contact counts. Follow-up letters of appreciation for action on an issue enhance relationships among elected officials and their constituents.

The following list outlines characteristics of an effective letter to an official:

1. Limit the letter to one page
2. Correctly address the letter, referring to the elected official as The Honorable (first name followed by surname)
3. Greet the official according to title (eg, Dear Senator _____, Dear Representative _____, Dear Congressman/Congresswoman _____, Dear Mr. Chairman or Madam Chairwoman _____, or Dear Mr./Madam Speaker_____)

text continues on page 284

TABLE 12-1

Helpful Resources to Stay Abreast of Legislative Activity*

Resource	Access Information
Legislative documents: bills, committee reports, conference reports, and public laws	Copies are available by writing the Senate Document Room or the House Document Room in Washington, DC. Please provide a self-addressed gummed label envelope. The House Document Room will accept telephone orders: (202) 225-1775. You will be asked to identify the organization you represent when you call.
Legislative Information System (LEGIS): a computerized information bank about legislation	
House Calendar: Contains a complete and accurate legislative history, including information on committee reports, conference committee actions, and new public laws.	Free from the House Document Room or by subscription from the Superintendent of Documents, Government Printing Office. Subscriptions may be placed on Visa or Master Card.
Daily Congressional Activities: A recorded message on the floor proceedings of each chamber is recorded daily when Congress is in session. This includes information on scheduling, voting, and floor debates.	Senate: (202) 224-8541 (Democrat) (202) 224-8601 (Republican) House: (202) 225-7400 (Democrat) (202) 225-7430 (Republican)
White House records and information on presidential signatures, vetoes, executive orders, presidential messages, and other official presidential actions.	The Office of the Executive Clerk of the White House: (202) 456-2226. Public law information: Office of the Federal Register, Presidential Documents Legislative Division: (202) 523-5230
Congressional Record: serves as a primary source of proceedings on the House and Senate floors, including an edited, substantially verbatim account of all debates as well as how each member voted on issues.	Contact your senator or representative. Each senator receives 40 free copies and each representative receives 25 free copies of The Record for distribution to constituents.
Digest of Public General Bills and Resolutions: Provides a list of all bills and resolutions in numerical order with a detailed description of each.	The Digest is published twice during each congressional session and is available from the Superintendent of Documents.
Committee prints and hearing records	Contact the publications clerk of the desired committee for free copies, but include a self-addressed label. Copies may be purchased through the Government Printing Office. Usually, the records are available for about 2 months after the hearings have concluded.
The legislative history provides the chronology of a law.	Contact the House or Senate Document Room or the Government Printing Office.
Congressional Quarterly Weekly Reports are published weekly and contain information about congressional action and developments; also contain articles on current legislative issues.	Published by Congressional Quarterly, Inc. 1414 22nd St. NW Washington, DC 20037.

The *Congressional Monitor* is a weekly publication that summarizes congressional activities including scheduled committee and subcommittee legislation. The cost is $1300 for an annual subscription, but subscribers get access to a telephone question-and-answer service as well as a 24-h tape recording of daily highlights.

Contact Congressional Quarterly, Inc.

The *National Journal* is a weekly publication that reports on various public policy issues and contains background information and issue analysis. The annual subscription rate is $775.

Some libraries subscribe to this journal. Published by National Journal, Inc. 1730 M St. NW, Suite 1100 Washington, DC 20036.

The *Compilation of Presidential Documents*, a weekly Governmental Printing Office publication, provides information on dates when the president vetoed or signed legislation.

Contact the Government Printing Office.

Congressional Caucus of Women's Issues Newsletter is a monthly publication that provides updates legislation affecting women.

Free to members of the Congressional Caucus for Women's Issues

Cable News Networks (C-Span & C-Span II)

Contact your local cable TV provider.

Daily newspaper

Contact your local newspaper.

The *Federal Register* officially announces regulations and legal notices issued by federal agencies and also includes acts of Congress, presidential proclamations and executive orders.

Published by the Government Printing Office every Monday through Friday, excluding holidays.

The *Code of Federal Regulations*, a quarterly publication of the Government Printing Office, publishes final federal regulations that are legally pending.

Contact the Government Printing Office or a local academic library.

Professional nursing journals frequently contain information on current legislative issues that affect nursing practice.

Contact journal publisher.

The Nurses' Strategic Action Team is a grassroots network of nurses coordinated by the ANA and individual state nurses associations to make the voice of nurses heard at the state and federal governmental levels. It publishes "Action Alerts" and "Legislative Updates" that detail specific legislative issues that affect nursing practice and the profession.

Contact the American Nurses Association
600 Maryland Avenue, SW
Suite 100 West
Washington, DC 20024-2571
(202) 554-4444.

The *Capitol Update* is a 20-issue legislative newsletter for nurses published by the ANA that highlights legislation that affects professional nursing practice.

Contact the American Nurses Association Publishing
PO Box 2244
Waldorf, MD 20604-2244
(800) 637-0323.

*See Appendix A for phone numbers and addresses.
Portions adapted from deVries, C., & Vanderbilt, M. (1992). *The grassroots lobbying handbook: Empowering nurses through legislative and political action.* Washington, DC: American Nurses Association.

TABLE 12-2

Lobbying Strategies

Direct Strategies: Through a Legislative Body	Indirect Strategies: Through Public Opinion
Participate in party platform development Contribute time and money to political campaigns	Publicize nursing organizational agendas Use the media, especially television broadcasts, to further the agenda
Influence legislative committees by personally visiting or writing committee members Contact agency regulators in writing or by personal visits	Write editorial pieces for written media such as the newspaper or news magazines Seek public opinion by polling members of the public and publishing the results
Engage in direct lobbying by visiting or writing elected officials or hiring a professional lobbyist Attend social event with elected officials Develop and understanding of elected officials' key positions on issues	Utilize paid media advertisements: television, radio and printed media Print and distribute books or pamphlets Develop and execute educational campaigns

Adapted from deVries, C., & Vanderbilt, M. (1992). *The grassroots lobbying handbook: Empowering nurses through legislative and political action.* Washington, DC: American Nurses Association.

4. Identify yourself as a constituent, health care expert, member of a large organization, and a credible source on the issue within the first paragraph
5. Refer to the specific piece of legislation by title (H.R. [number] for a House bill; S. [number] for a Senate bill) in the first paragraph if the letter pertains to a specific legislative proposal
6. Emphasize the local importance of the proposed issue
7. Be brief and specific and include key information
8. Handwrite the letter because computers can print many seemingly personalized letters in a matter of minutes
9. Use a professional letterhead if possible
10. Verify that the letter is neat and free of spelling, grammatical, or typographical errors (if typewritten)
11. Be specific about the desired action on the part of the elected official
12. Offer personal assistance or the organization's assistance in the closing
13. Thank the official for his or her action (deVries & Vanderbilt, 1992)

Using electronic mail (e-mail) to lobby an elected official has advantages and disadvantages. It is economical and quick. Use of this technology enables users to send messages at any time. The message is not dependent on postal delivery or a receptionist relaying the message to the official (Skaggs, 1997).

However, e-mail also has distinct disadvantages. The quality of messages sent depends on the software used to create them. Some software programs feature ways to emphasize specific message points. These programs cost more than other programs and users may find mastery of these features difficult. Therefore, the intended strength of the desired message may be impossible to achieve. Reading messages on the screen is not as easy as reading printed material. Printouts may not have as professional an appearance as a typed letter on a letterhead (Skaggs, 1997).

Because members tend to hear exclusively from dissatisfied constituents, they may be led to believe falsely that large numbers of their constituents disagree with a pending issue. A bill may be introduced for years before it is passed. "Persistence and patience are two key factors in lobbying" (deVries & Vanderbilt, 1992, p. 59). When nurses stay in regular contact with elected officials, the official is more likely to remember them and work to help support nursing's agenda.

Besides writing personal letters, other lobbying techniques may be used. Mailing a form letter is superior to sending nothing. If a nurse has no idea how to begin writing a letter, professional nursing organizations and nursing issue textbooks offer sample letters. If a specific piece of legislation is supported by a nursing organization, the organization may have a sample letter drafted for membership use.

A telephone call offers a way to deliver a brief and quick message to an elected official. Frequently, a legislator's staff members keep a tally of how many calls support and how many calls disapprove of pending legislation. Telegrams and e-mail messages are effective tools to send quick messages requesting prompt action. Petitions containing large numbers of signatures are usually effective only for public relations because it is difficult for staff to verify whether all signatures on the document represent constituents.

Besides written communication, a personal visit is an effective method of lobbying. Constituents are invited to meet with elected officials in the local or governmental offices. A personal visit lays the foundation for future contacts. A scheduled appointment usually ensures a personal meeting with an elected official. Frequently, visits are limited to 15 to 30 minutes. Because of legislative emergencies, appointments may be canceled, especially if a floor vote is scheduled during the planned meeting. The following suggestions will facilitate a personal visit with an elected official:

1. Confirm the appointment and arrive on time
2. Provide the official with a business card after greeting him or her with a firm handshake and a personal introduction
3. Open the meeting by informing the official of an established tie between you
4. Inform the official of the mission and how the visit represents it. Refer to pending legislation by bill number and title
5. Present statistics and personal stories when appropriate, while emphasizing the issue's importance to the local community

6. Request the name of the staff member who handles the issue and request follow-up
7. Be concise and focus totally on the issue of the meeting
8. Leave a one- or two-page fact sheet summarizing the issue and your position on it
9. Conclude the meeting by thanking the official for spending time with you
10. Write a thank you letter after the meeting (deVries & Vanderbilt, 1992)

Once reliable relationships are established with elected officials, nurses may be invited to testify at legislative committee hearings. When this happens, careful preparation is required and a witness may be accompanied by a technical expert or attorney. DeVries and Vanderbilt's *The Grassroots Lobbying Handbook*, published by the ANA (1992), outlines strategies to follow when testifying before Congress. The ANA president frequently testifies at committee hearings when issues regarding professional nursing practice are debated.

Writing letters and visiting legislators are the best-known lobbying techniques. Traditionally, persons lobby officials they have elected into office while ignoring powerful legislators such as party leaders and committee chairpersons.

Different lobbying strategies work more effectively during the various phases of the legislative process. Table 12-3 outlines specific lobbying strategies to be used during each phase of legislative and regulatory processes.

Obstacles to Effective Lobbying

Major obstacles encountered by nurses include not knowing whom to lobby, where to contact officials, and the best time for contact. Before contacting elected officials, nurses should find out about their personal biographies, committee memberships, voting records, and introduced or cosponsored legislative activity. Besides this information, knowledge of their personal causes or pet projects may be useful.

All members of the national legislative chambers maintain a Washington office as well as a local one in their district. Many have fax machines and e-mail systems that are connected to both offices. Much time and money can be saved by visiting elected officials while they are visiting their home districts when the legislature is out of session.

Staff Members

Because of their enormous responsibilities, all elected officials have staff. Much of the congressional work is handled by staff members. Good relationships with congressional staff at the national and local offices provide invaluable contacts and advantages when engaging in lobbying activities.

An elected official's personal staff may include an administrative assistant, a legislative director, legislative assistants, legislative correspon-

TABLE 12-3

The Legislative Process: Steps and Suggested Lobbying Strategies

Legislative Process Step	Suggested Lobbying Strategy
Legislation introduction	Hold a technical expert meeting to map out a strategy.
	Form a coalition of persons and organizations with the same goal.
	Identify a legislator in each chamber of Congress who would be likely to introduce the proposal.
	Schedule a staff meeting with the legislators' staff members.
	Initiate a letter-writing campaign to other congressional members who may wish to cosponsor the bill.
Immediately following introduction before committee assignment	Meet with interest groups to map out additional lobbying strategies.
	Create a one-page fact sheet to distribute to interested parties.
	Initiate a letter-writing campaign to elected officials to urge bill cosponsorship.
	Draft proposed amendments to bill.
Committee consideration	Write letters to all committee members to emphasize the need for a public hearing.
	Enlist letter-writing campaign by members of other interested organizations.
	Submit written information about oral or written testimony if a hearing is to occur.
	Have someone monitor the mark-up session and share information with letter writers.
	Conduct a letter-writing campaign to committee members either supporting or disagreeing with bill amendments added in committee.
	Conduct a letter-writing campaign to elected officials from local district outlining support or disapproval of the revised bill, or to enlist his/her support by contacting committee members or testifying at a committee meeting.
	Call a meeting of interested persons to verify if new amendments are tolerable or not.
	Work with committee staff in drafting the final draft of the bill.
	Notify the press about the bill.
Rules Committee action	Work with Rules Committee members to determine if amendments can be made while the bill is debated on the floor of either chamber.
Legislation on the floor of a chamber	Send short messages to all members of the chamber in great quantities (postcards, telegrams, e-mail messages, and telephone calls).
	Develop a swing list of officials.
	Initiate personal visits to officials on undecided, leaning no, and leaning yes lists.
Conference Committee action	Meet with other interested persons to verify which version (House or Senate) is to be supported.
	Write, visit, or call district officials and members of the Conference Committee.
Return to both chambers for approval	No lobby strategies needed if work has been consistent to now.
	Write or call elected officials from district.
Presidential or gubernatorial signature	Call the White House or governor's staff, leaving a message for veto or signature.
Veto override	Write or call locally elected official.
	Intensify lobbying efforts at those who appeared on the "leaning yes" list.

Adapted from deVries, C., & Vanderbilt, M. (1992). *The grassroots lobbying handbook: Empowering nurses through legislative and political action*. Washington, DC: American Nurses Association.

dents, a press secretary, case workers, a secretary, an office manager, and a receptionist. Nurses may be members of the staff. Staff members are responsible for scheduling appointments and activities. More importantly, officials fill staff posts with highly qualified persons who assist them in making decisions. For example, Sheila Burke, RN, MPA, FAAN, served as retired Senate Majority Leader Bob Dole's Chief of Staff (Goldwater & Zusy, 1990). During his tenure as majority leader, Burke advised Senator Dole on health care reform and other issues affecting public health, while directing all public activities of the Senator and his staff.

When nurses serve as staff members, they bring their expertise on health and safety issues to the team. To become a staff member, nurses should get to know political candidates, join political parties, donate time to work for election campaigns, contribute funds to campaigns, and market nursing expertise on issues related to health care and health promotion.

When lobbying for specific action on an issue, inviting an elected official for a personal tour of a local hospital or to participate in a local community service event may assist in advancing the cause. These activities increase the official's visibility and provide an opportunity for interaction with constituents. Because this may be viewed as an opportunity for press coverage, special attention to the press secretary at this time may increase chances of future access to the elected official (deVries & Vanderbilt, 1992).

Maintaining a Working Relationship

Expressing appreciation is frequently an overlooked step in the lobbying process. Elected officials should be acknowledged for introducing and supporting legislation that enhances the practice of professional nurses. Some SNAs bestow honors on elected officials who have developed records for supporting "nursing friendly" legislation. A thank you letter that includes a statement about informing other nurses living in the district about an official's action in supporting legislation increases support for an official running for reelection.

Honesty is perhaps the most important factor contributing to effective lobbying. When lobbying, nurses must be willing to spend the time to explore the issues and collect valid and reliable data surrounding them. When encountering questions that cannot be answered accurately with complete certainty, nurses should refer the question to another expert or offer to find the desired information and present it to the official at a later date. Attempts to "wing it" or inadvertently share untrue information could sabotage the personal relationships established with officials (deVries & Vanderbilt, 1992).

Without nurses' active participation in the legislative process, public policy may not remain friendly to the nursing profession or health care consumers. In the United States, public policy development and implementation is affected by money, power, and societal position. To maintain their position and power, elected officials frequently strive for reelection.

Because officials acknowledge the importance of pleasing their constituents, their acts are aimed at protecting and serving their voters. Politically astute persons acknowledge the importance of building coalitions and contributing resources to a political campaign to get their person elected to office.

COALITION BUILDING

Although difficult to establish and maintain, coalitions unite diverse groups, organizations, and people for a common specific purpose. Coalitions operate under the old assumption that "there is strength in numbers." Many coalitions begin with an informal structure that formalizes as the coalition evolves and becomes more active. Once formal structure has been established, employees may be needed to accomplish the coalition's goals. Before extending an invitation for membership, a background check verifies any strengths or weaknesses individuals or organizations bring to the coalition.

The goal of building a coalition is to capitalize on all members' strengths (Skaggs, 1997). Usually, the organization that started the coalition becomes its leader. However, if a goal is viewed as being self-serving for nurses, a member of another group should be designated as the coalition's official spokesperson. When the ANA and American Medical Association (AMA) work together to support a piece of legislation, they build a coalition of health care providers.

POLITICAL ACTION COMMITTEES

Political action committees (PACs) are created by existing organizations for the purpose of financing campaigns for political office. Federal election guidelines prohibit nonprofit groups from contributing to political campaigns. Funding for PACs is independent of its founding organization's funding.

Federal election guidelines mandate that PAC donations may be solicited from an organization's membership only for candidates for public office. However, general organizational funds may finance a political education program for members of the PAC's founding organization. Sometimes candidates for office receive political contributions from the PAC. However, some candidates may request only a public endorsement of their campaigns.

The ANA PAC, founded in 1972, is the sixth largest health care PAC in the United States and supports political candidates with "nursing friendly" agendas. The AMA PAC is the largest health care PAC, followed by the American Psychological Association PAC. The American Hospital Association PAC ranks fourth in size.

The ANA PAC raised over $1 million during the 1993–1994 and 1995–1996 election cycles. Of the 270 congressional candidates the ANA

PAC supported during the 1995–1996 election cycle, 77% became members of the 105th Congress. Membership of that House of Representatives includes nurses: Eddie Bernice Johnson, RN, the Democratic representative from the 30th Congressional District of Texas; and Carolyn McCarthy, LPN, the Democratic representative from the 4th Congressional District of New York (Schumacher, 1997).

◎ Current Political Issues Affecting the Practice of Professional Nursing and Health Care

Nursing practice and health care delivery are regulated by laws. Each state regulates nursing practice by its Nurse Practice Act. Health care access and indigent health care service reimbursement is regulated by federal and state governments. Many issues confronting legislators affect citizen safety, health care policy, and the control of nursing practice.

Hundreds of bills addressing health care are introduced into Congress and state legislatures annually. If a bill is not passed during the session of Congress when it was introduced, it dies. However, the bill may be introduced during each successive session of Congress until it passes. Issues that are current at the time of the writing of this chapter may become tomorrow's history. Through lobbying efforts and by serving as elected officials, nurses influence the future of health care delivery, public safety, and nursing practice. The following pending legislative issues may be of interest to professional nurses.

THE PATIENT SAFETY ACT

Since 1995, the ANA's "Every Patient Deserves a Nurse" campaign has heightened public awareness of the trend to reduce the numbers of RNs staffing acute care institutions. This campaign has demonstrated the benefits of patient care quality and safety when RNs, instead of unlicensed assistive personnel (UAP), assume patient care responsibilities.

This public campaign resulted in the introduction of the Patient Safety Act of 1997 (H.R. 1165), which aims to ensure safe patient care in hospitals and other health care institutions, and to provide "whistle blower" protection for RNs who speak out about patient care issues. The bill also advocates the development of nursing "report cards" that would identify and promote nursing quality indicators to measure and monitor health care quality. Besides this, each health care institution would have to make the following information available to the public:

1. Numbers of RNs and UAP providing direct patient care
2. The mean number of patients per RN who is providing direct patient care

These pieces of legislation were pending as of September, 1997.

3. Patient mortality rates
4. Numbers of adverse patient care incidents
5. Methods used to determine and adjust nursing personnel staffing levels according to patient care needs

A Patient Safety Act was not passed during the 1996 congressional session, but was reintroduced to Congress in 1997 by Representative Maurice Hinchey (D-NY). As client advocates, nurses should support this legislation because the quality of health care suffers when UAP are substituted for RNs as direct caregivers in acute care facilities (Reed & Franklin, 1997).

THE GENETIC INFORMATION NONDISCRIMINATION IN HEALTH INSURANCE ACT OF 1997

Representative Louise Slaughter (D-NY) and Senator Olympia Snowe (R-ME) sponsored the Genetic Information Nondiscrimination in Health Insurance Act of 1997 (H.R. 306/S. 89). This legislative act would protect American consumers from being denied health care insurance coverage based on high-risk genetic information. Besides denying health care insurance based on genetic testing results, the bill also prohibits insurance providers from requesting genetic testing information or requiring individuals to disclose results of genetic testing without prior written consent (Reed, 1997).

Advances in genetic research provide critical information for effective screening for diseases for persons at high risk for terminal and chronic illnesses, especially cancer. As client advocates, nurses should support this legislation.

THE HIV PREVENTION ACT

Representative Tom Coburn (R-OK) introduced the HIV Prevention Act of 1997 (H.R. 1062), which includes the following provisions:

1. Mandatory human immunodeficiency virus (HIV) testing of all sex offenders
2. Mandatory partner notification of persons testing positive for HIV
3. Allowing health care professionals to perform HIV testing without informed consent on any person undergoing an invasive medical procedure
4. Withholding Medicaid federal funding to states not complying with the Act

As client advocates, nurses should be concerned about any testing done without informed consent. In addition, this proposed legislation is inconsistent with much of the scientific research performed on HIV prevention (Gonzales, 1997a).

VICTIMS OF ABUSE INSURANCE PROTECTION ACT

Representative Bernard Sanders (I-VT) introduced The Victims of Abuse Insurance Protection Act of 1997 (H.R. 1117). This legislation was introduced in response to an informal 1994 survey by the Subcommittee Staff of the Crime and Criminal Justice Committee of the House Judiciary Committee, which revealed that eight of the 16 largest insurance companies in the United States were using domestic violence as a factor to determine insurance coverage and rates. This bill would prohibit the use of this information by insurers for refusing to insure persons or for charging higher premiums based on previous history of, or high risk for, domestic violence (Gonzales, 1997a).

As client advocates, nurses must support any legislation that prohibits access to, or increases the cost of health care for, any specified population.

THE TELEHEALTH BILL

Senator Kent Conrad (N-ND) introduced the Comprehensive Telehealth Act of 1997 (S. 385), which would provide Medicare reimbursement for telehealth services used by persons residing in rural and undeserved areas. Telehealth is the use of computer technology to link rural and underserved areas to large medical centers. This enables consultants with specialists for consumers without traveling to large medical centers. The bill also would provide loan and grant funding to establish telehealth networks in rural areas, and renames the Joint Working Group on Telemedicine as the "Joint Working Group on Telehealth." The name change recognizes the contributions of nurses and other health care providers to telehealth, and shifts the focus from physicians as the only providers of telehealth. Besides providing funding and acknowledging a team approach to telehealth, the bill would require the Department of Health and Human Services to conduct a study to provide telehealth services to home-bound persons or nursing home residents (Franklin, 1997).

As change agents, nurses should support this legislation, which may revolutionize the way persons access health care services.

WORKING FAMILIES AND FLEXIBILITY ACT

The Working Families and Flexibility Act (H.R. 1) has been introduced to assist parents meet family and work obligations. This bill proposes that employers compensate hourly-rate employees for overtime by offering them a choice of overtime pay or compensatory time off, at a rate of 1.5 times the hourly wage. The employee and employer would schedule compensatory time.

Proponents state that this bill would increase the flexibility of hourly-waged employees. Employees could use their compensatory time off to attend their children's activities, take a child or relative to a health care appointment, or stay home with an ill child. Opponents of the bill view its passage as providing employers a method to exploit their employees by forcing them to take compensatory time at times convenient to the employer. If the bill is enacted into law, opponents argue, workers who hope to increase their annual income through overtime pay may be coerced by their employers to select compensatory time off instead of overtime salary (Peterson, 1997).

Many nurses work for an hourly wage. Some nurses are single parents who may be dependent on overtime pay to meet their financial obligations. Other nurses may embrace the opportunity to spend more time with their families. With declines in inpatient length of stays, will hospitals require nurses opting for compensatory time off to use it when the patient census is low, instead of at a time when it is convenient for the nurse? Currently, the ANA opposes this piece of legislation.

EXAMPLES OF NURSES INFLUENCING PUBLIC POLICY

Although politics is frequently equated with corruption and power abuse, the combination of political activity and nursing does not create cognitive dissonance. Nurses bring a caring perspective to the political process. Health care delivery and access are greatly affected by the political process. Becoming politically active is one way to assume the roles of client advocate and change agent. The following examples provide evidence that nurses have fulfilled these roles by becoming politically active.

The ANA PAC endorses candidates at the state and national levels. Before candidates are endorsed, the ANA PAC Board of Trustees reviews their records and considers recommendations from SNA members. The SNA PAC presents checks to state political candidates (deVries & Vanderbilt, 1992). During the 1996 presidential election, the ANA PAC sent surveys to the Clinton and Dole campaigns to discover where each candidate stood on health care issues. The Dole campaign failed to respond. Considering the information received from the Clinton campaign and the legislative records of both candidates, the ANA PAC endorsed the reelection of President Clinton.

Besides influencing legislation, nurses have assumed responsibility in the legislative process by becoming members of legislative bodies. The right to run for and hold public office is guaranteed by the First Amendment of the United States Constitution (Tammelleo, 1990).

Elected to Congress with 74% of the popular vote from her district in 1992, Representative Eddie Bernice Johnson, RN (D-TX) serves as the Democratic Deputy Whip and holds membership on the House Committee on Transportation and Infrastructure, the House Committee on Science, and House subcommittees on surface transportation; public buildings and economic development; technology; and the environment. These committees and subcommittees frequently address issues related to public health, including transportation, roadways, and environmental safety. The U.S. Committee on Science frequently drafts legislation regarding funding for scientific research. In addition to these appointments, Johnson also serves as the Secretary of the Congressional Black Caucus. In Congress, passage of legislation frequently relies on members voting along party or special group positions.

Carolyn McCarthy, LPN, represents the 4th Congressional District of New York. Although she had no previous political experience, she ran as a Democrat and won her election in a predominantly Republican district. McCarthy was spurred to challenge a Republican incumbent who supported the repeal of a ban on assault weapons after McCarthy's husband was killed and her son seriously injured in the 1993 Long Island Railroad massacre (Canavan, 1997). Congresswoman McCarthy serves on the Education in the Workforce and the Small Business Congressional committees (K. Schumacher, personal communication, May 12, 1997).

In April 1997, Beverly Malone, PhD, RN, FAAN, president of the ANA; Marta Prado, RN, a Florida Nurses Association member, senior vice president of InPhyNet Medical Management, and chief operating officer of InPhyNet's Managed Care and Corrections Division; and May Wakefield, PhD, RN, FAAN, a member of the North Dakota Nurses Association, and professor and director for health policy at George Mason University, were appointed to President Clinton's bipartisan Advisory Commission on Consumer Protection and Quality in the Health Care Industry. The goal is to protect health care consumers from changes in health care delivery that could jeopardize the quality of care received, and investigate ways of guaranteeing high-quality health care in the United States. A major task of this commission is to create a "Consumer Bill of Rights" aimed at ensuring that health care consumers have adequate appeals and grievance processes when insured under managed care organizations. The Commission is also supposed to serve as consultants when relevant legislative initiatives move through both chambers of Congress (*Malone appointed*, 1997).

Virginia Trotter Betts, JD, MSN, RN, completed postdoctoral studies in health policy at the Institute of Medicine at the National Academy of Sciences as a Robert Wood Johnson Health Policy Fellow. As a past president of the ANA, she engaged in political activities such as analyzing policy, lobbying at the grassroots level, testifying before congressional committees, and developing Nursing's Agenda for Health Care Reform. She has been instrumental in positioning nurses as insiders in the political process (Schumacher, 1997).

In Ohio, Ann Hamilton, RN, and Ron Hamilton, RN, brought attention to the plight of professional nursing as hospitals in Ohio engaged in work redesign. They had bumper stickers made with the statement "Nurses.

You'll miss us when we're gone," and, after being deluged with requests, buttons made using a black ribbon design similar to the red-ribbon symbol of AIDS awareness. They also founded the Concerned Nurse Coalition, an organization of nurses concerned about recent changes in professional nursing positions and their effects on patient care.

Their actions resulted in a Cincinnati City Health Commission formal investigation of local hospital use of UAP. The Cincinnati City Council passed a resolution publicly denouncing RN replacement with UAP in hospitals, an action which helped support the introduction of the Patient Safety Act of 1997 at the federal level.

Nurses can also influence government reimbursements for health care. Linda Aiken, PhD, RN, FAAN, has served on the White House Physician Payment Review Commission that was created to make recommendations about provider payments under Medicare and Medicaid. Carolyne K. Davis, RN, PhD, served as the administrator of the Health Care Financing Administration. She credited her appointment to her direct political involvement in Michigan politics (Goldwater & Zusy, 1990).

The Kansas State Nurses Association successfully lobbied for the addition of an RN position to the Health Care Data Governing Board in Kansas. The board's mission is to promote the availability of and access to health care data, and to guide its use. This board develops policies and procedures for the Kansas health care data base administered by the Kansas secretary of health and environment (Irwin, 1997).

Nurses in Missouri initiated a public "Every Patient Deserves an RN" campaign, in response to hospital replacement of nurses by UAP as the major bedside care providers in acute care facilities. In the summer of 1996, nursing students Kathleen Buben and Jesse Evans obtained a grant from the ANA for a media campaign in the St. Louis area to educate the public about the issue. The campaign's radio broadcasts resulted in many calls from concerned citizens to St. Louis-area hospitals inquiring about RN–patient ratios and the use of UAP. This media campaign is credited with slowing down work redesign efforts in St. Louis hospitals, and resulted in a bill that would require all health care personnel to wear identification badges that prominently display the caregiver's name, licensing credentials, and title while acting within their scope of employment (Buben, Evans, & Reno, 1997).

During the 1997 Missouri Nurses' Day at the capitol, nurses from all areas of Missouri visited their legislators in order to push the bill forward. At the end of the day, the bill was placed on the Perfection Calendar (bills approved without amendment by committees of the Missouri House and Senate), despite opposition from the American Hospital Association and Missouri Hospital Association. The lobbying efforts of these nurses focused around patients' rights to know who is treating them, and patients' and families' needs to know who the RN is responsible for their care (Huber, 1997). The bill was signed into law by Governor Mel Carnahan in April 1997.

OPPORTUNITIES TO LEARN THE ART OF INFLUENCING PUBLIC POLICY

There are many ways to learn the art of influencing public policy development and legislative activity. Kathleen Schumacher (personal communication, May 12, 1997) suggests that ANA membership and involvement provides an avenue to learn how to play the political game. The ANA has four political action specialists who educate nurses about the political process, communicate directly with elected officials about pending legislation, collect information about elected officials' voting records, identify politicians who are friends of nursing, and advise the ANA PAC Board on potential candidates for ANA endorsement (Kathleen Schumacher, personal communication, May 12, 1997). Besides active involvement in national politics, SNAs offer day-long or week-long internships in the art and science of influencing public policies.

Besides the ANA, fellowships and internships offer nurses an opportunity to learn the process of public policy development through actual experience. Fellowships and internships inform participants about the complexities of health care policy and legislative priorities, as well as providing knowledge and skills to function in the public policy arena. Nurses may participate in formal fellowships and internships, or create their own Washington internship. Some colleges and university graduate programs offer college credit to students who complete Capitol Hill practicums. Internships offer nurses the ability to professionally network with members of congressional staff. Besides this, personal experience working within the organizational structure and the legislative process demystifies political and legislative processes. An internship may start a long-term relationship with a legislator or an influential staff member.

Informal internships can be set up by sending a brief letter and resumé to an elected official. The letter should be sent to the member's administrative assistant or chief of staff. Formal public policy fellowships are offered by a number of groups, including:

The Robert Wood Johnson Foundation
The W. K. Kellogg Foundation
The Congressional Black Caucus Foundation
The White House Commission
The Women's Research and Education Institute
The Coro Foundation
The American Association of University Women Educational Foundation
The Business and Professional Women's Foundation
The Everett McKinley Dirksen Congressional Leadership Research Center
The Supreme Court of the United States

The Woodrow Wilson National Fellowship Foundation
The Employee Benefit Research Institute
The Office of Technology Assessment of the United States Congress (Sharp, Biggs, & Wakefield, 1991)

Information on fellowship opportunities may be found at the local public library or by writing the foundations directly.

◎ Conclusion

Each nurse brings to the profession different talents that can be used for political action. Speaking out on unfair issues or writing elected officials takes time and courage, because health care organizations tend to bestow rewards on personnel who do not rock the boat (Leavitt & Barry, 1993). However, nurses must make their voices heard in the political arena, to ensure public safety and to maintain a place in the delivery of health care.

Health care policies are developed through the legislative process at the national, state, and local levels. Developing expertise in influencing public policy requires dedication, time, practice, and a willingness to work with others. Issues affecting personal and public health are too important to be left to the politicians. Political involvement is a means to influence and control public policy while demonstrating ethical caring for all citizens in a democratic society.

THOUGHT QUESTIONS

1 In a large urban area, three major health care networks have agreed to use UAP to perform all aspects of acute inpatient care except for medication administration. According to the current state nurse practice act, a nursing license is required to administer medications, but not to engage in invasive procedures such as phlebotomy, Foley catheter and nasogastric tube insertions, tracheal suctioning, other aseptic procedures, and discharge teaching. The health care systems have agreed not to hire any professional nurses who speak out against this change in acute care. As a professional nurse and citizen, you are outraged by the change in the delivery of health care in this community.
  a. List the persons who are affected by this change and speculate possible results for these persons.
  b. Outline potential strategies that the professional nurses in this community might consider to counteract this change in acute care delivery. For each strategy, specify its consequences.
  c. Who is at greatest risk from this change, patients or nurses? Why?

2 Why do nurses avoid becoming active in politics?

3 How does being politically active enhance the nursing profession?

REFERENCES

Buben, K., Evans, J., & Reno, D. (1997). *Nursing students: A school project that made a difference.* Educational session 1997 MONA Nurse Lobby Day, March 4, 1997, Jefferson City, MO.

Canavan, K. (1997). Washington watch. Election results: Strong finish by nurse candidates and ANA-PAC. *American Journal of Nursing, 97*(1), 20.

deVries, C., & Vanderbilt, M. (1992). *The grassroots lobbying handbook: Empowering nurses through legislative and political action.* Washington, DC: American Nurses Association.

Franklin, K. (1997). Legislative update. ANA endorses telehealth bill. *Capitol Update, 15*(5), 3.

Goldwater, M., & Zusy, M. (1990). *Prescription for nurses: Effective political action.* St. Louis: Mosby.

Gonzales, R. (1997a). Legislative update. HIV prevention act introduced. *Capitol Update, 15*(4), 4.

Gonzales, R. (1997b). Legislative update. Domestic violence insurance protection act introduced. *Capitol Update, 15*(4), 5.

Huber, D. (1997). Missouri *Nurses Association bills of importance to registered nurses introduced in the 89th General Assembly 1st regular session.* Legislative guide distributed to Missouri Nurses at the 1997 MONA Nurse Lobby Day, March 4, 1997, Jefferson City, MO.

Irwin, L. (Ed.) (1997, April 21). On the board: Nurse will be appointed to state health care post. *Kansas City Nursing News,* p. 1, 4.

Leavitt, J., & Barry, C. (1993). Learning the ropes. *Imprint, 40*(4), 58–61.

Malone appointed to president's health quality commission. *Capitol Update, 15*(5), 1–2.

Mish, F. C. (Ed) (1994). Merriam Webster's Collegiate Dictionary. Springfield, MA: Merriam-Webster Inc.

Peterson, C. (1997). Legislative update. Compensatory time off bill. *Capitol Update, 15*(4), 2–3.

Reed, S. (1997). Legislative update. ANA endorses genetic anti-discrimination bill. *Capitol Update, 15*(4), 3.

Reed, S., & Franklin, R. (1997). Patient safety act introduced. *Capitol Update, 15*(4), 1–2.

Schumacher, K. (1996, October). Nurses running for Congress. *The Political Nurse,* p. 12.

Sharp, N., Biggs, S., & Wakefield, M. (1991). Public policy: New opportunities for nurses. *Nursing & Health Care, 12*(1), 16–22.

Skaggs, B. (1997). Political action in nursing. In J. Zerwekh & J. Claborn (Eds.). *Nursing today, transitions and trends* (2nd ed.). Philadelphia: Saunders.

Stanhope, M. (1996). Policy, politics, and the law: Influences on the practice of community health nursing. In M. Stanhope & J. Lancaster (Eds.). *Community health nursing promoting health of aggregates, families, and individuals.* St. Louis: Mosby.

Tammelleo, A. D. (1990). Nurse terminated for election to public office. *The Regan Report on Nursing Law, 31*(6), 1.

Professional Practice Strategies

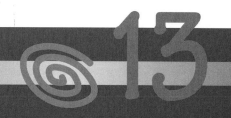

The Professional Nursing Role with Family and Community Clients

THE INDIVIDUAL AS CLIENT

THE FAMILY AS CLIENT
    The Family in the Change/Growth Models
        of Nursing
    The Family in the Change/Stability Models
        of Nursing

THE COMMUNITY AS CLIENT
    Definitions of Community
    A Systems Model of Viewing the Commu-
        nity as Client
    A Human Field/Environment Model of
        Viewing Community as Client

LEARNING OUTCOMES

By the end of this chapter, the student will be able to:

1 Define individual, family, and community as the client in nursing.

2 Understand the status of the development of nursing's conceptual models in terms of differentiating client systems in nursing.

3 Appreciate why nurses will be ineffective in nursing processes if they attempt to limit their view of the client system to individuals within the contexts of family and community.

4 Distinguish the commonalities and differences in the realms of family nursing in the change/growth view and the change/stability view.

5 Explain the differences in viewing communities as aggregates of people, human systems, and human field/environmental field process.

6 Begin to identify the gaps that exist in information that assists nurses to use nursing models in their practice with families and communities as clients.

Human systems are living systems open to interactions with other systems. Interacting systems are characterized by mutual change; that is, each human system can effect change in another and at the same time is influenced (changed) by that other system. Nurses are involved in professional practice with client systems, the health care delivery system, and their own professional self-systems—all of which are human systems. Clients are the recipients of nursing care. More significantly, they are participants with professional nurses in nursing processes.

This chapter explores the professional nurse's role with client systems. It presents a beginning differentiation of the client systems—individuals, families, and communities.

Traditionally, nurses have cared for individuals; conceptual models of nursing have developed their views of "the person" (individual); and nurses have practiced with families and communities. The traditional practice with families and communities usually has been practice with individuals in a collective setting; thus, family and community actually have been treated as contexts of the identified client. The major questions for the professional nurse are: How do I implement processes of nursing with the whole human being, the individual client? With the whole family unit, the family as client? With the community as client?

Change in human beings is lifelong, natural, and evolutionary. As human beings move through their lives, they establish themselves as integral elements of larger and more complex systems. The individual synthesizes the concept of "me" with "my family" and "my community." Sometimes it is entirely appropriate for the nurse to work with the "me" in professional relationships. In other instances, it is most appropriate for the nurse to work with "the family." Finally, in some instances it is most appropriate for the nurse to work with "the community."

According to the paradigm selected for application in this book—the growth or persistence views of change (Fawcett, 1989)—it is the client–environment relationship that is most important. In the change view, the outcome is growth. In the persistence view, the outcome is stability. The way the nurse thinks about change determines how she or he views the client. In the change/growth model, the client is seen as able to grow, and the change process is facilitated by the nurse focusing the client on the client's strengths and abilities. In the change/stability model, the client is seen as able to return to stability, and the process is facilitated by the nurse identifying and assisting with plans for resolving problems with the client.

All of the conceptual models of nursing were originally developed with "person" equated with the individual client. The developers of some models and other thinkers in nursing have attempted to explain how the models can be applied to family and community as client. Some nurse leaders believe that "person" has been redefined in the models to include families as clients, the recipients of care (Anderson & Tomlinson, 1992). Hanchett (1988) declares that community also can be defined as client; thus, "community" replaces "person" as the human being in some conceptual models.

The Individual as Client

The philosophy inherent in this book is that a person progresses through life. This progression is characterized by unique evolving patterns of interaction between the person and the environment. Such patterns of interaction determine the person's health. In general, the changes that occur in the developing human being are characterized by higher abilities to organize interactions and deal with more complex levels of interaction. The person's patterns are unique and are continuously evolving from earlier life experiences, including biologic, genetic, cultural, interpersonal, and social influences as well as current interactions and conception of the future.

The reader is referred to Chapter 8 for the view of the person and to Chapter 9 for full discussion of implementing nursing processes with the individual as client. Because the conceptual models of nursing were developed with the person defined as the client, the professional nurse's directives for working with individuals can be directly derived from the discussion of nursing processes according to both the integration and the interaction nursing models. The following sections reflect our efforts to differentiate professional nursing care of families and communities from care of individuals.

The Family as Client

Who is defined as family? This question has evoked many definitions of family, from the conjugal or nuclear family (the family of marriage, parenthood, or procreation) to the extended family (the kinships of biologically related persons—grandparents, aunts, uncles, and cousins). Such definitions have limited applicability and usefulness in today's society. Thus, the definition of *family* that is accepted is "two or more individuals who depend on one another for emotional, physical, and/or economic support. The members of the family are self-defined" (Hanson, 1996, p. 6).

How is family nursing care viewed today? Some call it family-centered care, some call it family-based care, others call it family-focused care, and others call it simply family nursing. These different terms reflect confusion about whether the family is the client (the recipient of care) or is the context of care (in which the individual family member is the recipient of care). Gilliss (1991) says that family nursing care traditionally has been offered from the perspective of the family as context.

According to Wright and Leahey (1988, p. 30), there is a trend toward the family as the unit of care (family systems care) in which the nurse focuses on interaction: "It is becoming more natural for nurses to accept the interaction between illness, the individual, and the family," and that interaction can be addressed at all levels of the system, "from the micro level of fluid and electrolytes to the macro level of the family and the community." For example, if the presenting problem of an individual is electrolyte imbalance, then the unit of care should be the individual. However, if the presenting problem is the husband and father's lack of compliance with his prescribed diabetic regimen, then the appropriate unit of care would be the family.

What are the indices and phenomena that represent the family as a holistic unit, on which the professional nurse must focus if the family is to be the client system? One approach is to view the family as a system interacting with subsystems and suprasystems. Artinian (1994) indicates that some of the assumptions of the family systems perspective are:

- A family system is an organized whole; individuals within the family are parts of the system and are interdependent.
- The family system is greater than and different from the sum of its parts.
- There are logical relationships (connectedness patterns) between the subsystems. In some families the connectedness patterns may reflect rigid and fixed structures and and relationships. In other families, the patterns of connectedness may reflect highly flexible structures and relationships.
- Using feedback from the environment, the family system responds (adapts) to change in ways that reduce strain and maintain a dynamic balance.

In the systems approach, the phenomena of interest are wholeness, relationships, belief systems, family rules, family needs, roles, and the tensions between individuation and togetherness. Two family theories that are congruent with the family systems model are the Calgary family assessment model (Hanson, 1996; Wright & Leahey, 1994), and the framework of systemic organization (Friedemann, 1995). A summary of the family systems model is presented in Display 13-1.

Another approach to family as client focuses on the family as a structural–functional social system (Artinian, 1994). The focus is the family structure and its effectiveness in performing its functions. Friedman (1992) identifies seven family functions:

1. Affective (meeting the emotional needs of family members)
2. Socialization and social placement (socializing children and making them productive members of society)
3. Reproduction (producing new members for society)
4. Family coping (maintaining order and stability)
5. Economic (providing sufficient economic resources and allocating resources effectively)
6. Providing physical necessities (food, clothing, shelter)
7. Health care (maintaining health)

The Friedman family assessment model (Friedman, 1992; Hanson, 1996) is congruent with a combination of the structural–functional model with the family systems model. A summary of the structural–functional model is presented in Display 13-2.

DISPLAY 13-1

The Family Systems Model

Overview: Focuses on interaction between members of the family system and on the family system with other systems. A change in one member of the family system influences the entire system.

Concepts: Subsystems, boundaries, openness, energy, negentropy (energy that promotes order), entropy (energy promoting chaos), feedback, adaptation, homeostasis, input, output, internal system processes.

Assumptions: Family system is greater than the sum of its parts. Subsystems are related and interact with one another and the whole family system interacts with other systems. Family systems have homeostatic features and strive to maintain a dynamic balance.

Clinical Application: Assess, diagnose, and intervene with family according to major concepts.

Sample Assessment Questions
- How did change caused by critical illness event effect all the members of the family?
- How are members of the family system relating with one another?
- How is the family system relating to the critical care environment?
- What is the "input" into the family system?
- Is the family system internally processing the input? What is the family system output?

- How open is the family system? Does the family system have homeostasis?
- Determine how family behavior affects the patient.
- Determine how the patient's behavior affects family.

Interventions
- Encourage nurse–family interactions through establishing trust and using communication skills to check for discrepancies between nurse and family expectations.
- Establish a mechanism for providing family with information about the patient on a regular basis.
- Foster the family's ability to get information.
- Listen to the family's feelings, concerns, and questions.
- Orient the family to the critical care environment.
- Answer family questions or assist them to get answers.
- Discuss strategies for normalizing family life with family members.
- Provide mechanisms for the patient and other family members to interact with one another through pictures, videos, audiotapes, or open visiting.
- Monitor family relationships.
- Facilitate open communication among family members.
- Collaborate with the family in problem solving.
- Provide necessary knowledge that will help family make decisions.

From Artinian, N. T. (1994). Selecting a model to guide family assessment. *Dimensions of Critical Care Nursing, 14,* 6. Used with permission of the publisher.

A third approach to family as client is the family stress model. Artinian (1994, pp. 277–278) lists the following assumptions of this model:

- The family is a system.
- Unexpected or unplanned events are usually perceived as more stressful than expected events.
- Events within the family that are defined as stressful are more disruptive than events outside the family.
- Lack of previous experience with a stressor leads to greater perceived stressfulness.
- Ambiguous stressor events are more stressful than nonambiguous ones.

Artinian (1994) indicates that assessment should include:

Family resources
The meaning of the situation to the family (eg, is it viewed as a threat or a challenge?)

The Structural–Functional Model

Overview: Focuses on family structure and family function and how well family structure performs its functions.

Concepts: Structural areas include family form, roles, values, communication patterns, power structure, or support network. Functional areas include affective, socialization, reproductive, coping, economic, physical care, and health care functions.

Assumptions: Family is a system and a small group that exists to perform certain functions.

Clinical Application: Assess, diagnose, and intervene with family according to major concepts.

Sample Assessment Questions
- What impact did critical illness event have on family structure and function?
- How did the critical illness alter family structure?
- What family roles were changed? What family functions have been affected?
- What are family member's physical responses to the illness event?

Interventions
- Assist family to modify its organization so that role responsibilities can be redistributed.
- Respect and encourage adaptive coping skills used by the family.
- Counsel family members on additional effective coping skills for their own use.
- Identify typical family coping mechanisms.
- Tell family it is safe and acceptable to use typical expressions of affection.
- Provide privacy for family to allow for family expression of affection.
- Provide for family visitation.
- Encourage family members to recognize their own health needs.
- Help family members find ways to meet their health needs while at the same time help them feel their concern for the patient has not diminished.
- Assist family to use existing support structure.

From Artinian, N. T. (1994). Selecting a model to guide family assessment. *Dimensions of Critical Care Nursing, 14,* 6. Used with permission of the publisher.

The level of crisis the family is experiencing
Coping mechanisms

Two theories that are congruent with a combination of the family stress model and the family systems model are the family assessment and intervention model (Hanson, 1996; Mischke & Hanson, 1995), and the resiliency model (McCubbin & McCubbin, 1993). A summary of the family stress model is presented in Display 13-3.

Anderson and Tomlinson (1992, p. 61) identify five realms of family experience that represent elements of the approaches identified above and that direct professional practice:

1. Interactive processes
   a. Family relationships
   b. Communication
   c. Nurturance
   d. Intimacy
   e. Social support
2. Developmental processes
   a. Family transitions
   b. Dynamic interactions between stages of family development and individual developmental tasks

---

DISPLAY 13-3

The Family Stress Model

Overview: Focuses on stressors, resources, and perceptions to explain the amount of family disruption due to a stressful event.

Concepts: "A"—stressful event with associated hardships; "B"—physical, psychological, material, social, spiritual, informational resources of family; "C"—family's subjective definition of the stressful event; "X"—crisis, the amount of disruption or incapacitation within the family due to the stressful event.

Assumptions: Family is a system. Unexpected and ambiguous illness events are more stressful. Stressful events within the family are more disruptive than stressor events that occur outside the family. Lack of experience with a stressor event leads to increased perceptions of stressfulness.

Clinical Application: Assess, diagnose, and intervene with family according to major concepts.

Sample Assessment Questions
- Identify the family's understanding and beliefs about the situation.
- What family hardships are associated with the critical illness event?
- What are other situational stressors for the family?

- Did the family have time to prepare for the event?
- Has the family had experience with the event?
- What resources are available to the family?
- Are the resources sufficient to meet the demands of the event?
- What are the family's perceptions of the event?
- Do they perceive the event to be a threat or challenge?
- Does the family blame themselves for the event?
- How incapacitated is family functioning?

Interventions
- Help family to cope with imposed hardships.
- If appropriate, provide spiritual or informational resources for family.
- Introduce the family to others undergoing similar experiences.
- Discuss existing social support resources for the family.
- Assist the family in capitalizing on its strengths.
- Assist family to resolve feelings of guilt.
- Help family visualize successfully handling all the hardships associated with the situation.
- If possible, encourage family to focus on the positive aspects of the situation or cognitively reappraise the situation as positive.

From Artinian, N. T. (1994). Selecting a model to guide family assessment. *Dimensions of Critical Care Nursing, 14,* 7. Used with permission of the publisher.

---

3. Coping processes
   a. Management of resources
   b. Problem-solving
   c. Adaptation to stressors and crisis
4. Integrity processes
   a. Shared meanings of experiences
   b. Family identity and commitment
   c. Family history
   d. Family values
   e. Boundary maintenance
   f. Family rituals
5. Health processes
   a. Family health beliefs
   b. Health status
   c. Health responses and practices
   d. Lifestyle practices
   e. Health care provision during wellness and illness

It is important to understand that the nurse needs to implement the nursing process in a way that facilitates exploration of all the realms listed above, not only the health processes. In all the conceptual nursing models, the client system is viewed holistically; thus, the professional nurse cannot extricate the health processes from the other processes (integrity, coping, development, and interaction).

How would nurse theorists explain the family as the client and the application of nursing to the nurse–family relationship? Following is a discussion of how the family may be understood in nursing models within the change/growth paradigm (Orem, Watson, Peplau, Rogers, Parse and Newman) and those nursing models within the change/stability paradigm (King, Neuman, and Roy).

THE FAMILY IN THE CHANGE/GROWTH MODELS OF NURSING

Orem's Self-Care Deficit Model

According to Taylor and Renpenning (1995, p. 356), Orem views family as a multiperson care system, which are

> those courses and sequences of action which are performed by the persons in multiperson units for the purpose of meeting the self-care requisites and the development and exercise of self-care agency of all members of the group and to maintain or establish the welfare of the unit . . . . The sub-systems of the multiperson system are the self-care systems of the individuals.

Whall and Fawcett (1991, p. 20) indicate that Orem's self-care conceptual framework primarily "views the family as only a backdrop for individuals." In her own words, Orem (1983, p. 368) directs the nurse to "first, accept the system of family living, the physical and social environment of the family, and the family's culture as basic conditioning factors for all the family members." She stresses that the family support system needs to be explored and "adjusted as needed and then incorporated into the system of family living" (Orem, 1983, p. 368).

Family is context in self-care, in which family members are able to take actions to create conditions essential for human functioning and development, and for dependent care, in which family members need their care provided by others. Both self-care and dependent care are directed toward creating and maintaining conditions that support life and integrated functions and promote human growth. Self-care and dependent care "are forms of deliberate action, learned behaviors, learned within the family and other social units within which individuals live and move" (Orem, 1983, p. 209). However, Orem also considers the family to be a unit, "a complex entity which can be regarded as a whole" (Taylor & Renpenning, 1995, p. 350). Thus, there is concern with the quality of interaction and outcomes of those interactions on the family as a whole.

Two realms of family care can be readily implemented in Orem's self-care model: the interactive processes, particularly the social support systems in the family, and the developmental processes, particularly in the understanding of dependent care needs at various stages of life. "Conditions which justify identifying the multiperson unit include a need for protection and prevention, regulation of a hazard, need for environmental regulation, [and] need for resources" (Taylor & Renpenning, 1995, p. 366).

Lapp and coworkers (1991) stress the concept of the family as partner in health care decision-making. In keeping with the self-care perspective, they see "the primary responsibility for health and life choices as ultimately resting with the client family" (Lapp et al., 1991, p. 306). They further suggest that the main responsibility of the nurse is "ensuring that those choices were made on the basis of the most complete information possible while facilitating self-discovery of strengths and resources already existing for a family" (Lapp, Diemert, & Enestvedt 1991, p. 306).

Watson's Human Science and Human Care Model

Watson's caring model lends itself to a view of the family as client if the nurse redefines the phenomenal field to be the family within the family system's environment. The nurse can assess family values by exploring the five realms of family experience (Anderson & Tomlinson, 1992)—namely, the integrity processes—through the family's shared meanings of experiences; its members' identity and commitment to that family identity; the family history; members' shared values and rituals; and their strategies for maintaining family boundaries.

Family *needs for information and problem-solving abilities* can be explored by identifying the family's coping processes, that is, how members obtain and manage resources and how the group solves problems. *Developmental conflicts* can be evaluated by studying the developmental processes, that is, the transitions of the family and the interaction of the family's stage of development with the individual developmental tasks. Losses and feelings about the human predicament can be analyzed through exploring the *interaction processes*, focusing on relationships and the family's communication patterns, patterns of nurturance, expressions of intimacy, and support networks. In the model of caring, the nurse would finally relate all of the aforementioned processes that occur in the family to the health processes, clarifying with the family their health beliefs, responses, and practices as well as the patterns of caring for each other during wellness and illness.

Peplau's Interpersonal Relations Model

Because Peplau's model of nursing is based on the central concepts of growth and development facilitated by relationships with significant others, it is proposed that the nurse could focus on the family as the unit of care if the patterns of interaction within the family, and the family developmental processes, replaced individual needs as the central area of concern. Forchuk and Dorsay (1995, p. 114) stated that Peplau's model and family systems nursing "both share a common focus on interactions, patterns and interpersonal relationships."

Perhaps Peplau's greatest contribution to the family nursing process is the stages of the nurse–client relationship. According to Friedman (1992, p. 42), "trust and rapport-building set the stage for and are the cornerstones of effective family nursing care." In the *orientation* stage, if the nurse and the family are to be effective in the relationship, each member of the family must be able to share his or her concerns so that the nurse and other family members may more fully understand the whole family and the meaning of its experience together. In the *planning* stage, mutual goal-setting—that is, jointly formulated among members and the nurse—and ways to meet commonly derived goals are directed toward reframing the need for help in the professional relationship to be a learning and growth experience.

It is proposed that, in the *intervention* stage (called the exploitation stage by Peplau) with families, Peplau's role behaviors originally designated as professional nursing roles could be developed as strategies for the entire family. Family needs replace individual needs, and the roles of resource person, teacher, leader, counselor, and surrogate may be played by both the nurse and various family members. Each role performance in the family should be fully explored in a way that the family learns about its interactive processes and the effect of those interactive processes on health processes.

Rogers's Science of Unitary Human Beings

Various analysts agree that Rogers's conceptual model of nursing science lends itself readily to the family as the recipient of nursing care—the client system. As Friedman (1992, p. 62) says, "Rogers's legacy is clearly associated with general systems theory, and because of this orientation there is a good fit between Rogerian nursing theory and family nursing." Rogers herself says that the family system is an energy field that can be the focus of study and interaction. She asserts that family fields and their respective environmental fields are engaged in a continuously evolving mutual process and that patterns identify this ongoing process (Rogers, 1983, p. 226). Some patterns may represent togetherness, others may represent activity/rest, and still others may represent rhythmicities in the family experience.

Whall and Fawcett (1991, p. 22) suggest that, in the Rogerian model, the family is "viewed as an irreducible whole that is not understood by knowledge of individual family members." Newman, Sime, and Corcoran-Perry (1991, p. 4) point out that, from the unitary–transformative perspective (the perspective first described by Rogers), a phenomenon (any client system) is "viewed as a unitary, self-organizing field embedded in a larger self-organizing field . . . [and] identified by pattern and by interaction with the larger whole." Given this perspective, the family can be described as a unitary phenomenon embedded in the larger environmental field, and a phenomenon that has patterns of energy exchange within its field and within its interactions with the larger environment.

Whall (1986) suggests that, despite the fact that Rogers has not been completely clear about what assessment strategies are used in the unitary model, she deserves credit for the idea that the family must be assessed as a whole by the nurse providing care. Other nurses have developed some of the assessment tools for assessing the whole family. For example, Smoyak developed the idea of using genograms and the identification of family rules of organization as approaches in the nursing process (Whall, 1986). The genogram records information about family members and their relationships over at least three generations. It involves mapping the family structure, recording family information, and delineating family relationships. According to McGoldrick and Gerson (1985, p. 1), genograms "display family information graphically in a way that provides a quick gestalt of complex family patterns and a rich source of hypotheses about how a clinical problem may be connected to the family context and the evolution of problem and context over time."

The genogram is one of nursing's most useful tools for studying family patterns. What does it do for the nurse? It maps relationships and patterns of functioning and thus "may help clinicians think systemically about how events and relationships in their clients' lives are related to patterns of health and illness" (McGoldrick & Gerson, 1985, p. 2). Using the historic data obtained by completing the genogram, the nurse can assess previous life cycle transitions. This assessment helps the nurse to "picture the important connections between the family and the world" (Wright & Leahey, 1994, p. 49). Readers are referred to McGoldrick and Gerson (1985) and Wright and Leahey (1994) for further details on constructing and interpreting the genogram as a tool for nursing assessment of the family.

All of the family realms described by Anderson and Tomlinson (1992) and discussed earlier in this chapter represent patterns of the family as a unitary phenomenon. Thus, these realms could be used as a basis for assessment, planning, intervention, and evaluation by nurses practicing on the basis of a Rogerian philosophy of nursing.

Parse's Human Becoming Model

Parse's and Newman's nursing models may be considered Rogerian-based. Thus, the nurse practicing within any of these models will incorporate Rogerian concepts in the caregiving process with the family.

For Parse, "since the abstract term 'human' includes all human phenomena, it encompasses family phenomena as inherent in being human" (Cody, 1995, p. 11). Parse, who views the person as an open being always in the process of becoming, probably would describe the family as open and always in the process of becoming. "Family health is cocreated by persons as they live family process" (Cody, 1995, p. 14). Nursing care probably would be directed at structuring meaning, cocreating rhythmical patterns of relating, and cotranscending with the possibles through the interpersonal processes occurring among family members and the nurse for the purpose of improving the quality of life for the family.

"For each participant family, a multiplicity of views cocreates the reality of the family situation as lived by each person" (Cody, 1995, p. 23). Clearly, the family realms (Anderson & Tomlinson, 1992) that characterize Parse's model are the interactive processes (family relationships, communication, nurturance, intimacy, and social support) and the integrity processes (shared meanings of experiences, family identity and commitment, family history, family values, boundary maintenance, and family rituals).

Newman's Theory of Health as Expanding Consciousness

Newman, who views the individual as a center of energy, views the family the same way—a center of energy in constant interaction with the environment. Newman (1983, pp. 169–170) makes five assumptions about families:

1. Health encompasses family situations in which one or more family members may be diagnosed as ill.
2. The illness of family member(s) can be considered a manifestation of the pattern of the family interaction.
3. Elimination of the disease condition in the identified ill family member will not change the overall pattern of the family.
4. If one person's becoming ill is the only way the family can become conscious of its pattern, then that is health (in process) for that family.
5. Health is the expansion of consciousness of the family. Consciousness has been defined as the informational capacity of the system, a factor that can be observed in the quantity and quality of responses to stimuli.

The nature of nursing with the family would be the repatterning of partnerships between the family and the environment that promote higher levels of consciousness. Newman (1983, p. 171) says that the purpose of nursing with the family is to facilitate the development of an increased range of responses of family members to each other and to the world outside the family and to facilitate the refinement of those responses (quality). She suggests that the first task is to assess the patterns of movement, space, time, and consciousness in the family (Newman, 1983, pp. 171–172). Movement is assessed through observing:

1. The coordinated movement of language between speaker and listener
2. Other coordinated movements (such as dancing, lovemaking, and sports)
3. The freedom of individual movement within the family
4. The movement outside the family

Time is assessed for the quantity and quality of private time, coordinated time, and shared time. Space is assessed for territoriality, shared space, and distancing. Finally, consciousness is assessed by collecting data on the informational capacity of the family system, the quantity and quality of interaction within the family, and the quantity and quality of the interaction of the family with the community.

By completing these assessments, the nurse providing care for the family would be able to analyze the patterns of energy exchange between the family and the environment, the transforming potential and life patterns of the family. These patterns will identify where the family energy is flowing and where it is blocked, depleted, or diffused and will determine whether there is overload or buildup of energy in the family. Newman (1983, p. 173) says that as these patterns emerge, the family's informational capacity will be increased in the nurse–client relationship. Assessment of these patterns will also reveal the family's evolving capacities, diversity, and complexity.

Consistent with Rogers's, Parse's and Newman's models is the fact that the family functions as a unitary, open, system integrated with its environment. Family functions may be organized around Anderson and Tomlinson's (1992) five realms of family experience; thus, the assessment, planning, implementation, and evaluation of the family as client by nurses practicing from any of the change/growth nursing models should reflect interactive, developmental, coping, integrity, and health processes and the relationship among all of these processes.

THE FAMILY IN THE CHANGE/STABILITY MODELS OF NURSING

This section presents a brief discussion of how the family may be viewed as the recipient of care in the nursing models in which the changes are directed toward restabilizing the client system.

King's Systems Interaction Model

King (1983, p. 179) views the family as "a social system that is seen as a group of interacting individuals." Thus, the family is an interpersonal system. In King's model, a theory of goal attainment in the family emphasizes interaction between the family members.

The major concepts in this theory of goal attainment are self, role, perception, communication, transaction, stress, growth and development, time, space, and interaction. Each of these concepts is assessed in the nursing process between the nurse and the family. Communication is the interrelating factor among these concepts. Nurses and families make transactions to attain goals. King says that family movement through space and time may be social (called vertical movement) or physical (called geographic mobility). She also states that family roles are related to growth and development and stress in the family.

To summarize King's perception of the family as client, the nurse assesses the family situation to identify real or potential problems. The nurse "assist[s] family members in setting goals to resolve problems

[and] provide[s] relevant information to help families make decisions about those factors that detract from or enhance healthy living" (King, 1983, p. 183).

Neuman's Health Care Systems Model
A stress/adaptation-based conceptual model for family nursing is Neuman's health care systems model. The nurse practicing with this model can modify assessment strategies to plan, implement, and evaluate primary, secondary, and tertiary interventions with families.

According to Neuman (1983, p. 241), "the concept of family as a system can be viewed as individual family members harmonious in their relationships—a cluster of related meanings and values that govern the family and keep it viable in a constantly changing environment." Stability is considered to represent the wellness state, instability the illness state, and transition the mixed wellness–illness state. The role of the nurse is "to control vigorously factors affecting the family, with special goal-directed activities toward facilitating stability within the system" (Neuman, 1983, p. 243). To understand influences on the stability of the family system, Neuman (1983, pp. 239–253) proposes the following points:

1. The nurse must deal with individual family member needs in terms of their developmental age, developmental state, their individual differences (their strengths and weaknesses), and environmental influences according to their perceptions of events.
2. The nurse must determine the structure and process of the family by studying the values and interaction patterns. The significant values and interaction patterns are the decision-making process (how power is distributed); coping style (how differences are negotiated in relation to stress); role relationships (the controlling or facilitating effects of roles in meeting individual and family needs); communication styles and interactions patterns (congruence of verbal and nonverbal messages and the effects of situational or entrenched defense mechanisms in the family); goals (the sharing and supporting of concerns and feelings between members); boundaries (rules that define the type of behaviors that are acceptable or unacceptable to the family); socialization process (the adequacy of resources to support cultural and structural factors in meeting family needs); individuation (the quality of individuality of each family member that defines the wellness or stability of the unit); and sharing (an index for family stability).
3. The nurse must facilitate the meeting of family needs by intervening in the intrafamily stressors (all things occurring within the family unit), the interfamily stressors (all things occurring between the family and the immediate environment), and extrafamily stressors (all things occurring between the family and distal or indirect external environment). These interventions occur as primary prevention, secondary prevention, or tertiary prevention.

Tomlinson and Anderson (1995) have described five areas of interface between Neuman's systems model and a general family health system paradigm:

1. Complexity of the system—"need to consider not only the individual stressor response in relation to the family but also the family's response relative to lines of defense and resistance" (pp. 138-139).

2. Conceptualization of the core of the family—"the core of the family is composed of its individual members, and assessment of the family is done in relation to the dynamics of individual member contributions to the whole within their environmental interactive context . . . [in comparison] the core of the family system is viewed as the interface of its members in interaction with the environment" (p. 139).

3. Goal of family health—"Neuman's central concern is to facilitate optimal client system stability or wellness in the face of change . . . [in comparison] from a family health system perspective, it is most desirable to facilitate family system wellness using strengths to reduce stressor effects and enhance family growth toward positive transformation" (p. 140).

4. Entry point in caring for families—the family becomes partners in health care. "According to Neuman, nursing functions to conserve system energy" (p. 140).

5. Nursing interaction—in the Neuman model, "the nurse role creates an explicit cooperative alliance with the client . . . [in comparison] based on a family systems perspective . . . in the family caregiving situation there may be considerable boundary ambiguity" (p. 141).

The nurse's prevention activities are the heart of Neuman's model of care. Primary preventions are those activities aimed at preventing stressors from invading the family. Secondary preventions are those protective activities following stressor invasion. Tertiary prevention are those activities during the family's reconstitution from stressors. All of these preventions are aimed at reestablishing stability within the family.

Roy's Adaptation Model

Roy's adaptation model can be used by the nurse dealing with the family as client. Roy (1983) believes that the family as an adaptive system can be analyzed, and that interventions can be organized around enhancing stimuli to the family.

Inputs for family include individual needs and changes within members and among members, and external changes in the environment. These inputs serve as focal stimuli for the family system. Processes handling the inputs are the control and feedback mechanisms. The control mechanisms—supporting, nurturing, and socializing—serve as contextual and residual stimuli to the family system. The feedback mechanisms are the transactional patterns and member control.

Outputs of the family system are the behaviors manifested. Roy (1983) has chosen three goals as proposed output of the adaptive family system: (1) survival, (2) continuity (role function), and (3) growth (the system's self-concept). At the current stage of development, Roy (1983, p. 275) simply says that "family behavior can be observed as it relates to the general family goals of survival, continuity, and growth."

The nurse observes for the outputs of survival, continuity, and growth and for the transactional and member controls that serve as feedback to the family to signal the need to adjust the behavior of a member or the group. Nursing practice emerges from the assessment of the previously described family factors. The nursing process continues to:

1. Identify and validate with family members the factor that is most immediately affecting their behavior
2. Identify individual family member needs as focal stimuli
3. Make nursing diagnoses and set goals
4. Intervene to enhance stimuli configuration in the family

Friedman (1992, p. 61) supports Roy's suggestion that "nursing problems involve ineffective coping mechanisms, which cause ineffective responses, disrupting the integrity of the person" and suggests that "this notion could easily be broadened to the family unit, where ineffective family coping patterns lead to family functioning problems." Whall and Fawcett (1991, p. 24) acknowledge the potential contribution of Roy's model of nursing care to care of the family as an adaptive system, but note that "theories of family adaptation and nursing practice theories of family need to be generated and tested." Family adaptation theories need to be elaborated by identifying specific and concrete inputs, processes, and outputs of the family system.

It can be clearly seen that the family as client rather than context is a significant new conceptual basis for nursing. Although the attribution "of wellness and illness to the family unit is a recent phenomenon" (Gilliss et al., 1989, p. 5), we anticipate that an eclectic view of family incorporating both the nursing conceptual models and other social systems approaches will continue to be refined.

Nurse leaders already are integrating approaches to caregiving with families. Examples for further study are Friedman's (1992) structural–functional model, and Wright and Leahey's (1994) Calgary family assessment model. Although these models are not specific to a particular nurse theorist, they are not inconsistent with elements of many of the theories. The structure provided by Anderson and Tomlinson (1992), cited earlier in this chapter, serves as an eclectic model for the implementation of caregiving in nursing according to nursing's conceptual models. The conceptual models derived from the change/growth paradigm probably will exhibit a better fit with these five realms of family experience than will the models derived from the change/stability paradigm.

◎ The Community as Client

In this book, the emerging philosophy of the community is that it is a so-cial system with open communication networks between structural and functional subsystems and the greater societal systems. Vertical bureau-cratic relationships tie the community to the larger society. A community always has a sense of common identification, even if it does not exist as a common geographic location. Thus, the boundaries of a community can be determined in terms of role relationships as well as geography. As with all open systems, the nurse influences change in the community. The change is directed toward higher levels of wellness in the system.

Several concepts from community health nursing are basic to the care of the community as client (Capuzzi, 1996, p. 358):

- Health promotion—improving the well-being of the community
- Risk—probability that the community will be affected by a health problem
- Disease prevention—protection of the population from diseases and disabilities and their consequences
- Primary prevention—preventing the occurrence of health problems
- Secondary prevention—activities to identify and treat health prob-lems early
- Tertiary prevention—activities to correct health problems and pre-vent further deterioration

DEFINITIONS OF COMMUNITY

Because community has been thought of primarily as a setting for care, it is important to explore the various definitions of community to determine how the community may be seen as a client for nursing services. Shaman-sky and Pesznecker (1991) identify no less than 100 definitions for the term *community*. Clark (1996, p. 6) defines a community as a "group of people who share some type of bond, who interact with each other, and who function collectively regarding common concerns." From a nursing perspective, Hanchett (1988, p. 7) says that community can be considered as an aggregate, a system, or as a human–environmental field: "As an ag-gregate, the individual is the basic unit of the community; that is, the com-munity is a number of separate individuals." As a system, one must consider the "relationships among the individuals or groups who consti-tute the community" (Hanchett, 1988, p. 8). As a human–environment field, the community represents a human field integral with its environ-ment and "manifesting correlates of the patterning of that field process" (Hanchett, 1988, p. 8).

If the nurse views the community as an aggregate, then nursing is really organized around the concept of the community serving as a context for individuals. Clark (1996, p. 56) defines community health nursing as "a synthesis of nursing knowledge and practice and the science and practice of public health, implemented via systematic use of the nursing process and other processes, designed to promote health and prevent illness in population groups. The focus of care is the aggregate." Clark (1996, p. 57) indicates that community health nursing is characterized by the following attributes:

Health orientation—health promotion and prevention of disease rather than cure of illness

Population focus—emphasis on aggregates rather than individuals or families

Autonomy—greater control of health care decisions

Continuity—continuing comprehensive care rather than on a short-term, episodic basis

Collaboration—nurse and client interacting as equals

Interactivity—awareness of interaction of a variety of factors with health

Public accountability—accountability to society for public health

Sphere of intimacy—greater awareness of the reality of client lives and situations

Christensen and Kenney (1990) have proposed a comprehensive model for implementing the nursing process focusing on the aggregate within the context of a geopolitical environment.

Zotti, Brown, and Stotts (1996, p. 211) differentiate between community-based nursing and community health nursing. *Community-based nursing* "means a philosophy of nursing that guides nursing care provided for individuals, families, and groups wherever they are, including where they live, work, play, or go to school." In contrast, *community health nursing* "represents a systematic process of delivering nursing care to improve the health of an entire community" (Zotti et al., 1996, p. 212). Characteristics of community-based nursing and community health nursing are compared in Table 13-1.

Bullough and Bullough (1990, p. 19) prefer to use the term "community health nursing" for preventive services, and the term "home health nursing care" for the work of nurses providing direct care to individual clients in their homes. They define community health nursing as the delivery of nursing services to population groups, families, and individuals in the community setting. The population groups are aggregates of people who share a common identity or have common interests.

If nurses view the community as a system, then they seek to introduce changes in the community systems and base interventions on their understanding of the impact of these changes on system functioning (Spradley, 1990). Christensen and Kenney (1990) have also proposed a general systems assessment model for directing the nursing process with families. Considerable work on viewing the community as a system that is the recipient of nursing care has emerged from Neuman's conceptual model of

TABLE 13-1

Community-Based Nursing Compared With Community Health Nursing

Component	Community-Based Nursing	Community Health Nursing
Goals	Manage acute or chronic conditions	Preserve/protect health
	Promote self-care	Promote self-care
Client	Individual and family	Community
Underlying philosophy	Human ecological model	Primary health care
Autonomy	Individual and family autonomy	Community autonomy
		Individual rights may be sacrificed for good of the community
Client character	Across the life span	Across the life span, with emphasis on high-risk aggregates
Cultural diversity	Culturally appropriate care of individual and families	Collaboration with and mobilization of diverse groups and communities
Type of service	Direct	Direct and indirect
Home visiting	Home visitor	Home visitor
Service focus	Local community	Local, state, federal, and international

From Zotti, M. E., Brown, P., & Stotts, R. C. (1996). Community-based nursing versus community health nursing: What does it all mean? *Nursing Outlook, 44,* 212. With permission of the publisher.

nursing. This model is discussed later in this chapter. Hanchett (1988) postulates that Roy's adaptation model of nursing and King's general system framework also offer the nurse the opportunity to practice nursing with the community as a client system, in which the focus is on the pattern of relationships among the elements of the system.

Following are brief discussions of a *systems* model of community as client based on Neuman's conceptual model, in which change is directed toward restoring stability to the system; and a *human field/environment* model of community as client based on Rogerian nursing science, in which change is directed toward increasing capacities and evolving growth. In both models, the emphasis is on health promotion and the characteristics of space, interaction, and population (McCarthy, 1990, p. 134). The community has geographic and interactional aspects in both models.

A SYSTEMS MODEL OF VIEWING THE COMMUNITY AS CLIENT

Anderson, McFarlane and Helton (1986) adapted the Neuman health care systems model in an effort to provide a way for nurses to conceive of the community as the recipient of care. This effort was their way of synthesizing public health with nursing. In their systems approach, the community has eight subsystems:

1. Recreation
2. Safety and transportation
3. Communication

4. Education
5. Health and social services
6. Economics
7. Politics and government
8. The physical environment

The boundaries of a community are generally geopolitical. The interactive nature of these eight subsystems result in a whole that is more than the sum of its parts. Other nurse leaders have expanded views on this model in terms of the nursing process (Christensen & Kenney, 1990). For example, Beddome (1995) stresses the need to clearly define the client system that is the target of data collection and nursing intervention (geopolitical or aggregate).

The application of Neuman's model to the development of the nursing process with the community as the recipient of care is built around the redefinition of person, environment, health, and nursing. Anderson and coworkers (1986) define the person/community as "all persons who reside within a defined geopolitical boundary or who share a common characteristic" (Saucier, 1991, p. 59). They redefine the environment to include all conditions, circumstances, and influences that affect the development of the community. Health is equated with competence to function and "a definable state of equilibrium in which subsystems are in harmony so that the whole can perform at its maximum potential" (Saucier, 1991, p. 59).

Nurses participate in the care of the community by participating in community assessment; identifying and diagnosing problems amenable to nursing interventions; planning for and implementing interventions that enhance the interacting forces within the system; and evaluating the outcomes of the interventions on the community's health.

Perhaps the most significant contribution of this model (Anderson et al., 1986) to the care of the community is the focus on prevention. Primary prevention strategies for the professional nurse include (Saucier, 1991, p. 64):

1. Increasing the public's awareness of health problems
2. Increasing the public's knowledge of the available community resources and services to resolve the problems
3. Preparing the public to self-refer to appropriate resources
4. Preparing the public to become involved in preventing the factors that lead to the problem

Secondary prevention strategies include facilitating people to do self-screening and to refer people to appropriate community resources. Tertiary prevention strategies include lobbying for adequate services and resources to meet the particular community health problems. An example is "health care reform by rethinking health policy and writing new health legislation at many levels of government" (Beddome, 1995, p. 571).

Adding the perspective of planned change to the Anderson, McFarlane, and Helton model may assist in the further development of that model.

McCarthy (1990) suggests that the assessed community be analyzed by reviewing the health clues from the emerging structures and patterns, delineating the strengths and concerns of the community, and finally validating a nursing diagnosis of the community. The population structure includes as a minimum requirement the total population in terms of age and gender. The patterns include health perception patterns derived from interviews and measurement data, value and belief patterns derived from interview data, role and relationship patterns derived from media data, and coping and stress tolerance patterns derived from both interview and observational data (McCarthy, 1990, p. 150).

A HUMAN FIELD/ENVIRONMENT MODEL OF VIEWING COMMUNITY AS CLIENT

From the paradigm of nursing in which change is directed toward growth, the following brief discussion uses the Rogerian framework for viewing the community as client.

Hanchett (1988, p. 128) says that, in this view, the community is seen as an energy field in process with the environmental energy field, and health is viewed as the dynamic well-being of the community–environmental process. Manifestations of these energy fields in process may be reflected in visible expressions such as motion, rhythms of quiet and activity, and the togetherness of the community people in participating in change.

For example, motion that is observable by the nurse is the speed of persons and traffic in daily life. Rhythms of quiet and activity may be seen in the sleep–wake patterns of the community. Everyone has heard about how the streets are "rolled up at night" in some communities. Gatherings of people in community settings can be observed to analyze togetherness. Other pattern manifestations of this energy process include the "number of cultural and ethnic groups of the community, the variety of lifestyles and ideas that flourish, and the pragmatic, imaginative, and visionary approaches to change evidenced by the community" (Hanchett, 1988, p. 129).

The goal of nursing is to help the community achieve maximum well-being. According to Hanchett (1988), this is done by the nurse participating in the process of change, assisting community groups to move toward well-being. Rogers's definition of health as "dynamic well-being" means that the community must become more aware of factors that maximize well-being, and minimize conditions that limit actualization or realization of full potential.

This view of health directs the actions of the nurse in this model. These actions all center around facilitating persons to become more aware of their patterns of energy exchange with the environment, and the evolving outcomes of these exchanges. Manifestations of field patterning include "diversity, rhythms, motion, the experience of time, sleep–wake and beyond-waking states, and pragmatic, imaginative, and visionary approaches to conscious participation in change" (Hanchett, 1988, p. 128).

The nurse attempts to facilitate evolutionary change in the human field/environmental field process from lesser diversity, longer rhythms, slower motion, experiencing time as slower, pragmatic foci, and longer sleeping to greater diversity, rhythms that seem continuous, motion that seems continuous, experiencing time as timelessness, visionary foci, and longer waking, perhaps even beyond waking (Hanchett, 1988, p. 127).

The essence of this model for community nursing is that the community as group/environmental field process determines the health of the community. In each community, the process unfolds at a unique pace and in unique patterns. The community's health is an expression of the mutually evolving process. Nursing's approaches to enhance the well-being of people/environment speak of community well-being. Influencing public policies to provide improved shelter, food, and clothing for all people are examples of approaches to improve community well-being. Nursing is "the science that the art of nursing uses in the conscious participation in the human–environmental field process toward the goal of maximum well-being" (Hanchett, 1988, p. 132).

In the Rogerian model of nursing, the community field/environmental field process integrates all other definitions of community; that is, it validates the community as a social system, as a place (space), and as a people. The resultant health of the client system (community) is more than the sum of these identified parts. Well-being is an integral process in which human beings/environment evolve toward greater awareness of their being. Respect for both diversity and sameness in patterns of energy exchange is essential for the professional nurse to operate out of this conceptual model of nursing.

It is evident from the general nature of the discussion of this model that much research is needed to assist further development of the Rogerian model. Determining manifestations of patterning of life, identifying patterns that maximize health, and developing strategies that focus on the community field/environmental field process are necessary for fuller implementation of this model in community nursing practice in which the community is the recipient of the care.

◎ Conclusion

Conceptual models of the client-environment relationship provide frameworks to guide practice with family and community clients as well as individuals. Views of change reflected by the models underlie strategies to promote growth of the family or community, or to facilitate their return to stability.

THOUGHT QUESTIONS

1 How can the professional nurse use conceptual models to guide family and community care?

2 What are the significant differences in care when guided by change/stability or change/growth models?

3 How does care differ when family or community are considered the client in contrast to the context for care?

REFERENCES

Anderson, E., McFarlane, J., & Helton, A. (1986). Community-as-client: A model for practice. *Nursing Outlook, 34,* 220.

Anderson, K. H., & Tomlinson, P. S. (1992, Spring). The family health system as an emerging paradigmatic view for nursing. *Image 24,* 57–63.

Artinian, N. T. (1994). Selecting a model to guide family assessment. *Dimensions of Critical Care Nursing, 14,* 4–12.

Beddome, G. (1995). Community-as-client assessment: A Neuman-based guide for education and practice. In B. Neuman (Ed.). *The Neuman systems model* (3rd ed., pp. 567–575). East Norwalk, CT: Appleton & Lange.

Bullough, B., & Bullough, V. (1990). *Nursing in the community.* St. Louis: Mosby.

Capuzzi, C. (1996). Families and community health nursing. In S. M. H. Hanson & S. T. Boyd (Eds.). *Family health care nursing: Theory, practice, and research* (pp. 351–368). Philadelphia: Davis.

Christensen, P. J., & Kenney, J. W. (1990). *Nursing process: Application of conceptual models* (3rd ed.). St. Louis: Mosby.

Clark, M. J. (1996). *Nursing in the community* (2nd ed.). Stamford, CT: Appleton & Lange.

Cody, W. K. (1995). The view of family within the human becoming theory. In R. R. Parse (Ed.). *Illuminations: The human becoming theory in practice and research* (pp. 9–26). New York: National League for Nursing.

Fawcett, J. F., (1989). *Analysis and evaluation of conceptual models of nursing* (2nd ed.). Philadelphia: Davis.

Forchuk, C., & Dorsay, J. P. (1995). Hildegard Peplau meets family systems nursing: Innovation in theory-based practice. *Journal of Advanced Nursing, 21,* 110–115.

Friedman, M. M. (1992). *Family nursing: Theory and practice* (3rd ed.). East Norwalk, CT: Appleton & Lange.

Friedemann, M. L. (1995). *The framework of systemic organization.* Thousand Oaks, CA: Sage.

Gilliss, C. L. (1991, Spring). Family nursing research, theory and practice. *Image, 23,* 19–22.

Gilliss, C. L., Highley, B. L., Roberts, B. M., & Martinson, I. M. (1989). *Toward a science of family nursing.* Reading, MA: Addison-Wesley.

Hanchett, E. S. (1988). *Nursing frameworks and community as client.* East Norwalk, CT: Appleton & Lange.

Hanson, S. M. H. (1996). Family assessment and intervention. In S. M. H. Hanson & S. T. Boyd (Eds.). *Family health care nursing: Theory, practice, and research* (pp. 147–172). Philadelphia: Davis.

Hanson, S. M. H., & Boyd, S. T. (1996). *Family health care nursing: Theory, practice, and research.* Philadelphia: Davis.

King, I. M. (1983). King's theory of nursing. In I. W. Clements & F. B. Roberts (Eds.). *Family health: A theoretical approach to nursing care.* New York: Wiley.

Lapp, C. A., Diemert, C. A., & Enestredt, R. (1991). Family-based practice. In K. A. Saucier. Perspectives in family and community health (pp. 305–310). St. Louis: Mosby-Year Book.

McCarthy, N. C. (1990). Health promotion and the community. In C. L. Edelman & C. L. Mandle (Eds.). *Health promotion throughout the Lifespan* (2nd ed.). St. Louis: Mosby.

McCubbin, M. A., & McCubbin, H. I. (1993). Families coping with illness: The resiliency model of family stress, adjustment, and adaptation. In C. B. Danielson, B. Hamel-Bissell, & P. Winstead-Fry (Eds.). *Families, health, and illness: Perspectives on coping and intervention* (pp. 21–63). St. Louis: Mosby.

McGoldrick, M., & Gerson, R. (1985). *Genograms in family assessment.* New York: Norton.

Mischke, K. M., & Hanson, S. M. H. (1995). Family health assessment and intervention. In P. J. Bomar (Ed.). *Nurses and family health promotion: Concepts, assessment, and interventions* (2nd ed.). Philadelphia: Saunders.

Neuman, B. (1983). Family interventions using the Betty Neuman health-care systems model. In I. W. Clements & F. B. Roberts (Eds.). *Family health: A theoretical approach to nursing care.* New York: Wiley.

Newman, M. A. (1983). Newman's health theory. In I. W. Clements & F. B. Roberts (Eds.). *Family health: A theoretical approach to nursing care.* New York: Wiley.

Newman, M. A., Sime, A. M., & Corcoran-Perry, S. A. (1991). The focus of the discipline of nursing. *Advances in Nursing Science, 14,* 1–6.

Orem, D. E. (1983). The self-care deficit theory of nursing: A general theory. In I. W. Clements & F. B. Roberts FB (Eds.): *Family health: A theoretical approach to nursing care.* New York: Wiley.

Rogers, M. E. (1983). Science of unitary human beings: A paradigm for nursing. In I. W. Clements & F. B. Roberts (Eds.). *Family health: A theoretical approach to nursing care.* New York: Wiley.

Roy, C. (1983). Roy adaptation model. In I. W. Clements & F. B. Roberts, Family health: A theoretical approach to nursing care (pp. 255–278). New York: John Wiley & Sons.

Saucier, K. A. (1991). *Perspectives in family and community health.* St. Louis: Mosby-Year Book.

Shamansky, S. L., & Pesznecker, B. (1991). A community is . . . . In B. W. Spradley (Ed.). *Readings in community health nursing.* Philadelphia: Lippincott.

Spradley, B. W. (1990). *Community health nursing: Concepts and practice* (3rd ed.). Glenview, IL: Scott, Foresman/Little Brown Higher Education.

Taylor, S. G., & Renpenning, K. M. (1995). The practice of nursing in multiperson situations, family and community. In D. E. Orem (Ed.). *Nursing: Concepts of practice* (5th ed., pp. 348–367). St. Louis: Mosby.

Tomlinson, P. S., & Anderson, K. H. (1995). Family health and the Neuman systems model. In B. Neuman (Ed.). *The Neuman systems model* (3rd ed., pp. 133–144). East Norwalk, CT: Appleton & Lange.

Whall, A. L. (1986). *Family therapy theory for nursing: Four approaches.* East Norwalk, CT: Appleton-Century-Crofts.

Whall, A. L., & Fawcett, J. (1991). *Family theory development in nursing: State of the science and art.* Philadelphia: Davis.

Wright, L. M., & Leahey, M. (1988). *Family nursing trends in academic and clinical settings.* Paper prepared for International Family Nursing Conference, Convention Centre, Calgary, Alberta, Canada, May 24–27, 1988, Conference Proceedings, pp. 29–37.

Wright, L. M., & Leahey, M. (1994). *Nurses and families: A guide to family assessment and intervention* (2nd ed.). Philadelphia: Davis.

Zotti, M. E., Brown, P., & Stotts, R. C. (1996). Community-based nursing versus community health nursing: What does it all mean? *Nursing Outlook, 44,* 211–217.

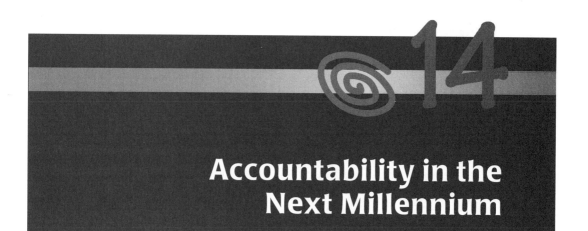

Accountability in the Next Millennium

LEARNING OUTCOMES

By the end of this chapter, the student will be able to:

1. Know what differentiates accountability from autonomy and authority.

2. Understand the essential questions the professional nurse must answer to be accountable to the client and public.

3. Describe the relationship between the educational level of the practitioner of nursing and accountability in practice.

4. List some current developments in nursing and health care that demonstrate an increased emphasis on accountability now and for the future.

5. Appreciate some of the positive outcomes of the nurse becoming accountable to clients, profession, self, employing institution, managed care networks, and third-party payers.

6. Evaluate oneself on accountability, using the checklist provided.

Chapter author: Susan E. Gordon, R.N., Ed.D.

Accountability is a concept that has been present in nursing for a long time, although the use of the word itself is relatively recent. In its simplest sense, accountability is synonymous with responsibility and, in this regard, permeates the writing of Florence Nightingale. When she discusses the nurse's responsibility for the state of the sick room (Nightingale, 1859, p. 45) or the need for careful observation on the part of the nurse to avoid patient accidents (Nightingale, 1859, p. 66), or the fact that "I have often seen really good nurses distressed, because they could not impress the doctor with the real danger of their patients" (Nightingale, 1859, p. 68), she is expressing the responsibility or accountability of that nurse to the patient.

Perhaps the epitome of the accountable nurse is the private-duty nurse of the past, who took a "case" and remained with it until the patient had no further need of nursing care. The patient was very much this nurse's responsibility and, in turn, the nurse was very much in charge of and accountable for the nursing care, life, and space of that patient.

However, after the Depression of the 1930s, the percentage of nurses choosing private-duty nursing decreased; more turned to staff nursing (Dachelet & Sullivan, 1979, p. 15) with its highly functional orientation at that time. Accountability became harder to pinpoint, with the care of the individual patient split among several different nurses and support staff. Accountability became limited to the provision of isolated treatments, any of which, if overlooked or performed improperly, might have severe repercussions for the nurse.

The notion of accountability, therefore, became tied to negative situations and picked up a punative connotation. Nurses were legally liable for their actions or the omission of necessary actions but often were unaware of this. The belief of many was that the ultimate liability remained with the institution, which would "cover" them in the event of a lawsuit. Accountability in a professional sense was not functioning and the entire concept certainly had no positive attributes as far as the individual nurse was concerned. This has remained the situation until relatively recently (Clifford, 1981, p. 20).

In the 1980s, there was an increased interest in accountability. Now, at the turn of the century, accountability has come to the forefront and assumed an importance and visibility it never before possessed. Why is accountability the byword of the future for the nursing profession? Why was it added in 1980 to the subject headings in the *Cumulative Index of Nursing and Allied Health Literature*? Why is it the subject of countless articles (Silver, 1986) and workshops? What evidence is seen today demonstrating the emerging centrality of the concept of accountability? Why is it so inextricably caught up with the emerging professional status of nursing?

◎ Definition of Accountability and Related Concepts

Before embarking on the answers to the above and other questions, it is necessary to define the word *accountability*. It is a term that is increasingly confused with and used in place of autonomy and authority, although it is synonymous with neither, but related to both (Batey & Lewis, 1982, p. 13). The meaning of this trio of terms must be clarified.

RESPONSIBLITY AND ANSWERABILITY

Accountability continues to retain its original meaning of responsibility but has an added dimension, that of answerability, the necessity of offering answers and explanations to certain others. That answerability can be to the public, to the other members of one's profession and allied professions, to the agency in which one is employed, to managed care networks, to third-party payers, and to oneself. As the American Nurses Association (ANA) Code for Nurses states, this accountability

> refers to being answerable to someone for something one has done. It means providing an explanation to self, to the client, to the employing agency, and to the nursing profession. (ANA, 1985)

An additional dimension of accountability is its reporting aspect, embodied in the following definition:

> (accountability is). . . the fulfillment of a formal obligation to disclose to referent others the purposes, principles, procedures, relationships, results, income and expenditures for which one has authority. This disclosure is systematic, periodic, and carried out in consistent form . . . . Initiating the disclosure is the responsibility of the one accountable and not of others. (Batey, 1982, p. 10)

In today's language this refers to the relationship between interventions (the care given), outcomes (results), and cost (expenditures), which is in the forefront of so many current discussions of accountability (Wilson, 1996, pp. 24–28).

Today, greater emphasis is placed on the documentation aspect of accountability than ever before. Because of legal factors, as well as the requirements of accrediting organizations, third-party payers, and managed care networks, nurses are being held accountable and liable based on the evidence found or not found in their reporting or documentation.

Accountability, then, is the state of being responsible and answerable for those behaviors and their outcomes that are included in one's professional role, as it is reflected in the periodic written reporting of those behaviors and their outcomes.

AUTONOMY AND AUTHORITY

In distinction to this, *autonomy* refers to the independence of functioning. Autonomy means that one can perform one's total professional function on the basis of one's own knowledge and judgment, and further, that one is recognized by others as having the right to do so. Obviously, this concept is related to accountability, as one who functions autonomously must be accountable for his or her behavior (Holden, 1991, p. 398; Hylka & Shugrue, 1991, p. 55).

The last of these three terms is authority. *Authority* can be defined as being in a position to make decisions and to influence others to act in a manner determined by those decisions. Again, this term is certainly related to accountability because those who are in authority are accountable for the decisions they make and for the actions of themselves and others who act on the basis of their decisions. Further, authority is related to autonomy because those in authority often act autonomously in performing all or part of their respective roles.

One can see these relationships further developed in the nursing literature. According to Batey:

> Responsibility, authority, autonomy, and accountability are inextricably related. Responsibility and authority are necessary conditions for both autonomy and accountability. It is illogical and inappropriate for an organization to hold a department or an individual accountable for those activities over which the department or individual has no authority . . . . Autonomy within the areas in which nursing service has responsibility is also a necessary condition for accountability . . . . Accountability is an exercise in futility and an experience in failure unless it is linked to nursing service's autonomy. The process of fulfilling nursing's formal obligation to disclose requires that nursing services have the formal and legitimate power to carry out relevant actions. Without the opportunity to make binding decisions, accountability is a hollow concept. (Batey, 1982, p. 13)

Bergman sees this relationship somewhat differently by considering responsibility and authority (along with ability) as preconditions leading to accountability. As she states:

> The basic precondition is to have the ability . . . to decide and act on a specific issue. One must be given or take, the responsibility to carry out that action. Next, one needs the authority, i.e. formal backing, legal right to carry the responsibility. Then, with the preconditions, one can be accountable for the action one takes. (Bergman, 1981, pp. 54–55)

Webb, Price, and Van Ess Coeling (1996) discuss the relationship of accountability and several other concepts in a more contemporary forum:

> The professional elements of practice are authority, accountability, responsibility and decision-making; therefore, the professional nurse is described as one who is autonomous and who desires responsibility and accountability. (Webb et al., 1996, p. 29)

What can be seen developing here, then, is a grouping of concepts, all related but not synonymous, projecting an image of a responsible, independent individual, who is able to make decisions and influence others to act on them, and who is answerable for his or her behavior and the behavior of associates. This image is clearly that toward which the profession of nursing is striving for its members, and provides part of the reason for the current upsurge in interest and relevance of the concept of accountability.

As the selected watchword for the International Council of Nurses for the quadrennium 1977 to 1981, "accountability" is an inherent part of the image of the professional nurse of the 1980s and beyond (Bergman, 1981, p. 54). This was reiterated in 1996 by Donnelly (1997), who stated, "Accountability is the watchword of the day." In fact, it is part of the image of any professional person. Accountability is a necessary attribute in all those who wish to exercise authority and act autonomously—and this characterizes nurses today.

Accountability of a Profession

As nursing has come closer to being a true profession, it is to be expected that its concern with accountability has increased. Accountability has always been acknowledged as one of the hallmarks of a profession. This view is supported in Flexner's work characterizing a profession, in which he indicates that a profession is likely to be more responsive to public interest than are unorganized and isolated individuals (Flexner, 1915).

In terms of nursing's involvement with its own professionalization in the 1950s and 1960s, it is evident in the conviction of Bixler and Bixler (1959, p. 1142) that a profession functions autonomously in the formulation of professional policy and in the control of professional activity. McGlothlin explains that a profession undertakes tasks that require exercise of judgment in applying knowledge to the solutions of problems, and accepts responsibility for the results (McGlothlin, 1961, p. 214). Today, other emerging professions such as social work and medical records professionals are addressing the issue of accountability (Abramson, 1984, pp. 35–43; Thompson, 1988, p. 59).

However, to be accountable, a profession must know that for which it is accountable. To do this, the profession must establish professional standards and attempt to enforce them. The ANA, nursing's major professional organization, has, in fact, done this, with its *Standards of Nursing Practice, Service, and Education.* In doing so it has complied with one of the functions of a professional organization, according to Merton (1958, p. 50), that is, of providing the means by which members of the profession can judge the competency of its members. Through its standards, the ANA has contributed greatly to the ability of the nursing profession to be accountable.

By using the *Standards of Nursing Practice* (ANA, 1991a) as a guide, the individual nurse can see, clearly laid out, the scope and the limits of practice. Nurses can internalize that for which they are accountable. In addition, a nursing service organization can monitor its collective accountability.

This monitoring has, in fact, increased radically in the last 10 years, through the introduction of systematic nursing quality assurance activities with active participation by staff nurses, in many institutions and agencies. The recent mandate by the Joint Commission on Accreditation of Health-care Organizations (JCAHO) indicating that quality assurance programs are requisite for accreditation, has hastened the process of operationalizing the concept of accountability as quality assurance at the nursing service department level (JCAHO, 1991, p. 94).

Nurses have another document to guide them in practice, the Code for Nurses, also developed by the ANA. More in the nature of an ethical code, this provides a clear framework within which the nurse can seek to uphold the standards of care. Should there be any further doubt about accountability of the nursing profession, the Code lays this to rest by confronting the issue head on. As stated in item 4 of the code, "The nurse assumes responsibility and accountability for individual nursing judgments and actions" (ANA, 1985).

Other items in the code do not address the area of accountability directly but, by discussing various factors that are necessary underpinnings for accountability, indirectly support the concept. These factors include the presumed competence of the nurse, use of informed judgment, and participation in nursing research.

It should be apparent by this point that nursing is accountable as a profession and that its individual practitioners are accountable as well. It has been implied throughout this discussion that nurses are accountable to the public and to the profession itself. Additionally, with most nurses remaining employed by health care agencies, rather than being independently employed, one must also consider the area of accountability to the institution (Copp, 1988, p. 42; Vaughn, 1989, p. 4). In the present climate of cost control, the notion of accountability to managed care networks and third-party payers of health care has emerged. Finally, in light of current emphases on self-actualization and growth, it is important to add that the professional nurse must be accountable to oneself as well.

ACCOUNTABILITY TO THE CLIENT AND PUBLIC

A profession exists to provide service to the public. Although it may be intellectually stimulating, gratifying, and exciting to a professional to perform a role, ultimately the reason for that role lies in its relationship with the public. Therefore, almost by definition, a profession must be accountable to that public. The consumer has the right to receive the best possible quality of care, care grounded in a firm knowledge base and performed by those who can make use of that knowledge base through the application of sound judgment and a clear and appropriate value system.

As consumers are becoming more knowledgeable through formal education and access to informal education as provided by a vast array of mixed media, they are able to know more about what the professions are supposed to be doing. They are able to demand more, and to make those demands more effectively and visibly.

Nursing must be aware of this increased consumer knowledge and sophistication, and must be prepared to respond to it in an equally knowledgeable and sophisticated manner. The nurse must be able to demonstrate clearly those principles and concepts on which practice is based. The nurse must be able to demonstrate an ability to call into play a problem-solving method to properly use those principles and concepts. The nurse must be able to evaluate the outcomes of care to determine if goals have been met, and be able to alter interventions if the goals have not yet been achieved.

The nurse must know the importance of documenting all work and the processes used in accomplishing goals, and the place served in the demonstration of abilities by this documentation. The nurse must be able to formulate and present to others the bases for the judgment exercised in the performance of the role by indicating the depth and breadth of nursing science and of educational preparation.

Nurses must be able to formulate and present to others the ethical code or value system to which they refer when making judgments and using their knowledge base. They must be able to answer the questions from consumers and others of "Why did you do that?," and "How did you come to that decision?," and "What makes you believe that is the most effective course of action?" Furthermore, they must be able to answer these questions without becoming defensive about them or about the questioner, because the consumer has the right to know and, if nurses are truly professionals, it is their responsibility to give the answers.

As a knowledgeable professional, the nurse should ultimately be accountable for health care delivery nationally (Lane, 1985). When nurses blame others such as physicians, administrators, or politicians for the state of the health care delivery system, or constantly look to others for improvement of this system, they weaken their position and power base. By accepting an appropriate degree of responsibility for the current situation and actively pursuing methods of improving it, nurses act on a more professional level and make their claim for a piece of the health care pie.

Nursing is also accountable to the public in guarding against ill-prepared coworkers being certified to give nursing care under the guise of a new category of health care worker (Wilkerson, 1988). Unlicensed assistive personnel, such as nursing technicians, are providing complex nursing care. Attempting to disguise this fact to attract potential caregivers and then to prepare them in hospital-based programs too short to do justice to the present complexities of care, and which will be at great cost to the hospitals, is simply not for the public's benefit. The quality of care is being seriously compromised. Nurses must raise their collective voice to educate and inform on this issue. There can be no doubt, they are accountable to the public.

ACCOUNTABILITY TO THE PROFESSION

The profession of nursing is exercising its accountability toward itself in the performance of its duty to formulate its own policy and control its activities. Its standards for licensure and certification, as well as those that exist for entry into a variety of professional groups and associations (such as the Association of Operating Room Nursing, the Association of Critical Care Nurses, and the American Academy of Nursing) all attest to nursing's attempts to set policy for its organization and performance. Further, the committees on professional conduct and discipline that exist on the state level, and are heavily staffed by nurses, are testimony to the profession's work in terms of controlling its activities and the work-related activities of its practitioners.

In connection with this aspect of accountability, the individual nurse must understand the necessity of being aware of and accountable for not only the nurse's own actions, but also those of colleagues. Often the professional nurse is the only one who is present to observe the behaviors of another nurse, or the only one competent to evaluate a coworker's care. Although sharing apparent evidences of poor practice or substance abuse with the appropriate authorities (within the agency or outside) may not be an attractive course of action, it is the only possible one if nursing is to strive toward ensuring quality care to all its recipients and toward functioning in a truly professional manner. Approaching the culpable individual first with the evidence of failure would serve to emphasize the observing nurse's empathy for and concern about the person, while eliminating the secrecy or spying aspect so detestable in our society.

Nurses are also accountable to the profession when they consider which educational system will prepare its members most satisfactorily for practice (and the level of entry into that professional practice). It is not enough to let nursing be buffeted by winds of change external to it or by individuals and forces outside its perimeter. The individual nurse must, through careful thought, be accountable on these crucial issues.

ACCOUNTABILITY TO SELF

Although professional people are perhaps more committed to their careers as a source of satisfaction and as a lifelong pursuit than are those who are following an occupation or who are working only to earn a living, it is now accepted that a professional life is but one aspect of life. Nurses are no longer expected to live on the premises in which they work, they are no longer expected to work most of their waking hours without time away from duties, and they are no longer considered a piece of property belonging to the agency in which they work. They are seen as free and independent persons with other aspects and facets to life beside the professional side.

However, the exigencies of the job situation often cause nurses and others to overlook these basic facts. Additionally, nurses' activities in other life roles often bear on professional performance in some way. Thus, nurses must be accountable to themselves for their own actions both on the job and off, because of the ways in which these actions will affect themselves and others.

The nurse who appears on the job still suffering the effects of too much celebrating on days off is not prepared to function in the manner expected. Fatigue, jet lag, minor illness, or the effects of alcohol or drugs make the nurse a liability rather than an asset in the work situation. Nurses who put in too much overtime; who allow themselves to be placed in a position far beyond their ability and knowledge, and are always functioning in a highly stressed state because of it; those who constantly fill in for those in the next tour who fail to show up; are not prepared to function in their social and personal life in the ways expected of them.

Significant others cannot always be expected to take second place to one's work, while work cannot always be expected to take second place to social and personal relationships. A certain balance is needed. Overdoing the amount of time and energy expected on the job will often lead to burnout, with the nurse no longer able or willing to do adequate work. This burnout can extend into the nurse's personal and social life as well, with relationships suffering (Chaska, 1983, pp. 874–875).

The nurse's accountability to self comes across clearly. Nurses must be responsible for their own mental and physical health, for ensuring that they keep all aspects of life in a balanced perspective. They must decide when to give more energy to work and when to give more energy to other areas, never sabatoging wholeness as a person by allowing one aspect of life to become overwhelming. They must be at fullest capacity when on the job and yet set a pace to avoid the staleness and despair that come when the throttle is constantly at full speed ahead.

The nurse's accountability to self includes refusing to work in situations that he or she considers unsafe. This may be by virtue of a lack of knowledge or experience of the area, or because of insufficient staffing or some other problem inherent in the situation itself. Nurses must be able to see this as ultimately of service to the consumer and the profession, although they must also be aware of the sanctions that may be applied.

Accountability to self also involves acknowledging one's own limitations and knowing when further education is needed to more fully and safely perform one's role. Decisions by others (perhaps to promote to head nurse only those with the bachelor's degree) should not be the controlling factor in this; the nurse's personal accountability is on the line here.

The nurse's accountability to self is being tested dramatically in the 1990s as those nurses infected with human immunodeficiency virus are forced to look at their place in the health care system. Able to effectively prevent transmission of the disease to their patients with the use of appropriate precaution techniques, they must use these constantly and conscientiously. However, they must also be aware of the danger to themselves of secondary infections and adjust work time, setting, and duties accordingly. In an area where accountability to the public and self overlap, they must recognize when they are too ill to continue to practice safely for either their clients or themselves.

Finally, nurses are accountable to themselves to do their own personal best (Styles, 1985). Factors outside nursing can influence this aspect of accountability. Government can aid or hinder nurses' ability to do their best through legislation, funding (or lack of it) of education and research, reimbursement policies, and health care priorities. Managed care networks and third-party payers also play a role in this area. The nurse must consider political activism a means to the end of accountability to self, as a method of bringing public policy and the most expert care into congruence.

ACCOUNTABILITY TO THE EMPLOYING AGENCY

Yet another domain of the nurse's accountability is the agency in which that nurse is employed. Contrary to the thinking of some, this is not the primary area of the nurse's accountability. Although not unimportant, accountability to the agency has received too much emphasis in the past. It more rightfully takes a back seat to the client and public, the profession, and nurses themselves—but it does have a place.

The agency is accountable to the public for the care provided under its auspices. Therefore, in turn, it has the right to expect the nurse to be accountable to that agency.

Quality of work is one aspect in which nurses must be accountable to the agency. This includes their own preparation for the job, as well as their fitness each time they appear on the job. The agency has contracted with the nurse for a specific job to be done at a specific time and place, for a specific wage. Nurses, then, must uphold their end of the bargain in all of these areas. They are accountable, as well, for the nature of peers' performance. Further, they are accountable for those over whom they have authority in the work setting (about which more will be said shortly), and must be aware of what they are doing and how they are doing it, to exercise that accountability.

Nurses must refuse to work in areas and situations that they consider unsafe. This further fulfills accountability to the agency (as well as self) because they are saying, in effect, "I will not put the agency in the position of giving unsafe care."

An additional aspect of the nurse's accountability to the agency involves the attitude toward that agency that the nurse projects to the client. The attitude should be one of objectivity and honesty. It is appropriate to promote the agency's strengths, to the extent that it has them, in a realistic manner, and not to exaggerate its shortcomings. Sometimes, in the heat of the moment, when particularly taxed or following a disagreement, the nurse may denigrate an agency to a far greater extent than is deserved. The nurse has not, then, acted maturely or accountably, and is probably unaware of the impact of such statements on the client and on the agency.

New concerns have arisen recently regarding accountability to the employer, because of a large and growing number of nurses employed by nursing agencies and then essentially "rented" to hospitals on a per diem basis. Another middleman has been introduced. What, then, is the order of accountability? Are nurses more accountable to the agency, thus diminishing some of the support they might be offering the hospital, or are they primarily accountable to the hospital, running the risk of being dropped by the agency?

Nurses have, for too long, maintained their accountability to their employing agency above their accountability to all others. This has detracted from a desirable image of nurses as working primarily in the public interest. It has, instead, fostered the impression of the nurse as being subservient to and totally under the control of the employing institution. It is time to fully recognize and implement nursing's accountability toward its primary foci: the client and public, the profession, and the self, without losing sight of the nurse's accountability toward the employing agency.

The Groundwork for Accountability

From this description of accountability, it should be evident that this quality cannot appear overnight and without adequate preparation in either a profession or its practitioners. It is necessary to provide a substantive service about which to be accountable as well as to possess a variety of skills and attributes that enable one to exercise that accountability. A definite foundation or groundwork must be laid.

RESEARCH AND THE ESTABLISHMENT OF A THEORETICAL BASE FOR NURSING

One of the major factors in the accelerating pace of nursing's movement toward professional status is the growth of its theoretical and conceptual base for practice. It is this growth that allows the nurse to be truly accountable in this technological and scientific era (Copp, 1988, p. 44). Theory-based knowledge is now available, in some instances, and will be available increasingly in others, as the result of nursing research.

However, it is not sufficient for research to be done and knowledge to be available if they are ignored by nurses in their practice. Although those involved in doing research, as well as nurses enrolled in nursing educational programs, are highly cognizant of the amount, quality, and distribution of nursing research, this is not universal among nurses.

The dissemination of the results of nursing research to those in the front lines, from whom accountability in practice is most commonly demanded, is not occurring rapidly enough. It is the rare nurse who introduces a new component into practice because of research findings. It is the rare nurse who justifies, or accounts for, actions or judgments on the basis of research findings. It is the rare supervisor or administrator who calls on those under her or his authority to institute change based on the findings of nursing research.

Among the reasons for this problem is the inability of many of these individuals to comprehend and evaluate the research studies they may read. This leads to a general "uncomfortableness" around nursing research and causes these nurses to bypass research literature altogether when planning change or implementing practice. Programs are urgently needed to help the practicing nurse understand available research reports and apply the findings to work situations. These can be provided under the auspices of staff development departments, nursing associations, continuing education departments, or degree programs, but they are a necessity.

COMPETENCE IN PRACTICE

If there is one attribute that has always been expected of professional nurses, it is that they be competent in their practice. Just what that practice encompasses has been a matter of discussion and dissension at various times, and just what the "professional" before the word nurse really means has also been hotly contended. However, everyone on all sides of these issues has always agreed that whatever it is that any type of nurse does, it must be done well.

Currently, with many levels of nursing being reflected in the makeup of the health care team, it is imperative that nurses at each level have a clear idea of the scope of practice at their level, and responsibly perform to the maximum limit of that level. The nurse's accountability may be called into question if he or she is functioning beyond the limits of a particular level. It is no more appropriate for nurses who have been educated at the baccalaureate level to restrict professional activities to those they may have exercised at the associate degree level, than it is for them to assume the role of the master's-prepared practitioner.

The key to expertise in practice lies in both knowledge and skill, a somewhat artificial distinction which, nevertheless, allows for more clarity in this discussion. Nursing has always had a strong manual skills component. To the extent that the nurse is in a role that calls for these skills, activity, gentleness, quickness, and accuracy remain hallmarks of excellence. Where the skills required are in the areas of communication, teaching, leadership, management, and research (the so-called "hands-off" skills), the matter of expertise is no less pressing.

Underlying all skills is excellence in terms of command of "nursing knowledge." Nurses can never expect to contribute significantly to health care in its assessment, planning, implementation, and evaluation aspects if they do whatever they do in a mediocre manner. Competence is an absolute prerequisite for accountability.

LEADERSHIP SKILLS

Leadership development frequently brings questions and puzzlement when first introduced to nursing students. A frequent response is, "Not everyone can be a head nurse or a supervisor, or wants to be an instructor. I don't want to be a leader; I just want to be a nurse." The fact is that, inherent in the "nurse" role, the elements of leadership are deeply imbedded.

Leadership ability is one of the most important areas in laying the groundwork for accountability. The nurse's accountability extends into the areas of health maintenance and promotion, as well as the area of promoting self-care by the ill, as long as possible. The nurse is a constant catalyst in the process of change, at this highly individual level at the very least, especially if she or he is "just" a nurse.

To satisfactorily fulfill this portion of the role, a nurse must be well versed in the theory and practice of change, which is practically synonymous with saying a nurse must be able to exercise leadership. Nurses are leaders in working with patients, their families, and significant others. They are leaders in regard to health care in contacts with friends and acquaintances in the community. They are leaders in performing and making certain that they are permitted to perform their roles as professionals involved in health promotion, maintenance, and restoration. Accountable nurses cannot function without leadership skills.

ETHICAL FRAMEWORK

Nurses are accountable within an ethical framework. They cannot be accountable in a moral vacuum. They must have as their guide standards and values in which they believe and to which they refer. To some extent these are determined by the collective values of the profession—and these in turn are partly determined by what the public expects of that profession and partly by what the profession demands of itself.

In nursing, these professional values are formalized by the Code for Nursing (ANA, 1985). However, in large measure, this ethical code is a personal one, developed in the course and context of the individual's total life experience. It includes those values learned in the home, in the schools, from social groups, during religious training, in the work setting, and from the activities and contacts of daily life. It is influenced by the nurse's ethnic and religious background, the area of the country in which he or she lives, and the nurse's own personality. It is highly individual.

A person's ethical code is often something of which he or she is relatively unaware. It is unconsciously used in making decisions and running one's life, but is rarely, if ever, pulled out and scrutinized, or even acknowledged as existing. It is this code that is so essential in the professional nurse. A nurse must be aware of his or her own code, how it affects decisions and actions, and where it is congruent with or departs from standard codes of the profession. These conflicts, then, must be worked through and compromise sought, so that the nurse can feel comfortable with and confident in the ethical basis in which the practice is rooted.

EDUCATION TO THE BACCALAUREATE AND BEYOND

It is obvious from the discussion thus far on laying the groundwork for accountability that this is neither a simple nor a short-term task. It is not one that can be accomplished in a weekend or, for most individuals, on one's own. Rather, it is a task that continues over a long period of time, during which various ideas are explored, analyzed, tested, and absorbed into the individual's makeup. It is a task that is partially contributed to, at times guided by, and discussed and shared with others. It is a task most ideally accomplished within the context of a higher education (Hegyvary, 1991, p. 8).

This educational experience should provide opportunities for the student to take responsibility and to exercise accountability. It should be an education toward an ability to make decisions and be accountable for them (Lanara, 1982, p. 10). In reviewing the areas requiring attention in the preparation for accountability, the desirability for addressing them within a baccalaureate or higher degree program in nursing becomes evident.

Although most educational programs in nursing are based on a conceptual framework, it is at the baccalaureate level that significant time is devoted to understanding some of the outstanding conceptual and theoretical frameworks for nursing practice. It is also at this level that the relationship between these frameworks and the research process is explored. The research course often included in a baccalaureate program provides an opportunity for learning how to read research, adequately evaluate it, and judge its potential applicability within a work setting. It is only after nurses can knowledgeably read and interpret research findings that they can use them to improve practice. It is at the point of usage and reference to research findings that this area of nursing activity adds immeasurably to the nurse's accountability.

Leadership truly comes into its own in the baccalaureate and higher degree program. It is here that styles of leadership behavior, health care delivery systems, the economics of health care, characteristics of bureaucracies, and change theory are explored. Here nurses who in practice may already be in leadership positions, learn how to function more effectively and more accountably in their roles, why some of their programs have succeeded and other have not, and how to inculcate greater levels of accountability in staff. It is here that they begin to learn something of the institution's accountability (or lack of it) in regard to the care they and others are providing. It is here that they will both work with and analyze the professional behavior of leaders in nursing, role models from whom they can learn accountability—for it is a learned behavior (Clifford, 1981, p. 20).

Finally, in the area of ethics and values, it is at the university level that the nurse can and is encouraged to contemplate his or her own value system, to uncover it and see its relationship to practice and to the other aspects of life. Through the liberalizing influence of baccalaureate and higher degree programs, nurses can learn of different value systems and how other nurses have sought to make their own ethical codes complementary to those of the profession.

In summary, it takes all of what the nurse is and does as a person to prepare for functioning in an accountable manner (Lanara, 1982, p. 10). It is a lifelong process engaged in with others in both structured and unstructured ways, and is interwoven with the nurse's preparation as a professional person.

Accountability in an Era of Cost Containment

The price tag associated with health care is soaring. Diagnosis-related groups are being used increasingly as the basis for payments to hospitals for patient care. Insurance costs are skyrocketing. The notion of imposing controls on these costs is also growing. Managed care is rapidly expanding to become the primary mode of delivering cost effective health care. That which is ineffective is to be decreased or discarded; that which is effective is to be increased and retained.

All too often, "effective" seems to mean "cost-effective." The idea of a universal right to top quality care for all is being diluted to a standard of adequate care to those who meet specific criteria set by the payers of care. Nurses are now asked to be accountable for the care they give, as well as for giving that care in the least expensive manner possible, and often in a setting or time frame severely limiting the comprehensiveness of that care.

THE NONLICENSED WORKER

Professional nurses have always been held accountable for the work performed by those with lower level credentials whom they supervise, such as the licensed practical nurse (LPN) and the nurse's aide (NA). In the past these, workers performed functions that, for the most part, the RN felt were within the workers' range of capability and for which their relatively short training programs had adequately prepared them. In the current climate of cost containment, however, there is an expanding infusion of unlicensed workers into areas and functions in which they have not practiced in the past. The nursing technician, nursing assistant, or NA is being "trained" to do and is performing functions that nurses are not comfortable having them perform.

There is great concern among RNs at having these workers perform "under" the RN's license, carrying out the implementation phase of many complex nursing functions, without having the concomitant assessment or evaluation skills to maintain a safe, low-risk situation. Further, there is genuine uneasiness that this will, inadvertently, be harmful to clients.

When more closely examined, however, this situation is not very different than in the past. The unlicensed worker has always worked under the supervision of a professional nurse who has always performed the assessment and evaluation aspects of care. The RN has always instructed the NA as to who needed the care and when. The RN has always been accountable for the care given.

Additionally, the NA has always been accountable for knowing how to properly perform his or her segment of assigned care and for knowing when other workers must be called into the picture, because it is beyond the limits of the NA's knowledge and training. Although the legal doctrine of *respondeat superior* is alive and well, unlicensed workers do carry some accountability of their own and always have.

Therefore, principles that have guided nursing care for years are still applicable, although perhaps with some additional caution. The RN is still accountable for the patient's overall care. However, the present does require that the RN broaden the scope of supervision and be more vigilant. The RN must be more aware of the NA's minute-to-minute activities and be more available for consultation.

The ultimate accountability the nurse carries is the same as it has always been. These are responsibilities that go along with the professional status nurses have always sought and must be made clear to every prospective nurse and new graduate, while being reinforced for those already holding the professional credential.

MANAGED CARE AND THIRD-PARTY PAYERS

Managed care is spreading throughout the United States with unbridled speed. This method of health care delivery has been seen as one that will monitor access to services, eliminate redundancy and overuse of services, and keep health care costs down. Nurses and other health care professionals are finding that the decision-making inherent in achieving these goals is impinging on their professional domains. Those without the appropriate knowledge base, or with cost containment as the driving force, are actually governing the type and amount of health care the client can receive (Leininger, 1994, pp. 94–95).

The nurse's role as a client advocate must include attention to and action in those instances where clients are being denied access to care, or seem to be short-changed by policies and actions directed primarily at cost containment (Aroskar, 1992, pp. 201–205; Stevens, 1992, pp. 185–200). The issue of access to care has been a legitimate one for nurses to address for years, as succinctly stated in the Code for Nurses:

> The nurse assumes the responsibility and accountability for individual nursing judgments and actions . . . . The nurse collaborates with members of the health professions and other citizens in promoting community and national efforts to meet the health needs of the public. (ANA, 1985)

More currently, this notion has been reiterated and emphasized by its inclusion in the ANA (1995) policy statement and agenda for health care reform (1991b). There can be no doubt that the nurse's accountability extends into exerting efforts to respond to the health care needs of the public in a collective sense.

Possible dichotomies are emerging, potential conflicts between effective, professional comprehensive nursing care and quick, inexpensive nursing care, between care for only a portion of the population or for the totality. The nurse of today is challenged to do it all. Accountability must function in all areas so as to promote the delivery of effective, professional, comprehensive, but inexpensive and fast, nursing care to all. Can nurses meet this challenge?

◎ Accountability in the Future

The future is on us. The changes being wrought by the new interest in accountability are already being seen. New directions are emerging more clearly.

Primary nursing, with its increased autonomy, demands increased accountability from its practitioners. In various forms, "modified" and "pure," sometimes tied in with other models of care, primary nursing seems likely to continue, as nurses taste the increased benefits of this more independent role, to both themselves and their clients.

Team nursing is being resurrected in some settings because the staff mix is changing to include fewer RNs and more LPNs and unlicensed personnel (Begany, 1994, p. 38). Here, too, however, professional nurses are and will be ultimately accountable for the care rendered by those they supervise.

Models of shared governance have developed, which respond to the nurse's call for increased participation and accountability (Brodbeck, 1991, p. 21). These models incorporate unit-based quality assurance activities that are the cornerstone of accountability, and further the staff nurse's autonomy (Brodbeck, 1991, p. 21).

The emphasis by the JCAHO on quality assurance, and, specifically, its goal of an outcome-oriented evaluation system in agencies under its jurisdiction, is a sure sign of the entrenchment of accountability. This emphasis denotes the recognition by the entire health care community that nurses are accountable for their practice (*American Journal of Nursing*, 1991, p. 39).

Advanced technology has provided the means for nursing to become more accountable. Nursing must clearly show what it does—the care nursing delivers, its cost and outcomes. Nursing must be rescued from burial in the category of "room and board" in budgets and on bills. The technological systems to do this already exist. Then, nursing must control its own budget because those with the financial control are typically those with the power. Only then can nursing hope to advance toward its goals of further autonomy and accountability (Simpson & Waite, 1989, p. 75).

Some are prepared for the accountability autonomy brings, but others are not. In some instances, significant shifts in attitude are necessary before this readiness exists (Holden, 1991, p. 398; Vaughn, 1991, p. 55). Education is consistently emphasized as the path to that readiness (Hegyvary, 1991, p. 8).

Nurses must ultimately decide that for which they want to be accountable. How much will nurses shoulder individually and as a group (Hegyvary, 1991, p. 8)? The concept of ownership has entered the scene. Jackson (1989, p. 4) suggests that nurses not take on problems that do not belong to nursing, but fully own up to others that are currently being avoided, and work through the means now available to improve the quality of that which is nursing's to improve. However, the recent thrust toward more multidisciplinary cooperation, planning, documentation, action, and evaluation may further cloud attempts to define that area for which nurses, and nurses alone, are truly accountable. Nursing may have to learn to be accountable within a more ambiguous, multidisciplinary framework.

◎ The Positive Aspects of Accountability

The image conjured up in the mind of the average nurse when accountability is mentioned is often a negative one, permeated with punishments, negative sanctions, reprisals, and "being called on the carpet" for tasks undone or done incorrectly (Clifford, 1981, p. 20). This is indeed an unfortunate state of affairs. Quite the contrary, accountability should be looked at as a highly positive concept, permeated with visions of respect, reward, effectiveness, control, and action. Concepts such as power, leadership, accomplishment, choice, and even professionalism are associated with it. Most fundamentally, it has been demonstrated that when nurses are given greater responsibility, quality of care seems improved (Simpson & Sears, 1985).

Nursing is striving for a voice in setting policy for health care delivery at every level, from that of the individual and institution, to those national in scope. Nursing is increasingly seeking to define the extent of its own practice and then to practice to the limits of that definition. Nurses act as vice presidents of hospitals, influence legislators in Washington, determine what kind of teaching their patients should receive, and decide when beds must be closed because of inadequate staffing. But to have the autonomy, the authority, and the power to make these kinds of decisions and perform these kinds of activities, nurses must be ready to be accountable.

Nurses must be willing to allow "the buck to stop with them." They must stop blaming others for the weaknesses and problems in health care (Schorr, 1981, p. 9). They must be willing to take the risks of accountability.

However, and this is what is often overlooked, they will also reap the rewards. Nurses will be the ones responsible and commended for maintaining safe standards for clients. They will be the ones responsible for and acknowledged as the vehicle for the client's increased level of knowledge and understanding of the health situation. They will be responsible for more progressive health care legislation and recognized as such, and will be responsible for and respected for determining what nursing is and what it does in a particular institution. They will reap many benefits and rewards. They will gain self-respect. They will finally have control over their practice, and that practice will be truly professional in nature.

◎ A Checklist for Accountability

In attempting to prepare to act in an accountable manner, and to evaluate one's actions, the following questions may serve as guides to the nurse. The list is not all-inclusive; it is merely a beginning tool for working the concept of accountability into one's life and work.

ACCOUNTABILITY TO THE CLIENT

- Am I providing the best care of which I am capable?
- Is that care sufficient to meet the needs of the client in this situation?
- Is this client entitled to more than I can offer, and am I turning elsewhere to obtain that additional dimension?
- Am I incorporating what I know of nursing theory and research into my practice in this situation?
- Am I using my leadership skills to encourage others to function at their optimal ability levels in the care of this patient?
- Am I acting in accordance with my own ethical code and that of the profession?
- If, by meeting the needs of this client, I am in conflict with my ethical code, am I seeking some alternative method or person to satisfy those needs?
- Have I given clients information that they want or need to know about their health status, while considering the effect on them of that knowledge?

ACCOUNTABILITY TO THE PUBLIC

- Am I seeking to improve health and nursing care?
- Am I speaking out against abuses I see in health and nursing care?
- Am I acting as a community resource in the areas of health and nursing?
- Am I remaining an active and contributing member of the profession after using public funds to finance my education?
- Am I attempting to increase the knowledge of the public to enable it to make more knowledgeable choices about health and nursing care?

ACCOUNTABILITY TO THE PROFESSION

- Am I fulfilling my professional role in accordance with the requirements of the profession?
- Are other nurses in my setting doing the same?
- If I am not performing satisfactorily, or if others are not, am I taking steps to remedy that situation?
- Am I a participant in professional meetings, organizations, seminars, conferences, and so forth, so that I may express my views on nursing to those in nursing?
- Am I working within the profession to improve practice, education, or research?
- Am I complying with the ethical code of the profession?

ACCOUNTABILITY TO SELF

- Am I satisfied with my chosen profession?
- Am I performing my professional role in the best way I can?
- Should I seek further preparation for that role?
- Should I withdraw from that role until I receive further preparation?
- In those areas where I am dissatisfied, am I seeking alternative modes of action or thought?
- Am I comfortable, ethically, with the way in which I am performing my professional role?
- Am I shortchanging my patients, my significant others, or myself in the way I am performing my professional role?
- Am I satisfied with the position this role assumes within my total lifestyle?

ACCOUNTABILITY TO THE AGENCY

- Am I performing in accordance with the job description for the position for which I was employed?
- If I am not satisfied with that job description, am I seeking appropriate ways to change it?
- Am I seeking to ensure that I am practicing under safe, if not optimal, conditions?
- Am I giving the institution its money's worth in terms of my work?
- Am I working in accordance with the policies and procedures of the institution?
- If I am not satisfied with those policies and procedures, am I seeking to change them using principles of leadership and change, and with the total mission of the institution in mind?

It would be quite the superperson, indeed, who could look through this checklist and confidently say he or she currently is carrying out all the above activities. Some activities are more appropriate than others for nurses in different settings and at different times. However, these and other questions must be considered by nurses who are to act in an accountable manner or increase the accountability of their decisions and actions. They must be considered by those who wishes to call themselves professional nurses.

Conclusion

After a brief discussion of the history of accountability in nursing, accountability and the related concepts of autonomy and authority are defined. The idea of accountability as a characteristic of a profession is then presented. The nurse's accountability to the client and public, the profession, the self, and the employing agency is discussed at some length.

The necessary groundwork for nurses to act in an accountable manner is presented, along with specific areas to be covered during this educational process. Accountability in an era of cost containment, the impact of the heavy use of unlicensed workers and of managed care, and a look at accountability in the future, are discussed. Finally, the chapter notes the positive aspects of being accountable, gives a checklist which can be used by nurses in determining if they are, in fact, acting as, or developing into, accountable professionals.

THOUGHT QUESTIONS

1 Explain the differences in, and relationships between, accountability, autonomy, authority, and responsibility.

2 What is the nurse's accountability when working with unlicensed assistive personnel?

3 What current developments in nursing and health care demonstrate the increased emphasis on accountability?

4 Discuss the nurse's accountability to the patient in the following vignette, both during the inpatient experience and after discharge.

VIGNETTE

Mrs. Joanna Morse is a 28-year-old newly diagnosed insulin-dependent diabetic. After a brief inpatient stay at Smithtown Hospital, she was discharged to her home. Her continuing care requires a 1,800 calorie diabetic diet, blood and urine testing, insulin administration, and regular exercise. Neither Joanna nor her husband have had any previous experience caring for a person with diabetes.

REFERENCES

American Journal of Nursing. (1991). New JCAHO standards: Nod to nurses. *American Journal of Nursing, 91*(5), 39.

American Nurses Association. (1985). *Code for nurses with interpretive statements.* (1985). Kansas City: Author.

American Nurses Association. (1991a). *Standards for nursing practice.* Kansas City: Author.

American Nurses Association. (1991b). *Nursing's agenda for health care reform.* Washington, DC: Author.

American Nurses Association. (1995). *Nursing's policy statement.* Washington, DC: Author.

Aroskar, M. A. (1992). Ethical foundations in nursing for broad health care access. *Scholarly Inquiry for Nursing Practice, 6*(3, 201–205.

Batey, M. V., & Lewis, F. M. (1982). Clarifying autonomy and accountability in nursing service: 2. *Journal of Nursing Administration, 12*, 10–15.

Begany, T. (1994). Layoffs: Targeting RNs. *RN, 57*, 37–38.

Bergman, R. (1981). Accountability—definition and dimensions. *International Nursing Review, 28*, 53–59.

Beyers, M., Bright, C., et al. (1996). Nursing in health networks: Direction and development. *Nursing Administration Quarterly, 21*(1), 7–13.

Bixler, G. K., & Bixler, R. W. (1959). The professional status of nursing. *American Nurse, 59*, 1142.

Brodbeck, K. (1991). Professional practice actualized through an integrated shared governance and quality assurance model. *Journal of Nursing Care Quality, 6*(2), 20–31.

Chaska, N. L. (1983). *The nursing profession: A time to speak.* New York: McGraw-Hill.

Clifford, J. C. (1981). Managerial control vs. professional autonomy: A paradox. *Journal of Nursing Administration, 11*, 19–21.

Copp, J. (1988). Professional accountability: The conflict. *Nursing Times, 84*(43), 42–44.

Dachelet, C. Z., & Sullivan, J. A. (1979). Autonomy in practice. *Nursing Practice, 4*, 15.

Donnelly, G. F. (1997, January). *How many faculty does it take to change a light bulb? Change???*

Flexner, A. (1915). Is social work a profession? *Proceedings of the National Conference of Charities and Correction* (pp. 576–590). Chicago: Heldman.

Hall, L. M. (1997). Staff mix models: Complementary or substitution roles for nurses. *Nursing Administration Quarterly, 21*(1), 31–39.

Hegyvary, S. T. (1991). Education: Freedom and responsibility. *Journal of Professional Nursing, 7*(l), 8.

Holden, R. J. (1991). Responsibility and autonomous nursing practice. *Journal of Advanced Nursing, 16.* 398–403.

Hylka, S. C., & Shugrue, D. (1991). Increasing staff nurse autonomy. *Nursing Management, 22*(5), 54–55.

Jackson, B. S. Ownership imbalance. *Journal of Nursing Administration, 19*(9), 4–5.

Joint Commission on Accreditation of Healthcare Organizations. (1991). *Nursing care accreditation manual for hospitals, 1991* (p. 94). Chicago: Author.

Lanara, V. A. (1982). Responsibility in nursing. *International Nursing Review, 29*, 7–10.

Lane, C. A. (1985). Exercising professional accountability. *Oncology Nursing, 12*, 12.

Leininger, M. (1994). Nursing's agenda of health care reform: Regressive or advanced-discipline status? *Nursing Science Quarterly, 7*(2), 93–94.

Matrone, J. (1996). How to move into the next era of health care. *Nursing Administration Quarterly, 21*(1), 1–6.

McGlothlin, W. J. (1961). The place of nursing among the professions. *Nursing Outlook, 9*, 214.

Merton, R. K. (1958). The functions of the professional association. *American Journal of Nursing, 68*, 50.

Nightingale, F. (1859/1946). *Notes on nursing: What it is and what it is not.* Philadelphia: Lippincott (facsimile of lst ed, London, Harrison & Sons, 1859).

Salmond, S. W. (1997). Delivery-or-care systems using clinical nursing assistants: Making it work. *Nursing Administration Quarterly, 21*(2), 74–84.

Schorr, T. (1981). Unity, authority, accountability—nursing's imperatives for the 80's. *Washington State Journal of Nursing, 53,* 7–10.

Silver, J. I. (1986). Management readings. *Journal of Nursing Administration, 16,* 43.

Simpson, K., & Sears, R. (1985). Authority and responsibility delegation predicts quality of care. *Journal of Advanced Nursing, 10,* 345–348.

Simpson, R. L., & Waite, R. (1989). NCNIP's system of the future: A call for accountability, revenue control, and national data sets. *Nursing Administration Quarterly, 14*(l), 72–77.

Stevens, P. E. (1992). Who gets care? Access to health care as an arena for nursing action. *Scholarly Inquiry for Nursing Practice, 6*(3), 185–197.

Styles, M. (1985). Accountable to whom? *Nursing Mirror, 160,* 35–37.

Vaughn, B. (1989). Autonomy and accountability. *Nursing Times, 85*(3), 54–55.

Webb, S. S., Price, S. A., & Van Ess Coeling, H. (1996). Valuing authority/responsibility relationships. *Journal of Nursing Administration, 26*(2), 29.

Wilkerson, I. (1988, June 30). AMA backs new category of hospital workers. *New York Times,* p. B8.

Wilson, A. A. (1996). The quest for accountability. Patient costs and outcomes. *Caring Magazine, 15*(6), 24–28.

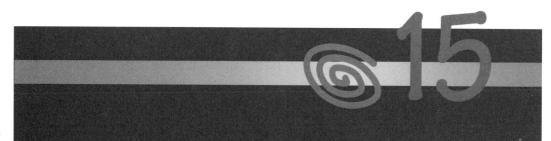

Communication:
Helping Relationships

LEARNING OUTCOMES

By the end of this chapter, the student will be able to:

1 Appreciate why communication is considered an essential element of nursing.

2 Know the major purposes of communication and be able to cite the significance of each purpose for nursing.

3 Know principles in the nurse–client relationship that ensure helpfulness in communication, and be able to define each principle and describe its significance to the nursing process.

4 Understand the outcomes of mutuality in helping relationships.

5 Understand how anxiety affects the nurse–client relationship.

6 List examples of therapeutic and nontherapeutic communication techniques.

7 Appreciate how nurses can use a relationship to promote healing.

The long-supported axiom of the helping professions—that behavioral change occurs by way of emotional experience—serves as the basis for emphasizing communication in nursing practice. The human need for relatedness binds people together, and communication serves as the exchange medium in these relationships. The verbal and nonverbal messages exchanged in human relationships determine, to a large extent, the structure and function of feelings. Indeed, the whole existence and the health status of human beings depend on communication because the affective component of life cannot be separated from the biologic component.

◎ Communication as Interaction

THE INTERPERSONAL COMPONENT OF THE NURSING PROCESS

In the nursing process, the client and the nurse both undergo emotional experiences as a function of the communication process between them. Because the ultimate goals of the nurse are to maximize the client's potential for health and to actualize the nurse's best professional abilities, the nurse must clearly understand the power of communication in shaping relationships.

The quality of communication between the nurse and the client is, therefore, an essential determinant of the success of the professional relationship. Mutual goals cannot be defined or achieved in the relationship without effective communication that positively influences the emotions of both the client and the nurse. This chapter focuses on communication as the interpersonal component of the nursing process and the essential component of helping relationships.

Assuming that humans possess all the characteristics of an open system, the nurse concludes that people are influenced by and influence all human beings with whom they are associated. Indeed, this reciprocal process suggests that the most important human attributes are not only openness to interpersonal experiences but also power to influence self and others. Sullivan (1953, p. 32) assumes that "everyone is more simply human than otherwise."

Human beings influence others primarily through communication. Communication is described as the "exchange of meanings between and among individuals through a shared system of symbols that have the same meaning for both the sender and the receiver of the message" (Vestal, 1995, p. 51). Through communication during nursing processes with a client, the nurse hopes to create new situations with the client that will influence the person to live in a healthier manner. This goal can be achieved only if the nurse is knowledgeable about the content and process of the nurse–client relationship.

To understand content in the nursing process, the nurse must have knowledge of the person as a human system interacting with the environment and striving for health, and of specific factors that promote positive change in human systems. To understand the process in the nurse–client relationship, the nurse must have both knowledge of communication and experience in developing helping relationships. Therefore, to participate effectively in nurse–client relationships, intradisciplinary or interdisciplinary relationships, and personal relationships, the nurse must understand both the structure and the functions of communication.

Nursing, as an organized body of professionals, has not always been successful in portraying an image of an autonomous professional discipline. Disagreement among nursing theorists, practitioners, and educators about the meaning of the "diagnosis and treatment of human responses to actual or potential health problems" (American Nurses Association [ANA], 1980) has led to multiple and sometimes conflicting images of nursing. Now there is general agreement among all parties that the essential features of contemporary nursing practice (ANA, 1995, p. 6) are:

- Attention to the full range of human experiences and responses to health and illness without restriction to a problem-focused orientation
- Integration of objective data with knowledge gained from an understanding of the patient or group's subjective experience
- Application of scientific knowledge to the processes of diagnosis and treatment
- Provision of a caring relationship that facilitates health and healing

Nursing's unique business is dealing with the human responses in health and illness. These responses are the substance of communication. Thus, professional nursing's business is communication and the purposeful use of communication in nurse–client relationships. The relationship should be "characterized by compassion, continuity, and respect for the client's choice. The focus is on the process: the process of the client–environment interaction and the process of the nurse–client relationship" (Newman, Lamb, & Michaels, 1991, p. 406).

THE STRUCTURE OF COMMUNICATION

Human communication is not only involved in conveying information and influencing another throughout a relationship, but "communication *is* the relationship" (Sundeen, Stuart, Rankin, & Cohnen, 1994, p. 94). It is dynamic interaction between two or more persons in which ideas, goals, beliefs and values, feelings, and feelings about feelings are exchanged. Experiencing even a minute communication exchange effects change in both communicants in the process.

It should be noted that communication is defined only in the context of process. Because human beings are continually and irrevocably exchanging energy with the environment, and life is continually being repatterned, it can be assumed that the individual human being reflects only dynamic actions. Each person is always affected by others and is always affecting others. One constantly communicates, thereby generating change in others and experiencing change in self.

Although communication is a dynamic process, it is possible to identify components and to analyze the interrelationships among the components. Berlo (1960), a noted authority on communications, traced the various models of communication from Aristotle to the 1960s. Aristotle identified the related components as the speaker, the speech, and the audience. After analyzing behavioral science research and several points of view, Berlo (1960, pp. 30–32) postulated a communication model generally accepted today:

1. An (interpersonal) source: some person(s) with ideas, needs, intentions, information, and a reason for communicating
2. A message: a coded, systematic set of symbols representing ideas, purposes, intentions, and feelings
3. An encoder: the mechanism for expressing or translating the purpose of the communication into the message (in human beings, these are the motor mechanisms—ie, the vocal mechanism for oral messages, the muscles of the hands for written messages, and the muscle systems elsewhere in the body for gestures)
4. A channel: the medium for carrying the message
5. A decoder: the mechanism for translating the message into a form that the recipient can use (in human beings, the sensory receptor mechanisms)
6. A receiver: the target or recipient of the message

In this model, the transmission of meaning occurs via a dynamic process in which

1. A person has an intention or purpose (the communication source)
2. That purpose is translated into communicable form by the person's set of motor mechanisms and skills (encoder)
3. The message is transmitted through a channel
4. The message is translated into receivable form by the recipient's sensory mechanisms and skills (decoder)
5. The recipient receives the message (the communication receiver)

Since this model was postulated, systems theorists have further explained the reciprocal relationship between the participants in the communication process. At any given time, the individual person is both an active initiator and a recipient of meanings in an interpersonal situation. Thus, it is important for nurses to understand that they are simultaneously acting and reacting in the nursing process, and that clients' meanings have an equal effect on the outcome of purposeful relationships. The process just described has been labeled "transactional."

The dynamic nature of the communication process dictates the need for the nurse to evaluate his or her own actions and reactions throughout the nursing process with a client. Without such awareness and evaluation, the professional will be less likely to experience successful communication with the feeling of satisfaction associated with transmitting clear meanings and the validation that the message intended was indeed the message received. Validation of meanings is essential to achieving any therapeutic goals in helping relationships.

FUNCTIONS AND TYPES OF COMMUNICATION

Synthesizing from several communication models, Cecchio and Cecchio (1982) propose four major purposes of communication: to inquire, inform, persuade, and entertain. The nurse may attempt to achieve any of these purposes with clients, the health care delivery system, peers, other personnel, and even the self. In attempting to achieve these purposes, the nurse transmits messages in the process.

Messages are transmitted verbally and nonverbally. Further, implicit in all models of communication is the concept that communication has two interacting components: (1) the content value of the message, and (2) the interactional or perceptual value of the message and its participants. The informational aspect of the message, the content value, is expressed in verbal or nonverbal forms. The interactional or perceptual value of the message (referred to as "metacommunication") identifies how the content is to be interpreted as well as how the relationship is perceived between the participants. Metacommunication may also be expressed in both verbal and nonverbal forms.

Verbal Communication

Verbal communication in nursing is primarily associated with the spoken word. It requires functional physiologic and cognitive mechanisms that potentiate speech production and reception. Although the greatest influence on communication is not the specific words (but rather, the nonverbal message), words are an essential tool of personal and cultural communication. Language comprises an elaborate system of symbols. Words are symbolic of actual objects or concepts. Lack of congruence in language between the nurse and the client usually interferes with initiating relationships and creates obstacles to validation of meanings—the essential characteristic of an effective message.

Two primary influences on verbal communications are developmental age and cultural heritage. Developmental age affects verbal abilities through the person's physiologic ability to change sounds into words and the cognitive ability to symbolize through language. Through the process of acculturation, the person develops culture-based variations from others in defining meanings for words. Although denotative meanings are equal among different persons (ie, the concrete representations of words are the same), connotative meanings often vary among persons of varying cultures and their accompanying acculturation.

Associated with the fact that words are the symbols of communication are three types of problems with which the nurse needs to be concerned (Cecchio & Cecchio 1982):

1. The technical problem: How accurately can one transmit the symbols of communication?
2. The semantic problem: How precise are the symbols in transmitting the intended message?
3. The influential problem: How effectively does the received meaning affect conduct?

The verbal content of communication can be used to evaluate the content theme of the communication process. If one evaluates the seemingly varied topics of discussion, the words that underlie or link together several ideas will reflect the what of the communication.

VIGNETTE

Margie is a staff nurse in the emergency room. A patient was brought in with severe chest pain. She noticed that the family members seemed very nervous, but when she asked them, they said they did not need anything. She wonders whether she should believe their verbal or their nonverbal communication.

Nonverbal Communication

The nonverbal component of the message is the greatest influence on communication. *Nonverbal communication* consists of all forms of communication that do not involve the spoken or written word. Perception of nonverbal communication involves all the senses, including hearing, which is used for the perception of verbal messages. Signs (gestures), actions or kinesics (all body movements that are not specific signs), objects (all intentional and nonintentional display of material things), and proxemics (the use of space) are all powerful nonverbal messages perceived by the senses.

A number of purposes of nonverbal communication have been identified (Sundeen et al., 1994, p. 99), including:

- Expressing emotion
- Expressing interpersonal attitudes
- Establishing, developing, and maintaining social relationships
- Presenting the self
- Engaging in rituals
- Supporting verbal communication

The tactile senses represent the most primitive sensory process developed by humans. Bonding between the infant and the parent figure (important to infant development) occurs largely through nonverbal tactile communication. Touch remains a powerful communication tool throughout life.

It is commonly accepted today that deprivation of tactile stimulation in infancy may impair the achievement of some developmental tasks. The young child orients himself or herself to space through touch. As the child develops into the adult, touch as nonverbal communication takes on specific cultural meanings.

Nurses must understand taboos concerning touch and distance if they desire to be purposeful in nonverbal as well as verbal communication. For example, to one person, a touch on the knee might mean concern, whereas to another it may be interpreted as seduction. Used sensitively at the proper time and within the context of the client's culture, touch is a powerful nonverbal tool for the nurse.

All the sensory processes become powerful components of the communication process as the human being exchanges nonverbal as well as verbal messages with others throughout life. For example, the olfactory (smell) and gustatory (taste) senses make it possible for the person to learn which odors and tastes are pleasant and which are not. Once that physiologic capacity is present, odor and taste are significant nonverbal messages in the communication process. The nurse needs to manipulate the environment in the health care delivery system in such a way that nonverbal messages such as odor are controlled.

Finally, in relation to the sensory aspects of nonverbal communication, the sense of hearing the spoken word has a nonverbal component: that of interpreting the qualities of the voice. Hunsaker and Alessandra (1980) state that the following voice qualities are strong determinants of effectiveness in communication:

Resonance: the intensity with which the voice fills the environmental space
Rhythm: the flow, pace, and movement of the voice
Speed: how fast the voice is used
Pitch: the highness or lowness of the voice, related to the tightening of the vocal cords
Volume: loudness
Inflection: change in pitch or volume of voice
Clarity: articulation and enunciation capacity of the voice

Motor or kinesic actions are perhaps most often performed with little or no awareness on the part of the communicant. Body movements are nonverbal communications that are largely determined through socialization. Developed in a particular psychosocial and cultural setting, motor actions vary according to gender, socioeconomic status, age, and ethnic background. It is generally accepted that misinterpretations of culturally variable kinesic behaviors produce barriers to effective communication. For example, eye motions involved with eye contact communicate culturally specific messages. If the nurse does not assign the same meaning to this nonverbal communication, the effectiveness of the nurse–client relationship may be limited.

Hunsaker and Alessandra (1980) suggest that 90% of meaning comes from nonverbal communication. Thus, nonverbal behavior has a significant impact on the recipient of the message communicated. Nonverbal behavior is, therefore, significant in leaders. It conveys the greatest meaning to the persons involved in the leadership process. For example, the following motor actions (which are commonly observed) may be highly influential in the communication process (Hunsaker & Alessandra, 1980):

1. Gently rubbing behind the ear with the index finger—interpreted as doubt
2. Casually rubbing the eye with one finger—interpreted that the recipient in the communication process does not understand what is being communicated
3. Cupping hands over the mouth—interpreted that the gesturer is trying to hide something
4. Leaning back with both hands supporting the head—interpreted as confidence or superiority
5. Pinching the bridge of the nose with eyes closed—interpreted as thoughtful evaluation
6. Moving eyeglasses to the lower bridge of the nose and peering over them—interpreted as a powerful negative evaluation

Kinesics, the meaning of motor actions, and *proxemics,* or the function of space in nonverbal communication, also play important roles in all aspects of life. Space is a constant. It may be perceived either as surrounding persons or as existing between them. Nurses must strive purposefully for congruence among their own nonverbal behaviors and the verbal communications they intend to convey. In addition, nurses must recognize that culture affects all aspects of nonverbal communication. The following examples have been modified from Vestal (1995, pp. 359–360):

■ Proximity/spacing. People from some cultures may tend to stand very close to a person with whom they are communicating. This can cause discomfort for someone with a different perspective on appropriate spacing.
■ Touching. Any physical contact or touching that is part of an individual's communication style can create problems or discomfort for people from many cultures. This does not mean that the nurse should abandon "hands on" a shoulder or arm to show support and caring. Rather, clients should feel empowered to tell the nurse if such touching makes them feel uncomfortable.
■ Gestures. People from some cultures may be more animated than others, using gestures and body language to communicate their

message. In addition, gestures that have a positive meaning in one culture may be insulting and rude in another.

■ Eye contact. Traditionally, Americans have valued direct eye contact as a sign of confidence and respect, whereas not making eye contact has negative connotations. However, in many cultures, making eye contact with an authority figure is considered an insult.

■ Use of silence. People from some cultures prefer active verbal interaction and are uncomfortable with silence. Other cultures may value periods of comtemplative silence, leading to the potential for misunderstanding of communication style and motivation.

■ Body language. The body is one of the more subtle ways people communicate meaning and sincerity. The nurse may say all the right things, but communicate tension through body language.

With an awareness of what a client perceives as acceptable use of space and how body position and direction affect the meaning of the relationship, the nurse can manipulate personal and environmental space for the benefit of the client in the nursing process. For example, the nurse attempting to teach a client how to give himself insulin cannot see the full picture of the client's nonverbal behavior if she sits side by side with him. In this position, the nurse's torso is not directed toward the client's, she must turn her head awkwardly to see his facial expressions, and so forth. This position gives the client a message that the nurse is not being with the client.

Metacommunication

Occurring on both verbal and nonverbal levels, *metacommunication* represents an integrative level that defines the "what," the "who," and the relationship between the "what" and the "who" of the communication process. Because this level of communication is influential in determining the effectiveness of relationships, the nurse must evaluate communication both in terms of its context and in terms of the relationships among its parts. Understanding themes of the relationship helps the nurse evaluate the metacommunication occurring in the nursing process. The nurse must search for the *content* theme (the central underlying idea or links), the *mood* theme (the emotion communicated—the how of the message), and the *interaction* theme (the dynamics between the communicating participants).

Knowing that change occurs more readily and more effectively if congruence exists between the verbal and nonverbal components of communication, the nurse must be alert to indicators of the degree of agreement on the meaning of the content and on the process of the relationship. When a discrepancy arises between verbal and nonverbal components, the nonverbal component is usually the more accurate indicator. However, nonverbal behavior is more open to subjective meaning and variations; thus, it must be verbally validated. This validation process plays an important part in effectively using metacommunication in the nursing process.

INTERPRETATION AND PERCEPTION

Communication is possible between human beings because they have the capacity for interpretation. Interpretation involves perception, symbolization, memory, and thinking. Perhaps the most important of these is perception, the basic component after which the others follow. Taylor et al. (1977) define *perception* as the selection and organization of sensations so that they are meaningful. They take the position that perceptions are learned and that what is learned depends on experience during socialization. Perceptual expectations are influenced by emotions, language, and attitudes, and they vary widely from one individual to another. One's interpretation ability, therefore, is highly dependent on perceptual ability.

Factors affecting perception in the nurse–client relationship are the capacity for attention (reception of sensations) by nurse and client, the perspective each brings to the relationship, and the physical condition of the receptors. Anxiety (the actual or anticipated negative appraisal by the other) in the nurse or the client limits the ability to be attentive in the communication process, interferes with the validation of individual perspectives, and decreases physical capacities. Thus, it is essential that anxiety be controlled in the nurse–client relationship. Validated perceptions between nurse and client are essential to goal-setting and achievement.

The evolutionary nature and significance of perception can be seen in the following statement of relationship:

> How we perceive and feel about the world is a force for and a result of our pattern of organization as a living system. This pattern affects our perception and feelings at any given time. Perceptions and feelings about them affect how we communicate.

The nurse must constantly be aware of the power and influence of perception on the outcomes of verbal communication, nonverbal communication, and metacommunication.

SELF-CONCEPT AND INTERPERSONAL RELATIONSHIPS

Another important factor affecting communication in the nursing process is the relationship between the participants in the process. The self-concept of each participant largely determines this relationship. Self-awareness and awareness of others depends on self-concept. Chapter 5 elaborates on the significance of the personal self-concept in developing professional abilities.

According to Brill (1990, p. vii), "In dealing with people it is essential that workers possess awareness of themselves, their own needs, the ways in which they satisfy these needs, the ways in which they use themselves in relationship with others." In addition to self-awareness, other factors involved in the self-concept are essential to effective communication:

- Ability to share with individuals (a function of achievement of interpersonal developmental tasks)
- Ability to establish, maintain, and terminate the kind of relationship in which one is comfortable (a function of the human need to perpetuate a personal self-concept)
- Ability to share power (a reflection of the person's view of self and others)

If the major reason for nurses' communication with clients is to influence clients toward better health, nurses must develop concepts of self that are most effective in actualizing the potential of the client for growth. These concepts include

> awareness of one's own perceptions of and feelings about self
> ability to derive satisfaction by sharing with the client the responsibility for the nurse–client relationship
> ability to view the self as the therapeutic tool for implementing the nursing process, and
> appreciation of the value of shared power in activities directed toward change

PRINCIPLES OF COMMUNICATION IN COLLABORATIVE RELATIONSHIPS BETWEEN NURSE AND CLIENT

Vital characteristics possessed by effective communicators are the abilities to empathize, to demonstrate respect, and to respond genuinely. The process for achieving each of these characteristics represents a principle on which to base communication in the nursing process. Collaborative relationships mandate that the nurse and the client mutually and equally share the responsibility and authority for planning, implementing, and evaluating the helping process. Such collaboration cannot occur without presence, empathy, respect, and genuineness.

Presence

Presence is an important part of several nursing conceptual models including those of Parse (1996), Paterson and Zderad (1988), and Watson (1996), as described in Chapters 8 and 9. "The core element in presence is 'being there'. . . . It is described as a gift of self and is equated with a use of self that is conveyed through open and giving behaviors of the nurse" (Osterman & Schwartz-Barcott, 1996, p. 24). Characteristics of four ways of "being there" are described in Table 15-1. These ways "reflect degrees of intensity in the context of another " (Osterman & Schwartz-Barcott, 1996, p. 29).

Presence is integrally related to genuineness and a necessary antecedent to empathy.

TABLE 15-1

Presence: Characteristics of Four Ways of Being There

Characteristics of Presence	Presence	Partial Presence	Full Presence	Transcendent Presence
Quality of being there	Physically present in context of another	Physically present in context of another	Physically present (there) (physical attending behavior—eye contact, leaning toward) Psychologically present (with) (attentive listening behavior)	Physically present Psychologically present (metaphysical beliefs) Holistic
Focus of energy	Self-absorbed	Objects or tasks in environment, relevant to the other individual but none of the energy is directed at the other	Self/Other (focusing on another influences response—reciprocal)	Centered—(drawing from universal energy) Subject/Subject—leads to oneness
	Personal, subjective reality	Mechanical/technical reality	Present oriented (here and now)—anchoring in present reality	Transcending and oriented beyond here and now—sustaining while at the same time transforming reality
Nature of Interaction	No interaction; self-absorbed, intrapersonal encounter	Interaction with part of other encounter	Interactive; essential communication; boundaries—role constraints; professional relationship; dyad caring	Relationship; high degree of skilled communication; role free; human intimacy/love; humanistic caring, no boundaries; monad relationship;
Positive outcomes	Reduce stress; reassurance that someone is there; may be quieting and restorative; facilitates creative thinking	Reduce stress; solving a mechanical problem; reduces amount of stimuli in an encounter	Solving of a human problem; relief of a here-and-now distress	Transformations decreased loneliness; expansion of consciousness; spiritual peace, hope and meaning in one's existence (love/connectedness); nice feeling generated in the environment; transpersonal (oneness)
Negative outcomes	No interpersonal engagement—missed communication; isolation, withdrawn, increased anxiety	Not interpersonal connectedness	May be too much energy for recipient or feel negative to a recipient; energy not always available for full presence; increased anxiety	Fusion and possible loss of objective reality; danger of taking on recipient's problems

From Osterman, P., & Schwartz-Barcott, D. (1996). Presence: Four ways of being there. *Nursing Forum, 31,* 25. Used with permission of the publisher.

Empathy

For effective change to occur in any helping relationship, the principle of empathy must be observed:

> To be helpful, the nurse must demonstrate the ability to participate in the client's feelings or ideas by sensing, sharing, and accepting the client's feelings.

According to Olsen (1991, p. 62), "empathy can reintroduce values and value-based decisions into nursing." He suggests that empathy occurs "when one person experiences a commonality with another . . . a feeling, an experience, a shared situation, or something unnameable" (Olson, 1991, p. 74).

Empathy is defined as "the art of communicating to others that we have understanding [of] how they are feeling and what makes them feel that way" (Keegan, 1994, p. 127). Defining attributes of empathy as described by Wiseman (1996, p. 1165) are:

See the world as others see it
Be nonjudgmental
Understand another's feelings
Communicate the understanding

Nurses possessing empathy show awareness of the uniqueness and individuality of clients. They are involved with sharing in clients' feelings. They care about clients as sentient beings like themselves. If clients perceive that nurses care about them and how they feel, benefits include (Keegan, 1994):

- Relationships will bring forth trust and open communication
- The feeling of being connected to another is increased
- Self-esteem is fostered in both nurse and client
- Genuine acceptance of others as they are is demonstrated
- Self-awareness is increased for both nurse and client
- Clients are allowed "to be less critical and increasingly caring toward themselves" (p. 130).

To really be empathic, helpers have to listen so well that they can act as intended, can perceive and accept the inner feelings and experiences of clients as the clients experience them, and can paraphrase feelings, ideas, and intentions to clients' satisfaction. If, on the other hand, clients are perceived as objects, they are immediately put on the defensive.

Two essential actions are necessary for a nurse to develop empathy: (1) awareness and acceptance of self as a feeling person open to one's own experiences, and (2) ability to listen to each message of the client, to identify the client's feelings associated with it, and to respond to these feelings. Thus, empathy involves far more than the cognitive or thinking part of the self. It involves the acceptance that we are feeling beings, commonly feeling multiple emotions simultaneously. In effective communication, the client's feelings perceived and accepted by the nurse are known to both nurse and client.

Respect

The following passage describes the principle of respect in the nurse–client relationship:

> In order for the client to experience his right to exist as an other, the nurse must demonstrate a receptive attitude that values the client's feelings, opinion, individuality, and uniqueness (Hammond, Hepworth, & Smith, 1977, pp. 170–203).

Respect is feeling or showing deferential regard or esteem (Soukhanov, 1992, p. 1536). "The behavior that demonstrates respect is acknowledgment" (Smith, 1992, p. 67). Respect is the nonpossessive caring for and affirmation of another's personhood as a separate individual. Respect builds self-esteem and positive self-image. In the nurse–client relationship, respect is demonstrated by equality, mutuality, and shared thinking about strengths and problems.

Smith (1992, p. 67) offers the following concrete actions nurses can follow in demonstrating respect to clients:

- Look at your client
- Give your undivided attention
- Maintain eye contact
- Smile if appropriate
- Move toward the person
- Determine how client likes to be addressed
- Call client by name and introduce yourself
- Make contact with a handshake or gentle touching

Clients who are members of a cultural group unlike that of the nurse may have special needs for respect. According to Bradley and Edinbergh (1990, p. 226), nurses may be "viewed as being powerful, one-up, and, if from a different racial group, nonempathic. . . . In addition, it can be the nurses who view the clients as powerless, one-down, and different." Respecting the client's dignity is critical to therapeutic communication, "even when the client is in dire social, economic, or health circumstances" (Bradley & Edinberg, 1990, p. 226).

Genuineness

Genuineness, used synonymously with authenticity, is supported in the following nursing principle:

> Positive therapeutic outcomes for the client are enhanced when the nurse in the helping relationship acts with genuineness.

In defining authenticity, phrases such as "being actually and precisely what is claimed," "genuine," "good faith," and "sincere" are used. "Being genuine means that you send the other person the real picture of you, not one distorted by being different than how you really think or feel" (Smith, 1992, p. 74). The genuine nurse acts in ways that are unrehearsed and noncontrived. It has been argued that neutrality is the essence of the nurse's behavior in a helping relationship (Rogers, 1951). Others argue that neutral behavior often has the appearance of being depersonalized and thus is ambiguous and leads to anxiety on the part of the client, who may not get a clear message of how he or she stands with the nurse.

It is a risk to be genuine because it may involve expressing negative thoughts and confronting others. However, there may be even more risk in incongruence. Negative effects of incongruence may include (Smith, 1992):

Distrust of the nurse
Suspicion of the nurse
Strained, tense relationship
Confusion
Questioning the credibility of the nurse
The client may believe only the nonverbal message.
Valuable information may not be shared.
Clients may "feel that the nurse is trying to impress, rather than reach or connect with them" (p. 80).

Guidelines for the effective use of genuineness applicable to the nurse in the nurse–client relationship include:

1. The nurse should avoid early self-disclosure until the client demonstrates a readiness to respond positively to such disclosure
2. As trust is established, the nurse can become more open and spontaneous while adhering to the principles of empathy and respect
3. The nurse should avoid using self-disclosure to manipulate, give advice, or influence for the nurse's own goals

"Being real does not mean being overly familiar" . . . What the client wants "is an emotionally available, calm, caring proficient resource that can protect, care about, and above all, listen to him or her" (Arnold & Boggs, 1989, p. 439).

Effective changes in clients occur when the nurse:

■ Speaks deep from within without apology (Smith, 1992)
■ Shows spontaneity
■ Conveys openness
■ Uses a high degree of positive regard
■ Demonstrates congruence between who and what he or she is
■ Demonstrates congruence between verbal and nonverbal communication
■ Infers accurately the inner world of the client by listening well and understanding the subjective and objective world of the relationship as it changes over time

Internalizing the principles of empathy, respect, and genuineness make it possible for the nurse to demonstrate these behaviors and experience satisfaction in the nursing process.

◎ Helping Relationships—The Nurse as Helper

The nurse–client relationship is a special helping relationship characterized by the following features (Smith, 1992, p. 28):

- It is a partnership between the client and the nurse
- It is purposeful and productive
- It can palliate the client's worries and fears
- It can be a psychic or morale booster
- It has phases
- It should be personally tailored to the needs of each particular client
- It is platonic
- It is a private relationship
- It can be a powerful relationship

The nurse as an authority in health care recognizes his or her expertise in health promotion, maintenance, and restoration and in illness prevention. The nurse also accepts a societal obligation to share these abilities with clients in need of nursing services. Although in the United States today a nurse usually is not directly employed by a client, the nurse nevertheless is professionally accountable first to the client who is the recipient of services and then to self and the employer and other health team workers.

It is the nurse's responsibility to fulfill a helper role regardless of the specific parameters and purposes of each relationship. The nurse must validate that the client knows the areas of concern for which he is ready to seek help and assume that they will mutually share the responsibility for the outcomes of the nursing process. The nurse further assumes that the client can achieve an improved state of health. The helping role is viewed as a facilitative one in which the nurse uses self and expertise as therapeutic tools to assist the client to more successfully develop responses to resist or overcome threats to health.

Rogers (1958) set the following essential conditions of a helping relationship, which are applicable to the nursing process:

1. The individual is able and expected to be responsible for himself
2. Each individual (nurse and client) has a strong drive to become mature and to be socially responsible
3. The climate of the helping relationship is warm and permits the expression of both positive and negative feelings
4. Limits, mutually agreed on, are set on behavior only, not on attitudes
5. The helper communicates understanding and acceptance

TABLE 15-2

Interchange of Knowledge, Attitudes, and Skills Between Client and Nurse in the Helping Relationship

What the Client Brings to the Client–Nurse Relationship	What the Nurse Brings to the Client–Nurse Relationship
Cognitive	
• Preferred ways of perceiving and judging	• Preferred ways of perceiving and judging
• Knowledge and beliefs about illness in general and his illness in particular	• Knowledge and beliefs about illness in general
• Knowledge and beliefs about health promotion and maintenance in general, and information about his own health care activities	• Knowledge about his/her clinical specialty
• Ability to problem solve	• Knowledge and beliefs about health behaviors which prevent illness and promote, regain, and maintain health
• Ability to learn	• Ability to problem solve
	• Knowledge about factors which increase client compliance with treatment regimen
Affective	
• Cultural values	• Cultural values
• Feelings about seeking help from a nurse	• Feelings about being a nurse–helper
• Attitudes toward nurses in general	• Attitudes towards clients in general
• Attitudes toward treatment regime	• Biases about nursing treatment regimen
• Values toward preventing illness	• Value placed on being healthy
• Willingness to take positive action about own health status at this time with this particular nurse	• Value placed on people actively preventing illness or enhancing well-being
	• Willingness to help client take positive action to improve his well-being
	• Ability to relate and communicate with others
Psychomotor	
• Ability to relate and communicate with others	• Proficiency in administering effective nursing interventions
• Ability to carry out own health care management	• Ability to teach nursing interventions to client
• Ability to learn new methods of self-care	

From Smith, S. (1992). *Communications in nursing* (2nd ed., p. 23). St. Louis: Mosby.

The characteristics of helping as developed by Rogers have positively influenced many health professionals and continue to be refined and reformulated in improving their practice.

Table 15-2 displays what the client and the nurse bring to their relationship (Smith, 1992, p. 23).

THE NATURE OF HELPING IN PROGRESSIVE STAGES OF THE NURSE–CLIENT RELATIONSHIP

The purposes and functions of the nurse–client relationship vary as interaction proceeds through predictable sequential stages. Although the nurse in a helping relationship always enacts the roles of facilitator, advocate, and coordinator, specific functions and purposes evolve throughout the relationship. The facilitator helps the client move toward greater health. The advocate protects the client from stress inherent in the petitioner role and acts on behalf of the client in promoting access to and use of health care delivery services. The coordinator attempts to organize and articulate all the services related to meeting the client's health care needs.

The knowledge base needed to act as a helper in the nursing process was largely developed and shared by Dr. Hildegard Peplau 40 years ago. Her book, *Interpersonal Relations in Nursing* (Peplau, 1952), presented a thorough analysis of Harry Stack Sullivan's interpersonal theory in psychiatry and gave nursing a sound conceptual model for practice. Although other nurse scholars have developed other models and changed forms of the interpersonal model, Peplau's contribution regarding the phases of the nurse–client relationship remains applicable. Following is a brief summary of the phases and their purposes, with associated functions of the nurse in each phase.

Phases of the Relationship
ORIENTATION PHASE
The purposes of the orientation phase include:

- Introduction of nurse and client
- Elaboration of the client's need to recognize and understand both his or her difficulty and the extent of a need for help
- Acceptance of the client's need for assistance in recognizing and planning to use services that professional personnel can offer
- Agreement that the client will direct energies toward the mutual responsibility for defining, understanding, and meeting productively the problem at hand
- Clarification of limitations and responsibilities in the delivery system environment

When the nurse and the client validate understanding of the client's need for help and acceptance of resources to meet those needs, and they do so with feelings of shared responsibility and a sense of trust, they move into a new phase of the relationship.

IDENTIFICATION PHASE
The purposes of the identification phase include:

- Provision of the opportunity for the client to respond to the helper's offer to assist
- Encouragement for the client to express feelings, to reorient those feelings and strengthen positive forces
- Provision of the opportunity for the nurse and the client to clearly understand each other's preconceptions and expectations

EXPLOITATION PHASE
The purposes of the exploitation phase include:

■ Full utilization of the nurse–client relationship to mutually work on the solution to problems and the changes needed to improve health
■ Provision of opportunities for the client to explore earlier experiences and behaviors and to have emerging needs met

RESOLUTION PHASE
The purposes of the resolution phase include:

■ Provision of opportunity to formulate new goals
■ Encouragement of gradual freeing of the client from identifying with the nurse
■ Promotion of the client's ability to act more independently

Changing Roles of the Nurse Throughout the Relationship

Overlapping in various stages, the following roles of the nurse tend to emerge as the nurse promotes growth (change) in the client:

1. Orientation phase
   Stranger
2. Identification phase
   Unconditional mother surrogate
   Resource person
   Teacher
   Leader
   Counselor
   Surrogate
3. Exploitation phase
   The adult support person in new enactment of the aforementioned roles
4. Resolution phase
   Same adult roles

It should be noted that the nurse moves back and forth in some of these roles in the various phases. Essentially, however, as the client's needs are met, more mature needs arise; thus the need for more mature roles.

In the role of *stranger*, the nurse is an individual unknown to the client. Peplau points out how it is essential for the nurse in this role to accord the client respect and positive interest to promote open communication. A *surrogate* is a substitute figure who, in the client's mind, reactivates the feeling generated in earlier relationships. The nurse's responsibility in this role is to help the client to become aware of likenesses and differences and to differentiate the nurse as a person. Permitting clients to reexperience old feelings, the nurse acting as surrogate sets up the opportunity for growth experiences.

The *resource person* role involves the nurse in providing specific information, usually formulated in relation to larger problems. The *teacher* role involves the nurse sharing information and promoting the client's learning through experience, and requires the development of novel alternatives with open-ended outcomes in the nurse–client relationship. The *leader* role involves the nurse facilitating the client's work on the solution of problems.

The *counselor* role incorporates all of the activities associated with promoting experiences leading to health. The counselor helps a client to become aware of health behaviors, to evaluate them, and to plan how to improve them. Counseling focuses primarily on how the client feels about himself and what is happening to him (Peplau, 1952).

MUTUALITY IN RESPONSIBILITY AND DECISION-MAKING

Reciprocity is a concept that has similarities with mutuality. *Reciprocity* "is characterized as an interpersonal exchange, customarily expected to be symmetrical or equivalent" (Mendias, 1997, p. 435). This concept, a part of Peplau's (1952) and Watson's (1996) conceptual models, addresses the mutual gain in a client–nurse relationship.

Developing these ideas of mutual exchange and gain, Marck (1990) discusses the concept of therapeutic reciprocity as

> one phenomenon of caring, [that] allows both the nurse and the client to benefit from their relationship in a mutually empowering manner . . . . Therapeutic reciprocity is a mutual, collaborative, probabilistic, instructive, and empowering exchange of feelings, thought, and behaviors between the nurse and client for the purpose of enhancing the human outcomes of the relationship for all parties concerned (p. 49, 57).

All of the previously specified roles represent elements of presence, empathy, respect, and genuineness. Communication in these role relationships will evolve from diagnostic interactions to therapeutic interactions and eventually to educative and supportive interactions as the client moves from illness to a higher level of health. The absolute element of all of these roles is mutuality in responsibility and decision-making if both the nurse and the client are expected to experience growth and satisfaction in the nursing process.

COMMUNICATION AND THE PHENOMENON OF ANXIETY

Social systems are characterized by continual interaction among their components. This means that every person involved in the communication process affects and is affected by every other person in the communication field. Rogers calls this phenomenon "reciprocy" (Rogers, 1970, p. 97).

Reciprocal relationships are the basis of the nursing process. The fact that the nurse has the potential to affect the client, as well as to be affected by the client, offers the nurse the potential to assist the client to change behaviors in the direction of improved health. Such nurse–client exchanges can be powerful in problem-solving and decision-making situations that determine the nature and direction of change.

The nature of change includes alternatives of cognitive repatterning (using new information to increase understanding), affective adjustment (using the relationship to become aware of, accept, and express feelings), and synthesis of cognitions and feelings in interpersonal repatterning (using the relationship to learn to interact with others in the social system). The direction of change can be toward greater or lesser health. Obviously, the nurse wants to affect the direction of change toward greater health.

Every social system has expected role behaviors from its constituents. The way a person communicates is greatly affected by his or her perceived role in the system. Roles "are structures that are imposed on behavior" (Berlo, 1960, p. 153). Three aspects of role must be understood in trying to positively affect the other person in a relationship: role prescription, role description, and role expectations. Berlo defines these aspects as follows:

1. Role prescription: the formal, explicit statement of what behaviors should be performed by persons in a given role
2. Role description: a report of the behaviors that actually are performed by persons in a given role
3. Role expectations: the images that persons have about the behaviors that are performed by persons in a given role (Berlo, 1960, p. 153; enumeration added)

In the ideal nurse–client relationship, there is congruence among role prescriptions, descriptions, and expectations. Together, the nurse and the client have agreed on the structure and dynamics of their purposeful communication. When there are differences regarding the prescriptions, descriptions, and expectations of role behavior between the nurse and the client, communication breakdowns occur.

Congruence in role relationships in the social system reduces uncertainty. Uncertainty and ambiguity lead to increased tension and discomfort in the system. Such tension in human systems leads to dissipation of energy and less ability to use the energy exchanged for purposes of improving health. In interpersonal systems, such tension is often called anxiety.

Anxiety is the tension state resulting from the actual or anticipated negative appraisal of the significant other in the communication process. Prolonged or intensive anxiety ties up available energy, making less energy available to the system for the decision-making or problem-solving necessary for purposeful change to healthier role behaviors.

A commonly accepted principle is that the tension state of anxiety in one person is readily communicated, thus engendering anxiety in the other person(s). Sullivan (1953) attributes great power to the tension of anxiety in a person's interpersonal growth, development, and ability in all stages of life. The actual or anticipated negative appraisals by others that lead to anxiety are perceived as threats to one's self-image. If the anxiety is limited in amount and duration, it simply leads to an increased state of alertness, mediated through physiologic reactions and behavior to reduce the tension. However, if the state of anxiety is not limited in amount or duration, the level of alertness and successful tension-reducing behaviors are decreased.

Sullivan (1953, pp. 151–154) postulates that learning occurs through an anxiety gradient extending from mild to severe. A client with mild anxiety can focus energy on most of what is really occurring. A client with moderate anxiety has limited ability to focus on what is really occurring and tends to distort reality. A client with severe anxiety cannot focus energy on what is really happening and thus cannot participate effectively in problem-solving or decision-making. Because the effective nursing process requires that both the nurse and the client focus on what is really happening, it is essential to control anxiety in the communication process.

The nurse has two primary responsibilities in controlling anxiety: (1) to be aware of his or her own feelings of anxiety, and to structure interactions in such a way that limited anxiety is empathized to the client, and (2) to use effective strategies for intervening in the client's anxiety. Such strategies are usually called "therapeutic."

Intervention in a client's anxiety is based on the nurse recognizing the client's anxiety. The nurse also has primary responsibility for monitoring his or her own anxiety and relieving personal tensions. The nursing profession often places nurses in stressful situations. In recent years, nursing leaders have begun to act on the need to help nurses learn to develop stress-reduction strategies for themselves as well as for clients.

Techniques to help clients recognize, gain insight into, and cope with threats of anxiety are discussed in the following section.

COMMUNICATION STRATEGIES THAT REFLECT CARING FOR CLIENTS

Listening is the most important therapeutic technique in the process of effective communication. Sundeen and coworkers (1994, p. 118) state that it is devastating to the formation of a helpful relationship if the nurse fails to listen. Listening transmits the messages "You are of value to me" and "I am interested in you."

Guidelines for listening might include (Pagano, 1992; Vestal, 1995):

1. Give the other person your full attention
2. Resist distractions and letting your mind stray
3. Listen for central ideas and validate with the client
4. Avoid gut-feeling traps that confirm prejudices and biases
5. Overcome defensiveness
6. Prepare yourself physically by standing or facing the speaker
7. Watch for nonverbal as well as verbal messages
8. Do not prejudge worth based on appearance or delivery of the speaker
9. Listen for ideas and underlying feelings
10. Do not interrupt
11. Try to see the situation from the other person's point of view
12. Do not try to have the last word

To listen effectively, the nurse must use verbal communication techniques that facilitate the client's verbal and nonverbal expressiveness. Such techniques are generally referred to as "therapeutic communication techniques" (Table 15-3).

To be helpful, the nurse must respond empathically, attempt to extend the client's meaning, and respond with respect and authenticity. What does the nurse do to show empathy? The empathic nurse attends carefully, listens intensely, responds reciprocally to verbal and nonverbal messages, uses appropriate language, times responses appropriately, clarifies and confirms ideas, explores the world from the client's viewpoint, and paces verbal and nonverbal behavior to the client's abilities.

TABLE 15-3

Summary of Therapeutic Communication Techniques

Technique	Definition	Therapeutic Value
Listening	An active process of receiving information and examining one's reaction to the messages received	Nonverbally communicates to client nurse's interest in client
Silence	Periods of no verbal communication among participants	Nonverbally communicates nurse's acceptance of client
Establishing guidelines	Statements regarding roles, purpose, and limitations for a particular interaction	Helps client to know what is expected of him
Open-ended comments	General comments asking the client to determine the direction the interaction should take	Allows client to decide what material is most relevant and encourages him to continue
Reducing distance	Diminishing physical space between the nurse and client	Nonverbally communicates that nurse wants to be involved with client
Acknowledgment	Recognition given to a client for contribution to an interaction	Demonstrates the importance of the client's role within the relationship
Restating	Repeating to the client what the nurse believes is the main thought or idea expressed	Asks for validation of nurse's interpretation of the message
Reflecting	Directing back to the client his ideas, feelings, questions, or content	Attempts to show client the importance of his own ideas, feelings, and interpretations
Seeking clarification	Asking for additional inputs to understand the message received	Demonstrates nurse's desire to understand client's communication
Seeking consensual validation	Attempts to reach a mutual denotative and connotative meaning of specific words	Demonstrates nurse's desire to understand client's communication
Focusing	Questions or statements to help the client develop or expand an idea	Directs conversation toward topics of importance
Summarizing	Statement of main areas discussed during interaction	Helps client to separate relevant from irrelevant material; serves as a review and closing for the interaction
Planning	Mutual decision-making regarding the goals, direction, and so on of future interactions	Reiterates client's role within relationship

From Sundeen, S. J., Stuart, G. W., Rankin, E. A. D., & Cohen, S. A. (1994). *Nurse–client interaction* (5th ed., p. 124). St. Louis: Mosby.

What does the caring nurse do to help the client understand or solve problems? The nurse identifies relationships and makes connections based on knowledge; states implicit assumptions; conceptualizes trends and patterns; verbalizes implied feelings, thoughts, goals, and attitudes; summarizes appropriately; explains purposes of activities; identifies non-verbal meanings; and assumes responsibility in the nursing process.

What does the caring nurse do to show respect? He or she verbalizes a clear commitment to understand, conveys acceptance, clearly affirms the client's worth as a unique person, and affirms the client's strengths and ability to assume responsibility for self. Such a nurse will help the client to strengthen self-identity. Strengthening self-identity is heard in phrases like "You have . . ." and "You do . . . ."

How does the nurse respond with authenticity? The nurse is consistent in responding with real thoughts and feelings and resists all urges to play-act; is clear on owning ideas and feelings; and permits himself or herself to share emotions with clients. The nurse who is authentic will say "I feel," "I think," or "I believe."

All of the preceding therapeutic professional nursing activities require the ability to listen. Listening demonstrates the nurse's ability to put the nurse's own needs after the client's needs (Sundeen et al., 1994, pp. 127–131). The use of therapeutic techniques is based on the nurse's belief that the client has the ability to be responsible for himself or herself, and to solve problems. The nurse facilitates the client's efforts at problem-solving, self-expression, and improvement in health status. The client shares equally in both the responsibility and the accountability for the nursing process.

COMMUNICATION STRATEGIES THAT REFLECT NONCARING FOR CLIENTS

The failure to listen is the most noncaring communication behavior the nurse can exhibit. When the nurse fails to listen, the message communicated to the client is "You are not of value to me" or "I am not interested—actually, I'm bored." Other nurse behaviors that are not helpful to clients are being judgmental (ie, putting personal values, beliefs, and perceptions above the client's); making stereotyped responses (ie, negating the uniqueness of the client by stating platitudes and cliches); and changing the subject (ie, stating nonverbally to the client that she will choose the topic and that what she thinks is more important than what he thinks). Blocks to therapeutic communication are summarized in Table 15-4.

Why do nurses use noncaring communication techniques with clients? Generally, one can assume that the nurse who communicates nontherapeutically has some need to behave regressively. This need, accompanied by increasing anxiety, sometimes leads to nurses seeing themselves as superior, and is expressed in negative actions such as moralizing, rejecting, or reacting with hostility.

Defensive behavior is common in regressive states. For example, a person might demonstrate denial, unconsciously evading or negating the real

TABLE 15-4

Summary of Nontherapeutic Communication Techniques

Technique	Definition	Therapeutic Value
Failure to listen	Not receiving client's intended message	Places needs of nurse above those of client
Failure to probe	Inadequate data collection represented by eliciting vague descriptions, getting inadequate answers, following standard forms too closely, and not exploring client's interpretation	Inadequate data base on which to make decisions; client care not individualized
Parroting	Continual repetition of client's phrases	The metacommunication is "I am not listening" or "I am not a competent communicator"
Being judgmental	Approving or disapproving statements	Implies that nurse has the right to pass judgment; promotes a dependency relationship
Reassuring	Attempts to do magic with words	Negates fears, feelings, and other communications of client
Rejecting	Refusing to discuss topics with client	Client may feel that not only communication but also the self was rejected
Defending	Attempts to protect someone or something from negative feedback	Negates client's right to express an opinion
Giving advice	Telling client what nurse thinks should be done	Negates the worth of client as a mutual partner in decision making
Stereotyped responses	Use of trite meaningless verbal expressions	Negates the significance of client's communication
Changing topics	Nurse directing the interaction into areas of self-interest rather than following lead of client	Nonverbally communicates that the nurse is in charge of deciding what will be discussed; possible to miss important topics for individual client
Patronizing	Style of communication that displays a condescending attitude toward the client	Implies that the nurse–client relationship is not based on equality; places the nurse in a "superior" position

From Sundeen, S. J., Stuart, G. W., Rankin, E. A. D., & Cohen, S. A. (1994). *Nurse–client interaction* (5th ed., p. 132). St. Louis: Mosby.

factors in a situation. Regressive states also may be marked by distortions, rote habitual actions, dogmatic responses, loss of control, unvalidated assumptions (jumping to conclusions), parroting, inappropriate timing, and poor judgment. These behaviors are important components of noncaring and nontherapeutic nursing strategies.

Because therapeutic communication is essential for effective professional nursing practice, it is imperative that nurses evaluate their communication techniques and seek help if a pattern of nontherapeutic behaviors is demonstrated. In actual nurse–client interactions, it is suggested that nurses let their own feelings be a guide to evaluation. The feeling of persistent anxiety or tension is perhaps the best cue that they may be unwittingly communicating in a noncaring and nonhelpful way.

Although there are different views on the advantages and disadvantages of nurses (as professionals) being characterized as caring persons, the fact has remained that nurses do care about their fellow humans. One dilemma for nurses is that they are not always permitted to care for clients to the best of their knowledge or ability. Benner and Wrubel (1988) note that when nurses can use their knowledge and ability to care for clients, stressors in nursing practice are reduced. Noting that "expert caring has nothing to do with possessing privileged information that increases one's control and domination of another," Benner and Wrubel (1988, p. 1075) postulate that "caring unleashes the possibilities inherent in the self and the situation" and that the one caring is also enriched in the communication process.

OUTCOMES OF HELPING RELATIONSHIPS

Two major client outcomes are desirable goals for the nurse–client relationship: (1) increased client understanding of how better personal responsibility and accountability for health can be achieved (learning), and (2) perceived satisfaction in the relationship. In terms of nurse outcomes, knowing that clients are adequately prepared to solve problems is the desired outcome. If clients are adequately prepared, they are free to choose, to put forth energy, and to assume greater responsibility for their own health.

In the nurse–client relationship, change occurs in two ways: (1) as an outcome of learning in terms of the information gained and understood, and (2) as an outcome of learning in terms of the interpersonal experience in the nursing process. The quality of communication plays the paramount role in change. When change and its effects are not communicated clearly, the change cannot be understood. Lack of understanding leads to resistance.

Kasche and Dine (1988, p. 323) propose that the profession needs a theory of nursing action "to account for the processes by which nurses effect changes in patients' health care status." The two aspects of communication that they identify as basic to this nursing action are "the ability to adopt a person-centered interpersonal orientation" and "to show perspective-taking ability" (Kasche & Dine, 1988, p. 324). They advise that a research agenda should be implemented on person-centered communication strategies and perspective-taking abilities. Such research would increase the nurse's understanding of communication and its significance in accomplishing nursing goals.

Hunsaker and Alessandra have proposed a schema for self-evaluation of communication patterns of persons in management positions. They raise a number of questions to ask oneself, which are clearly applicable to the evaluation of communication in the nursing process (Hunsaker & Alessandra, 1980, pp. 140–141, enumeration added):

1. Did I comprehend each point made?
2. Did I make judgments of the words before the speaker was through speaking?

3. Did I make decisions in my own mind while he or she was still speaking?
4. Did I hunt for evidence that would prove the speaker right? Wrong?
5. Did I hunt for evidence that would prove myself right? Wrong?
6. Did I become upset while listening?
7. Did I generally jump to conclusions while listening?
8. Did I let the client speak at least 50% of the time?
9. Did I understand the words in terms of their intended meanings?
10. Did I restate ideas and feelings accurately?
11. Did I study voice, posture, actions and facial expressions as the client talked?
12. Did I listen between the lines for unspoken meanings behind the words?
13. Did I really try to listen to the client?
14. Did I really want to listen to the client?
15. Did I really show the client I was, in fact, motivated and interested in listening to him?

Nurses should continually evaluate their own communication behaviors. In addition to self-evaluations by such schema as the preceding questions, the nurse should consistently evaluate the effectiveness of communication with the client. Feedback should be sought from the client about what has been said and about how the client feels the relationship is going. The value of the nurse–client interactions should be explored at intervals to promote mutual benefits to nurse and client. A focus on asking the client "How are we doing?" states to the client that the nurse values him and cares how the communication affects him.

VIGNETTE

Susan has recently accepted a position in an outpatient radiation oncology unit. Traditionally, nursing care in this unit has focused on relief of symptoms of the medical treatment, but Susan feels that many patients need more holistic care. She wants to promote healing in her patients, but she does not know how to start.

Healing Relationships—The Nurse's Role in Healing

A healing relationship might be considered a special type of helping relationship. As "to heal is the activity of becoming whole" (Kritek, 1997, p. 11), healing has been defined as "a process of bringing parts of one's self together at deep levels of inner knowing, leading to an integration and balance, with each part having equal importance and value" (Dossey, Keegan,

Guzzetta, & Kolkmeier, 1995, p. 62), and, as "an inner process through which a person becomes whole" (Lerner, 1994, p. 13). Healing occurs within the person, and external interventions mobilize the client's inner healing resources (Micozzi, 1996).

A number of types of healing have been described (Keegan, 1994, pp. 4–6), including:

- Faith healing based on prayer and religious faith (eg, charismatics)
- Mind cures based on changing mental states (eg, Scientology)
- Metaphysical healing based on the nonreality of matter (eg, Christian Science)
- Spiritualism based on intervention by spirits of the dead (eg, Shamanism)
- Mesmerism based on the movement of vital fluid
- Energy medicine based on unblocking energy fields (eg, Oriental medicine)
- Hypnotism based on power of suggestion (eg, behavior modification)
- Germ theory based on invading pathogenic organisms (eg, scientific medicine)

Lerner (1994) differentiates among universal, common, and unique conditions of healing. Examples of universal conditions are inner peace and a deep experience of love. Attention and care from friends and family, deeply enjoyed work, laughter, moving music, and great art are examples of common conditions. However, Lerner indicates that the unique conditions of healing are some of the most important. Thus, the nurse in a healing relationship needs to identify the particulars that are most meaningful for the individual client.

Given that healing occurs within the client, the nurse healer's role is to facilitate another person's growth and life processes toward wholeness or to assist with recovery from illness or with transition to peaceful death (Dossey et al., 1995, p. 62). The nurse assists and responds to the client who is the central force in the healing process. "Nurses assume that their actions, as professionals, aim to facilitate wholeness in others through an interaction based on a mutuality of purpose" (Kritek, 1997, p. 14). Kritek (1997, p. 21) states that four fundamental elements are always present in the healing encounter:

Nurse and client interact within a given context
The encounter is in response to a health experience
The nurse works in a pattern of mutuality with the client
Healing is facilitated in response to a client's elicitation of nursing involvement and expertise

Healing is facilitated within a helping relationship that is characterized by such principles as presence (being rather than doing), intention and purpose, empathy, guiding, creativity, imagery, and spirituality (Dossey et al., 1995; Keegan, 1994; Lerner, 1994).

The following guiding principles for nurse healers' practice have been identified (Keegan, 1994, pp. 211–212):

1. There is a unity and interdependence within the mind, body, and spirit
2. Health is a process that may include disease
3. One's attitudes and beliefs toward life (mental–emotional energy fields or consciousness) is a major etiologic factor in health and disease
4. One's health and disease are manifested in one's life-style, habits, and conscious awareness, as well as the body's physical being and energy
5. The self is empowered with the ability to create or maintain health/disease
6. Changes in health can occur through experiential learning. Experiential learning is defined as a change in behavior that occurs as a result of living through an activity, event, or situation
7. Experiential learning is essential to changing one's life-style for high-level wellness
8. Human beings are energy fields
9. Healing involves a tranformational change that encompasses the whole person; it requires the involvement of the spiritual, emotional, and intellectual domains, as well as the physical body
10. Energy fields can become unbalanced as a response to stress in any one of the three domains of body, mind, and spirit
11. The client–practitioner relationship is one of partnership—equal with differing responsibilities
12. Any modality or health system that supports healing should be valued
13. Each health system should be respected for the resources and the tools that it offers while being challenged to prove its credibility
14. Each person is an open system with the environment without separating boundaries
15. Energy fields are constantly interacting
16. Health is the dynamic evolution toward balanced integration
17. Health involves a sense of unity with the self and cosmos
18. Wellness encompasses increasing openness (acceptance of diversity) and increasing harmony (coherent, high-frequency energy fields)
19. Health is influenced by the environment (interpenetrating external energy fields) and genetics (transgenerational energy fields)
20. Healing, when viewed holistically, is not predictable in terms of time frame, cause, or outcome
21. The division of the whole person into three domains of body, mind, and spirit is an old-paradigm illusion
22. Body, mind, and spirit share one consciousness

23. The human spirit is the core of the person
24. Spiritual health is necessary for physical, mental, and emotional well-being
25. The Source is experienced or known primarily through joy, beauty, love, light, peace, power, and life

◎ Conclusion

All people have visions of what they would like to accomplish and noble intentions about acting on their dreams. Bennis and Nanus (1985, p. 33) state, however, that "without communication nothing will be realized." Mastery of communication is necessary for carrying out the agendas of life, and promoting health and healing.

THOUGHT QUESTIONS

1 Are you an effective listener? What can you do to improve your listening skills?

2 Monitor your therapeutic communication during one week. How many effective and ineffective techniques did you use? How can you improve your communication skills?

3 Are there differences between a helping and a healing relationship? Can you think of ways that you and Susan (see vignette) can get started?

REFERENCES

American Nurses Association. (1980). *Social policy statement*. Kansas City: Author.
American Nurses Association. (1995). *Social policy statement*. Kansas City: Author.
Arnold, E., & Boggs, K. (1989). *Interpersonal relationships: Professional communication skills for nurses*. Philadelphia: Saunders.
Benner, P., & Wrubel, J. (1988). Caring comes first. *American Journal of Nursing, 88,* 1072–1075.
Bennis, W., & Nanus, B. (1985). *Leaders: The strategies for taking charge*. New York: Harper & Row.
Berlo, D. K. (1960). *The process of communication*. New York: Holt, Rinehart and Winston.
Bradley, J. C., & Edinberg, M. A. (1990). *Communication in the nursing context* (3rd ed.). East Norwalk, CT: Appleton & Lange.
Brill, N. I. (1990). *Working with people: The helping process* (4th ed.). New York: Longman.
Cecchio, J. F., & Cecchio, C. M. (1982). *Effective communication in nursing theory and practice*. New York: Wiley.
Dossey, B. M., Keegan, L., Guzzetta, C. E., & Kolkmeier, L. G. (1995). *Holistic nursing: A handbook for practice* (2nd ed.). Gaithersburg, MD: Aspen.
Hammond, D. C., Hepworth, D. H., & Smith, V. G. (1977). Improving therapeutic communication. San Francisco: Jossey-Bass.
Hunsaker, P. L., & Alessandra, A. J. (1980). *Art of managing people*. Englewood Cliffs, NJ: Prentice-Hall.

Kasche, C. R., & Dine, J. (1988, June). Person-centered communication and social perspective taking, *Western Journal of Nursing Research, 10,* 317–326.

Keegan, L. (1994). *The nurse as healer.* Albany, NY: Delmar.

Kritek, P. B. (1997). Healing: A central nursing construct—Reflections on meaning. In P. B. Kritek (Ed.). *Reflections on healing: A central nursing construct* (pp. 11–27). New York: National League for Nursing.

Lerner, M. (1994). *Choices in healing.* Cambridge, MA: Massachusetts Institute of Technology.

Marck, P. (1990). Therapeutic reciprocity: A caring phenomenon. *Advances in Nursing Science, 13,* 49–59.

Mendias, E. P. (1997). Reciprocity in the healing relationship between nurse and patient. In P. B. Kritek (Ed.). *Reflections on healing: A central nursing construct* (pp. 435–451). New York: National League for Nursing.

Micozzi, M. S. (Ed.). (1996). *Fundamentals of complementary and alternative medicine.* New York: Churchill Livingstone.

Newman, M., Lamb, G. S., & Michaels, C. (1991, October). Nurse case management: The coming together of theory and practice. *Nursing & Health Care, 12,* 404–408.

Olson, D. P. (1991). Empathy as an ethical and philosophical basis for nursing. *Advances in Nursing Science 14,* 62–75.

Osterman, P., & Schwaartz-Barcott, D. (1996). Presence: Four ways of being there. *Nursing Forum, 31,* 23–30.

Pagano, M. P., & Ragan, S. L. (1992). *Communication skills for professional nurses.* Newbury Park, CA: Sage.

Parse, R. R. (1996). The human becoming theory: Challenges in practice and research. *Nursing Science Quarterly, 9,* 55–60.

Paterson, J. G., & Zderad, L. T. (1988). *Humanistic nursing.* New York: National League for Nursing.

Peplau, H. (1952). *Interpersonal relations in nursing.* New York: G. P. Putnam's Sons.

Rogers, C. R. (1951). *Client-centered therapy: Its current practice, implications, and theory.* Boston: Houghton Mifflin.

Rogers, C. R. (1958). Characteristics of a helping relationship. *Personnel and Guidance Journal, 37,* 6–16.

Rogers, M. E. (1970). *An introduction to the theoretical basis of nursing.* Philadelphia: Davis.

Smith, S. (1992). *Communications in nursing* (2nd ed.). St. Louis: Mosby.

Soukhanov, A. H. (Ed.) (1992). *The American Heritage Dictionary of the English Language* (3rd ed.). Boston: Houghton Mifflin.

Sullivan, H. S. (1953). *The interpersonal theory of psychiatry.* New York: Norton.

Sundeen, S. J., Stuart, G. W., Rankin, E. A. D., & Cohen, S. A. (1994). *Nurse–client interaction* (5th ed.). St. Louis: Mosby.

Taylor, A. (1977). *Communicating.* Englewood Cliffs, NJ: Prentice-Hall.

Vestal, K. W. (1995). *Nursing management: Concepts and issues* (2nd ed.). Philadelphia: Lippincott.

Watson, J. (1996). Watson's theory of transpersonal caring. In P. H. Walker & B. Neuman (Eds.). *Blueprint for use of nursing models: Education, research, practice and administration* (pp. 141–162). New York: National League for Nursing.

Wiseman, T. A. concept analysis of empathy. *Journal of Advanced Nursing, 23,* 1162–1167.

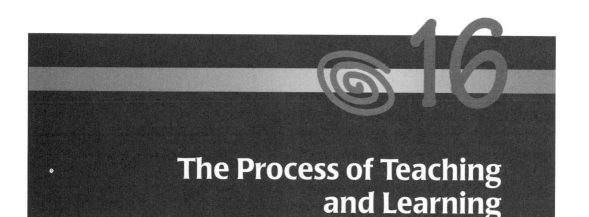

The Process of Teaching and Learning

LEARNING OUTCOMES

By the end of this chapter, the student will be able to:

1 Understand why it is important to think about teaching–learning as a process, not a product.

2 Cite the rationale for the declaration that both the client and the nurse are "experts" in the teaching–learning process.

3 List the three main communication concepts that facilitate teaching–learning.

4 Explain how mutuality enhances learning for the client.

5 Describe each step of the traditional teaching–learning process.

6 Relate the concepts of growth, change, and learning to each other.

7 State two important factors that the nurse must assess to determine the client's readiness for learning.

8 Explain the significance of validation in learning.

9 Know what the client should know about the nurse in the teaching–learning process.

VIGNETTE

Lillian has just completed her first 6 months as a staff nurse on a medical–surgical hospital unit. Her evaluations have been generally positive, but she has been urged to pay more attention to the teaching needs of patients. Lillian feels that she lacks the skills to provide effective patient teaching, and she feels that patient teaching is time-consuming and not feasible because of her heavy workloads and the usually inadequate staffing on her unit.

Teaching has been accepted as a leadership role for professional nurses for decades, even before the development of nursing models on which nurses could base their practice. When nurses based their practice on knowledge primarily borrowed from medicine and the physical and behavioral sciences, they agreed that it was important to share information with clients about their medical condition, their medications, and ways to implement the medical regimen when they were discharged from the hospital. Historically, patient teaching was "centered on a rather rigidly defined goal of compliance with the medical regimen" (Redman & Thomas, 1992, p. 304).

In the past two decades, nurses have continued to agree that clients need information from them; however, professional nurses have learned that the content of their teaching emerges from a mutually determined process between nurse and client and that it focuses on the health of the client, not on the medical diagnosis. Schlotfeldt (1988, p. 18) says that one specific function of a scholarly nursing practitioner is "teaching and guiding persons toward pursuit of their own health goals, stimulating and sometimes inspiring them toward knowledgeable pursuit of optimal health and recovery."

Teaching–learning has also been cited as a public duty of all professions. Nursing thus has an obligation to present organized educational activities and public discussions. Professional responsibility goes beyond individual professional–client teaching–learning relationships. Nursing as a professional entity has the opportunity and obligation both to educate the larger client system—the public—about the relationships between quality of life and health, and to influence the mission of health care delivery institutions regarding the social ends they should serve. Listening and learning from the public, the professional nurse grows in ability to provide information that promotes health. "During the past three decades, changing needs and mandates have increased the visibility, involvement, and expertise of nurses as patient teachers" (Rankin & Stallings, 1996, p. 18). This chapter focuses on nurses' responsibility in the teaching role and the mutuality in teaching–learning relationships in nursing processes.

Philosophic Assumptions About Teaching–Learning

The description of teaching–learning as a leadership function for professional nurses is based on the beliefs that (1) teaching–learning is a process, not a product; (2) the process is implemented in a relationship between experts; and (3) communication is the essential element of the process.

PROCESS–NOT PRODUCT

Believing in the significance of interpersonal relationships, the nurse must consider the possibility that the health of a person is determined to a large extent by the quality of the person's relationships with other people. Through relationships, growth can occur—that is, the person integrates new functions that lead to a more satisfactory life. Thus, the nurse needs to provide the client with educative experiences that increase the integration of functions that improve health. Teaching–learning in the nurse–client relationship is directed toward such growth.

Defined as development to a more complex form (Soukhanov, 1992, p. 801), growth includes the development of capacity for healthy behaviors. This development of capacity occurs in teaching–learning relationships between nurses and clients. "Learning is a process that is dependent on an interchange between the learning individual and the environment" (Babcock & Miller, 1994, p. 22). Learning may involve skills and performance (psychomotor), feelings or belief (affective), or thinking (cognitive), and is usually associated with a change in behavior.

Such operations cannot occur in the client if nurses simply offer information as a product of their trade. Rather, such operations require that teaching–learning be viewed as a process in which the nurse offers a professional relationship in which the new functions can be validated. Such validation is further discussed in Chapter 15, which presents the concepts of empathy, respect, and genuineness in communication. Therefore, teaching–learning is an interpersonal process in which both the teacher and the learner acquire new information, experience new relatedness, and behave in new ways as a result of the relationship.

Patient education is "a process of helping someone to learn through planned sequences of teaching, supportive activity, and directed practice and reinforcement" (Redman & Thomas, 1992, p. 304). Clients are encouraged to assume responsibility for improving their health and their own self-care. Argyris (1982, p. 94), who believes that human beings are "self-governing and personally responsible," says that people (1) have the ability to bring about certain consequences; (2) have ideas about how to accomplish their intentions; and (3) feel success or failure on the basis of their achievement or nonachievement of their intentions.

If professional nurses believe that clients have these abilities, they will view learning as far more than discovery by the client. They will define their teacher role as focusing on "learning that leads to new action and new problem-solving, which enable individuals and systems to continue to learn" (Argyris, 1982, p. 160). Teaching–learning thus becomes an ongoing dynamic process.

If learning is not the passive acceptance by the learner of information from the teacher, nurses must commit themselves to collaborative relationships with their clients to fulfill their teaching–learning role function. This means that the teaching enables clients to participate, to define their own strengths and problems, and to construct their own meanings. Teaching–learning thus is a collaborative process that is most effective when nurses fully engage clients as participatory learners.

RELATIONSHIP BETWEEN EXPERTS

Teaching–learning can be viewed as a relationship between experts. In the professional nursing process, we view nurses as the experts on health, and clients as the experts on their experience of health and the circumstances of their life. In the teaching–learning process, we view nurses as the expert on knowledge about health and the information that enables people to achieve health, and clients as experts on the context of their life and needs for information and experiences to achieve their intentions to maximize health.

Nurse—Information and Knowledge Expert

Teaching–learning may be seen as a part of the healing process. Nurses who have reported that they believed their interventions made a difference in their clients' progress described several steps in that healing relationship (Benner, 1984, p. 49):

1. Mobilizing hope for the nurse as well as for the client
2. Finding an acceptable interpretation or understanding of the illness, pain, fear, anxiety, or other stressful emotion
3. Assisting the client to use social, emotional, or spiritual support

Viewing teaching as a coaching function, Benner (1984, p. 77) says that "nurses become experts in coaching a patient through an illness. They take what is foreign and fearful to the patient and make it familiar and thus less frightening." The teacher needs to have expertise in helping. Helping the learner become aware of learning and thinking processes and helping the person understand the nature of the problems may be equally as important as providing information.

To be an expert in the teaching–learning process, the nurse must also be an enabler. Learning is facilitated when teachers treat learners as responsible people. It is interesting to note this idea of enabling clients is a recently developed belief. According to Fine (1988, p. 66), in the health care delivery system "the impetus to share information with patient consumers was almost unheard of until the beginning of the consumer movement in the 1960s." Because nurses are educated as health professionals, their knowledge endows them with expert ability to "increase the use of information flow to and from the consumer, thus facilitating the right and responsibility of the consumer to have a greater voice in health care decisions" (Fine, 1988, p. 72).

In addition to coach and enabler, several other roles have been proposed for the nurse–teacher, including (Forbes, 1995, p. 99):

- Learning facilitator, who breaks down barriers to learning by listening, probing, and being aware of feelings
- Authority, who sets up a teaching structure and rules
- Ego ideal, who serves as a role model for the client's "altered existence"
- Socializing agent, who acknowledges concerns and fears for the future
- Person, who relates to clients as people on the basis of much more than a disease diagnosis

Client—Context and Needs Expert

No one knows better the meaning of his or her own life, individual health status, and full circumstances integral to life experiences than does the client. Thus, clients are the experts on the context in which they will be attempting to implement new health behaviors. They are the experts on their need for information, support, and relatedness. If the nurse can appreciate both his or her own expertise and the client's expertise, then the teaching–learning process can truly be implemented as a mutual responsibility.

The Joint Commission on the Accreditation of Healthcare Organization (JCAHO) has developed standards for client and family education as an essential element of nursing. To "improve patient health outcomes by promoting recovery, speeding return to function, promoting healthy behavior, and appropriately involving the patient in his or her care decisions" (JCAHO, 1994), education should:

- Facilitate patient/family understanding of the patient's health status, health care options, and consequences of options selected
- Encourage patient/family participation in the decision-making process about health care options
- Increase patient's/family's potential to follow the therapeutic health care plan
- Maximize patient/family care skills
- Increase patient's/family's ability to cope with the patient's health status/prognosis/outcome
- Enhance patient's/family's role in continuing care
- Promote a healthy patient lifestyle

The standards, with targets and supporting evidence, are presented in Table 16-1. Knowledge about communication is a prerequisite to the nurse's development of teaching knowledge and associated clinical judgments and skills.

TABLE 16-1

JCAHO Standards for Patient/Family Education

Standard	Targets	Evidence*
Standard PF.1 Patient and family provided with appropriate education and training to increase knowledge of illness and treatment needs, and skills/behaviors to promote recovery and improve function	• Patient and family understanding of current health problem and reason for admission • Patient informed consent re: treatment • Patient and family understanding of treatment plan and the role they will play • Overview of survival skills needed for safe discharge	• All patients receive instruction • Priorities for education are identified by the organization
Standard PF.2 Patient and family receive education specific to patient's assessed needs, abilities, readiness, and appropriate to length of stay	• Safe and effective use of medications • Medical equipment • Potential drug–food interactions, modified diets • Rehab techniques • Community resources • How to obtain further treatment • Ongoing health care needs	• Patient assessment • Information understandable to patient • Teaching is culturally appropriate
Standard PF.3 Any discharge instructions given to the patient and family are provided to the organization responsible for patient's continuing care	• Written discharge instructions, understandable to patient, include targets for PF.2. • Continuing care provider identified • Instructions provided to continuing care providers	• Discharge planning involves patient and family • Discharge instructions clear: who is to do what
Standard PF.4 The organization plans and supports the provision and coordination of patient and family education activities and resources	• Classes • Community resources access • Closed circuit TV • Multimedia library • Patient education materials data base • One-on-one presentations • Interdisciplinary educational process	• Provision and coordination of patient education activities and resources • Resources selected based on patient needs • Health care team involvement • Educational formats based on specific needs

*Policies and procedures, progress notes, flowsheets, referral and consultation notes, interviews with staff, written information given to patients and families.

Adapted from JCAHO. (1994). *Comprehensive accreditation manual for hospitals*. Chicago: Author.

COMMUNICATION: THE CONDITION FOR TEACHING–LEARNING

The reader is referred to Chapter 15 for more extensive discussion of communication concepts essential for effective teaching–learning: empathy, respect, and genuineness. The nurse needs empathy to understand the client's situation and take full advantage of the expertise the client brings to the relationship. The client needs empathy to perceive that the nurse is sensitive to the client's human needs, and to reinforce that the client is able to act as a full human being.

If the teaching–learning process is to be accepted by both the nurse and the client as a mutual responsibility, respect must be experienced in the communication between the two. The perception of self-worth is based on this respect, and an enhanced sense of self-worth facilitates both teaching and learning.

Full exploration and analysis of health concerns and information needed to change health behaviors cannot occur unless both the nurse and the client perceive each other as real—as genuinely human, open, honest, and caring in their responses to each other. Thus, the characteristic of genuineness must be present in the relationship between the teacher and the learner.

Given the communication characteristics of empathy, respect, and genuineness, the nurse will exhibit the action of empowerment, which concerns perceived client ability to have control in his or her life. The nurse will empower the client by (Rankin & Stallings, 1996, p. 103):

■ Helping to establish critical thinking and analytical skills
■ Providing a framework for creative thinking
■ Assisting the client in raising questions
■ Establishing an environment where genuine dialogue can occur
■ Encouraging chosen actions
■ Evaluating the results of actions with clients

These functions are incorporated in the nursing process.

◎ The Traditional Teaching–Learning Process

The traditional process for organizing teaching–learning into a specific framework that has been accepted as both workable and traditional is presented first, followed by a discussion of other approaches implied in advocacy and change theory. The activities in this process are assessment, planning, implementation, evaluation, and documentation. The synthesis of the process in practice is diagrammed in Figure 16-1.

The first activity on the part of the nurse–teacher is assessment: to gather facts and information that will help the nurse meet the client's or the family's needs for learning. Rankin and Stallings (1996) indicate that there are four steps in the assessment process:

■ Selecting the areas to be assessed
■ Gathering the data

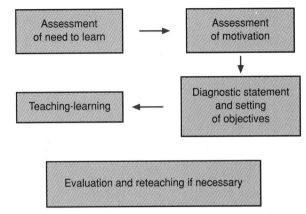

FIGURE 16-1 The process of teaching. (From Redman, B. K. [1993]. *The process of patient education* [p. 12]. St. Louis: Mosby-Year Book. Used with permission of the publisher.)

- Sorting and categorizing the data
- Writing a summary statement (nursing diagnosis)

Purposes of assessment include (Rankin & Stallings, 1996; Redman, 1993):

1. Identify what the client wants to learn
2. Identify what information the client needs
3. Establish a point of reference for learning (relate new information to preexisting knowledge)
4. Identify incorrect information and assumptions
5. Determine what factors in the environment may pose barriers
6. Identify what will need to be evaluated
7. Build trust and rapport
8. Provide for involvement of family
9. Prioritize needs and problems

The assessment may be conducted by using the following behaviors: listening and questioning, observing, reviewing records, collaborating with the health care team, and integrating the client's verbal description with the nurse's observation.

After determining the learning needs in the assessment stage, the nurse develops a plan that contains objectives for the client's learning that have been established together with the client and the family. These objectives clarify what is to be taught, what is to be learned, what and how to evaluate, and what to document. An objective must be (1) singular to be specific; (2) inclusive of all elements of content necessary to be understood; (3) measurable; and (4) realistic to the extent that it can be attained by the client.

After objectives are clarified and validated in the plan, implementation of the learning objectives is done by analyzing the information to be pre-

sented and selecting a method of presentation that maximizes the involvement of the client's senses. The nurse often can complement the presentation of information by using supplemental materials, such as audiovisual
aids. Another major function of the nurse in the implementation phase is
to observe the client's reaction to the teaching–learning.

In evaluation, the next activity in the teaching–learning process, the
nurse and client determine whether or not the client has achieved the objectives. The criteria used in evaluation are the specifications of what the
client will do and the particular behavior that the client will demonstrate
that are stated in each objective. The outcomes must be recorded on the
client's official record. Using the objectives as a basis, the nurse should
record client achievements and note client reactions on the record.

◎ Teaching–Learning as a Responsibility of the Advocate

The American Nurses Association (ANA, 1995) stresses that nurses provide care that promotes well-being in both healthy and ill people, individually or in groups and communities. Practicing within this scope,
professional nurses have agreed on the following statements:

1. Clients want and need to participate actively in the nursing process
2. Clients have the right to make decisions about their own health behaviors
3. Clients need cognitive and interpersonal support from professional
   nurses to make decisions that promote the highest level of health
4. Clients want and need to experience mutuality in the teaching–
   learning process that occurs in nurse–client relationships to offset
   feelings of helplessness, dependency, and submissiveness that commonly occur when they experience health concerns or illness

The belief in advocacy as an appropriate role of the nurse has evolved
in harmony with a larger social movement characterized by consumerism,
self-care, justice and human rights, equal opportunity for all, and individual accountability for health. People no longer believe that illness is an
event over which the person has no control. Given these values, nurses today readily accept the obligation to act as advocates in their relationships
with clients. See Chapter 17 for a fuller discussion of the advocate role.
One of the most significant activities of the nurse advocate is to provide
informational support to assist the client to make the wisest possible decisions in the pursuit of well-being.

THE PURPOSE OF TEACHING–LEARNING

The search for meaning in the nursing process should be focused on the
client's perception of his health situation. The phenomenologic model of
curriculum proposed by Diekelmann (1988) fits the role conception of the

nurse as an advocate for the client. In this model, "the central concern is the communicative understandings of meanings given by people who live within the situation" (Diekelmann, 1988, p. 142). Thus, the purpose for teaching–learning is to provide the opportunity for the nurse and the client to explore together the importance and meaning of the client's experience.

Applying Diekelmann's proposition, the essential aspect of the process is not transmitting or acquiring facts; rather, it is "making meaning and giving meaning . . . through the initiation and maintenance of dialogue" (Diekelmann, 1988, p. 143). Further, Diekelmann (1988, p. 143) proposes that the teacher's role is to "link the contextual and conceptual worlds of students," who are, in this discussion, clients participating in the nursing process. In this kind of dialogue, clients retain the authority and responsibility for their own decisions and their own health behaviors.

According to Babcock and Miller (1994), if we expect clients to take interdependent and independent responsibilities for decision-making, then we must have nurses who can:

Identify central issues
Recognize underlying assumptions
Recognize evidence of bias and emotion
Solve problems
Think creatively

The development of these abilities are the challenge for educational programs preparing new practitioners of professional nursing.

FUNCTIONS OF THE ADVOCATE IN THE TEACHING–LEARNING PROCESS

Providing the opportunity for dialogue to fully explore health concerns is the major function of the nurse acting as an advocate for clients, whether they are experiencing high or low levels of wellness. Within this exploration, nurses use their expertise to "not only offer information [but also] offer ways of being, ways of coping, and even new possibilities" for the clients (Benner, 1984, p. 78).

Benner (1984, pp. 78–93) proposes that teaching–learning transactions take on new dimensions when the learner (client) is ill. She cites the following competencies necessary for the nurse to assume the teaching–coaching function with a client who is ill:

1. Carefully time the interventions to capture the client's readiness to learn
2. Help the client integrate the implications of the illness and recovery into the client's lifestyle
3. Elicit and respect the client's interpretation of the illness
4. Respond fully and cogently to the client's request for explanation of what is happening (within the limits of both the client's and the nurse's own understanding)

5. Make approachable and understandable any culturally avoided or uncharted aspects of an illness by exploring ways of being and coping for the client and the family and by identifying new possibilities.

Growth through learning is maximized if the nurse fulfills these functions with the client.

MUTUALITY IN THE TEACHING–LEARNING PROCESS

One of the primary characteristics of an advocate–client relationship is mutuality. Watson (1988, p. 4), supporting the concept of mutuality, stresses that we must "shift from oppressive interactions to liberating interactions." In her view, both the teacher and the student should be learners rather than simply "givers of information" (Watson, 1988, p. 4). Learning would be mutual, characterized by anticipatory–participatory behaviors, shared power, and the absence of separation of "doing from knowing and being" (Watson, 1988, p. 2). Watson's model of nursing is cited as one example of a model that mandates mutuality in the nursing process and places high priority on teaching–learning as a significant intervention mode in a reciprocal nurse–client relationship.

Mutuality can be defined as "a connection with or understanding of another that facilitates a dynamic process of joint exchange between people. The process of being mutual is characterized by a sense of unfolding action that is shared in common, a sense of moving toward a common goal, and a sense of satisfaction for all involved" (Henson, 1997, p. 80). Mutuality balances power and respect, encourages accountability, and "facilitates active involvement of both nurses and clients in effectively working toward mutually identified goals" (Henson, 1997, p. 77). Mutuality is consistent with any learning theory used to guide the teaching–learning process.

◎ Learning Theories

The process by which learning occurs has been described in several different ways. Each of the multiple models explaining how people learn are considered to be potentially useful in specific circumstances when mediated through specific patterns of meaning to particular learners.

LEARNER MODELS

Bruner (1986) cites five popular models of how the learner learns: empiricism, hypothesis generator, nativism, constructivism, and novice-to-expert. *Empiricism* is considered the oldest model. It is based on the premise that "one learns from experience" and that "such order as there is in the mind is a reflection of the order that exists in the world" (Bruner, 1986, p.

199). A person is successful in learning in the empiricism model if he or she has experiences.

Unlike the rather passive view of the empiricism model, the *hypothesis generator* models include a major premise of intentionality. "The learner, rather than being the creature of experience, selects that which is to enter" (Bruner, 1986, p. 199). The characteristic of the learner is "active curiosity guided by self-directed projects" (Bruner, 1986, p. 199). A person is a successful learner in this model if the person has a good theory from which hypotheses are generated.

The *nativism* model proposes that the mind is innately shaped by "a set of underlying categories, hypotheses," both forms of organizing experiences (Bruner, 1986, p. 199). The task of the learner in this model is to develop a way of organizing perceived reality. Using the innate powers of the mind is the formula for successful learning in this model.

The *constructivism* model was largely developed by Piaget, who, according to Bruner (1986, p. 199), says that "the world is not found, but made, and made according to a set of structural rules that are imposed on the flow of experience." These structural rules provide boundaries for learning. The learner goes through stagelike progressions characterized by tension between previously assimilated structural rules and changes in the rules that come in later stage development. In accommodating these new rules, the learner is successful if his or her learning structure changes by moving to a higher system that subsumes the earlier structures.

The newest of the learner models, according to Bruner (1986), is the *novice-to-expert* model. It "begins with the premise that if you want to find out about learning, ask first about what is to be learned, find an expert who does it well, and then look at the novice and figure out how he or she can get there" (Bruner, 1986, p. 199). In this model, the formula for success is to be specific and explicit in taking the steps to attain expertise.

Bruner (1986, p. 200) suggests that there is not just one kind of learning and that we would be better served if we understood that "the model of the learner is not fixed but various." If we appreciate the diversity in learner models, teaching–learning becomes "more than a scripted exercise in cultural rigidity" (Bruner, 1986, p. 200).

TYPES OF LEARNING

Bevis (1988, p. 40) offers a helpful differentiation of six types of learning that may be useful in the teaching–learning process in nursing:

1. **Item learning:** simple relationships between separate pieces of information, as seen in mechanistic and ritualistic lists and procedures
2. Directive learning: rules, injunctions, and exceptions, as seen in safety requirements

3. Rational learning: use of theory to buttress action, enabling logical decision-making and logical judgments
4. Syntactic learning: seeing meaningful wholes, relationships, and patterns "addresses the lived moment and the relationships that ideas, concepts, have with each other" and enables the learner to develop insights and find meaning
5. Contextual learning: acceptance of culture, mores, folkways, rites, and rituals as ways of being; these learning transactions are "caring, compassionate, and positive"
6. Inquiry learning: investigating, categorizing, and theorizing in a way to generate ideas and develop a vision

Bevis (1988, p. 45) suggests that syntactic learning, contextual learning, and inquiry learning are necessary for change that can truly maximize the client's abilities to gain the best control of his health.

PRINCIPLES OF LEARNING

Principles identified by Babcock and Miller (1994, pp. 45–48) are considered useful in any of the aforementioned learner models or types of learning. These principles to guide the nurse in the teaching–learning process are:

1. Focusing intensifies learning.
2. Repetition enhances learning.
3. Learner control increases learning.
4. Active participation is necessary for learning.
5. Learning styles vary.
6. Organization promotes learning.
7. Association is necessary to learning.
8. Imitation is a method of learning.
9. Motivation strengthens learning.
10. Spacing new material facilitates learning.
11. Recency influences retention.
12. Primacy affects retention.
13. Arousal influences attention.
14. Accurate and prompt feedback enhances learning.
15. Application of new learning in a variety of contexts broadens the generalization of that learning.
16. The learner's biologic, psychological, sociologic, and cultural realities shape the learner's perception of the learning experience.

Further, because clients vary in individual learning preferences, the professional nurse needs to understand the multiple models and types of learning to personalize the teaching–learning process effectively. Effectiveness is measured by the success the nurse and client experience in changing the client's health behaviors in a positive direction.

◎ Implications of Change Theory for Teaching–Learning

Inherent in the definition of learning is growth. Growth implies that change occurs and is ongoing throughout life.

BEHAVIOR CHANGE AS A GOAL OF TEACHING: GROWTH

The mutually determined goal of the nurse and the client who are participating in the teaching–learning process is "becoming different than before" (Douglass, 1988, p. 226). Douglass notes that forces that influence change can be external or internal. The nurse is an intentional external force assisting the client to demonstrate different and better health behaviors.

In a series of sequential steps that are consistent with planned change theory, the nurse in the teaching–learning relationship needs to do the following (Douglass, 1988, pp. 226–232):

1. Explore the client's perceived need for change
2. Identify the forces for change with the client
3. Help the client state health concerns
4. Identify constraints and opportunities in the situation
5. Provide the information needed to analyze both the change needs and the potential strategies to achieve the desired change
6. Critique each of the possible change strategies on the basis of both the information understood and the situational factors
7. Select the change strategy to be attempted in the effort to achieve a different and better health behavior
8. Plan the implementation, filling in all of the informational gaps perceived by the nurse and the client
9. Design an evaluation process to determine success in changing health behavior
10. Client: Implement the planned behavioral activities. Nurse: Offer feedback and facilitate opportunities in the delivery system environment to promote success of the client
11. Evaluate the overall results of the teaching–learning interaction and the specific health behavior changes on the part of the client

OUTCOMES OF KNOWLEDGE ACQUISITION

The outcome of knowledge acquisition in the teaching–learning process is not always satisfying to the nurse and the client. If the information acquired is congruent with previously integrated functions, harmony is most likely to be perceived within the human system. If the information acquired is incongruent with the previously integrated functions, disharmony is most likely to be perceived within the human system. Nurses often need to help clients understand the long-term value of those planned changes that cause feelings of disharmony.

O'Connor (1986, p. 52) advises that the nurse and the client should analyze the "situational context of a proposed change," taking into account "the individuals involved, the institutional climate, and societal trends." She also suggests that the nurse and client need to analyze their motivation to work on the planned change in terms of "potential threats to or fulfillment of basic human needs" (O'Connor, 1986, p. 54). Both the situational context and the motivational aspects of planned change play a significant role in the client's ability to integrate information and develop new behaviors. The quality of the integration of new functions from the new information is affected by the perceived harmony or disharmony in the system.

READINESS FOR LEARNING

A central issue for professional nurses in implementing the teaching–learning process as a strategy for changing behaviors is the client's readiness for learning. Benner (1984, p. 79) notes that teaching–learning interventions are often dictated by schedules in the health care delivery environment: "Assessing where a patient is, how open he is to information, deciding when to go ahead even when the patient does not appear ready, are key aspects of effective patient teaching."

Sensing the pressure for nurses to decide what is essential when the clock is ticking, Hurxthal (1988, p. 1097) raises the question, "Where do you begin when you learn that Mr. Green, now on insulin with newly diagnosed type I diabetes, will be discharged in two hours?" The dilemma is that the client needs the information to safely control his blood sugar at home, yet in the acute situation he is experiencing, he is overwhelmed and unlikely to absorb more than a very limited amount of information. Quick assessment needs to be done to determine how simple or complex the teaching can be. Priorities have to be made, such as always keeping in mind that the client "must be safe until he can learn to be proficient [and that] meal timing is more important than meal content" (Hurxthal, 1988, p. 1099).

It is our hunch that illness trajectories are paralleled by anxiety trajectories. Readiness thus must be evaluated in terms of the degree of anxiety the client expresses. Minimal anxiety serves as a positive force for attention, alertness, or awareness, all of which are necessary for learning and integration of function to occur. Moderate anxiety is usually associated with selective inattention and decreasing awareness; extreme anxiety is associated with lack of attention and loss of awareness. Moderate or extreme anxiety is usually an indicator of the client's lack of readiness for learning. In these two anxiety states, the nurse's focus needs to be on reducing anxiety to enable the client to regain a sense of security and repossess the energy required for attention and awareness, which are prerequisites for learning.

VALIDATING LEARNING—FEEDBACK

Validation is a necessary element of teaching–learning. For a behavioral change to become well integrated, it must be validated by those persons significant to the client. Throughout life, a person requires validation through feedback from significant others to maintain the integrity of his or her self-system.

Through research, Milde (1988, pp. 432–433) found that groups who received both verbal and visual feedback on prescribed performance in a teaching–learning situation achieved at a higher level than those who received only verbal feedback. Although the subjects in this study were student nurses, nurses in practice might find value in replicating this study with clients to evaluate the significance of visual feedback on clients' integration of new health behaviors.

◎ Communication Strategies in the Teaching–Learning Process

FOCUS ON THE PARTICIPANTS

It is important for the nurse and the client in the teaching–learning process to know about each other. What does the nurse (teacher) need to know about the client (learner)? Fine (1988, p. 70), drawing from recommendations from a consumer health policy group, suggests that nurses individually and collectively provide "their standards of education and training, standards of practice, licensure standards, . . . anticipated treatment outcomes of health providers, as well as the varied classifications of health care providers." She specifically advises that "each primary care nurse should present the patient or patient's family with a professional card that has appropriate concise information, stating his or her professional degrees, certification, and scope of practice" (Fine, 1988, p. 70). In addition to providing these credentials to the client, the nurse should communicate clearly her intentions in the teaching–learning process, share a clear plan of the times she will commit to the client, and establish how additional contact can be established if the client feels the need to do so.

What does the nurse need to know about the client? The nurse needs to know:

1. How the client perceives the health situation
2. What limits or opportunities may be expected on the nurse's activities with the client in terms of other providers' plans for the client or other providers' assessment of the client's health status that may not be clear to the client
3. What the client's conscious intentions and desires are regarding health behaviors, and
4. What information the client perceives that is needed to achieve the client's health goals

Given these basic data about the nurse and clients, both should be able to work through the teaching–learning process.

MOTIVATIONAL STRATEGIES

There are many teaching strategies to enhance the client's motivation to participate in learning. This chapter attempts only to list some of these strategies. The reader is encouraged to seek further information from other books devoted to this topic.

Theis and Johnson (1995, p. 100), in synthesizing the existing body of research examining teaching strategies, found that "66% of subjects receiving planned teaching had better outcomes than did control group subjects receiving routine care." Structured approaches, reinforcement, independent study, and multiple strategies were found to be the most effective teaching strategies.

Other teaching strategies include (Babcock & Miller, 1994; Rankin & Stallings, 1996; Redman, 1992):

- Computer-based instruction materials
- Observation and assessment scales
- Demonstration
- Lecture/discussion
- Modeling
- Programmed instruction
- Role playing
- Group activities
- Use of media (posters, flipcharts, overhead projection, videotapes, audiotapes, film)
- Games and simulations

Motivation for learning is enhanced if (1) the student and the teacher trust and respect each other; (2) the teacher assumes and expects that the student can learn; (3) the teacher is sensitive to the student's individual needs; and (4) both the student and the teacher feel free to learn and make mistakes in their own unique styles. Boswell, Pichert, Lorenz, and Schlundt (1990) reinforce the idea that active participation in learning is a strong motivator. Bevis (1988, p. 45) lists the following as effective motivating strategies for learning:

- Engaging the learner in active analysis
- Raising questions
- Nurturing
  - The learner
  - The ethical ideal
  - The caring role
  - The creative drive
  - Curiosity and the search for satisfying ideas

- ■ Assertiveness
- ■ The desire to seek dialogue

CONTEXTUAL CONSTRAINTS AND OPPORTUNITIES

Some contextual constraints—such as the dilemma of insufficient time and great need on the part of the client—have already been mentioned. To attempt to control the environmental constraints that might be imposed on the teaching–learning process, the nurse should keep the following teaching strategies in mind:

1. Try to arrange learning experiences when the learner feels relatively healthy
2. Provide time for learning at a comfortable pace
3. Have sufficient grasp of the subject matter to translate concepts into different terms for different learners
4. Make sure expectations and standards are clear

Bruner (1986, p. 198) suggests that we need to assist learners to perceive the value of the rich diversity in the world. He encourages us to view the learner as "equipped to discriminate and deal differentially with a wide variety of possible worlds exhibiting different conditions, yet worlds in which one can cope." The nurse should perhaps heed this advice and have confidence in the client's ability to mutually participate in teaching–learning and to succeed in a diverse world, rather than trying to control all the contextual constraints that might interfere with learning. Power-sharing would be more likely by nurses with this confidence in clients. Perceived abilities and learning are more likely in such relationships.

◎ Conclusion

Teaching–learning is presented as a process between experts: the teacher and the learner, in which both acquire new information, experience new relatedness and behave in new ways as a result of the interaction. The nurse–teacher is an expert on health, and the client–learner is an expert on the client's experience of health and life circumstances. For teaching to be an empowering process for the client, the nurse must effectively use empathy, respect, and genuineness in communications.

Teaching is an essential role of the nurse as advocate. When the nurse acts as an advocate, mutuality characterizes the teaching–learning process. Growth occurs for both the client and the nurse if the teaching–learning process has been effective.

THOUGHT QUESTIONS

1 How can teaching–learning be incorporated within the nursing process? Do you have any suggestions for Lillian (see vignette)?

2 Why are communication, change, and advocacy principles so important in patient teaching?

3 Think of a recent client who needed teaching to promote a change in behavior. How could you have done a better job of implementing the teaching–learning process?

REFERENCES

American Nurses Association. (1995). *Social policy statement*. Washington, DC: Author.

Argyris, C. (1982). *Reasoning, learning, and action: Individual and organizational.* San Francisco: Jossey-Bass.

Babcock, D. E., & Miller. M. A. (1994). *Client education: Theory and practice.* St. Louis: Mosby-Year Book.

Benner, P. (1984). *From novice to expert.* Menlo Park, CA: Addison-Wesley.

Bevis, E. O. (1988). New directions for a new age. In National League for Nursing. *Curriculum revolution: Mandate for change* (pp. 27–52). New York: National League for Nursing.

Boswell, E. J., Pichert, J. W., Lorenz, R. A., & Schlundt, D. G. (1990). Training health care professionals to enhance their patient teaching skills. *Journal of Nursing Staff Development, 6,* 233–239.

Bruner, J. (1986, Summer). Models of the learner. *Education Horizons, 64*(4), 197–200.

Diekelmann, N. (1988). Curriculum revolution: A theoretical and philosophical mandate for change. In National League for Nursing. *Curriculum revolution: Mandate for change* (pp. 137–158). New York: National League for Nursing.

Douglass, L. M. *The effective nurse leader/manager* (3rd ed.). St. Louis: Mosby.

Fine, R. B. (1988). Consumerism and information: Power and confusion. *Nursing Adminstration Quarterly, 12*(3), 66–73.

Forbes, K. E. (1995). Please, more than just the facts. *Clinical Nurse Specialist, 9,* 99.

Henson, R. H. (1997). Analysis of the concept of mutuality. *Image, 29,* 77–81.

Hurxthal, K. (1988). Quick! Teach this patient about insulin. *American Journal of Nursing, 88*(8), 1097–1100.

Joint Commission on the Accreditation of Healthcare Organizations. (1994). *Comprehensive accreditation manual for hospitals.* Chicago: Author.

Milde, F. K. (1988). The function of feedback in psychomotor-skill learning. *Western Journal of Nursing Research, 10*(4), 425–434.

O'Connor, A. B. (1986). *Nursing staff development and continuing education.* Boston: Little, Brown.

Rankin, S. H., & Stallings, K. D. *Patient education: Issues, principles, practices* (3rd ed.). Philadelphia: Lippincott-Raven.

Redman, B. K. *The process of patient education* (7th ed.). St. Louis: Mosby.

Redman, B. K., & Thomas, S. A. (1992). Patient teaching. In G. M. Bulechek & J. C. McCloskey (Eds.). *Nursing interventions: Essential nursing treatments* (2nd ed., pp. 304–314). Philadelphia: Saunders.

Schlotfeldt, R. M. (1988). The scholarly nursing practitioner. In *Alternate conceptions of work and society: Implications for professional nursing* (pp. 15–30). Washington, DC: American Association of Colleges of Nursing.

Soukhanov, A. H. (Ed.) (1992). *The American heritage dictionary of the English language* (3rd ed.). Boston: Houghton Mifflin.

Theis, S. L., & Johnson, J. H. (1995). Strategies for teaching patients: A meta-analysis. *Clinical Nurse Specialist, 9,* 100–105.

Watson, J. (1988). A case study: Curriculum in transition. In National League for Nursing. *Curriculum revolution: Mandate for change* (pp. 1–8). New York: National League for Nursing.

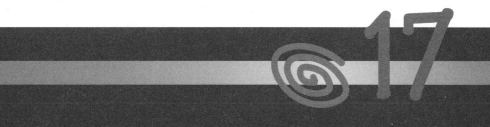

Leadership of Client Care

LEARNING OUTCOMES

By the end of this chapter the student will be able to:

1 Identify the characteristics of transformational leadership.

2 Identify the essential habits of an effective leader.

3 Appreciate the strengths that women bring to leadership.

4 Understand how the nurse can deal with the conflicting demands of relationships and task accomplishment.

5 Appreciate the value of empowering self and others in professional nursing relationships.

6 Understand how advocacy and change agency roles are integral to leadership.

7 Know how to use leadership behaviors to promote change within the nursing process.

VIGNETTE

Steven has been looking forward to learning more about leadership. He says, "Ever since I entered nursing school, I've wanted to be a nursing executive. That's where the money, prestige, and power are."

◎ Changing Views on Leadership

Older views of leadership include that it involves "interaction between members of a group that initiates and maintains improved expectations and the competence of the group to solve problems or attain goals" (Bass, 1981, p. 584) and that it is a process of "influencing individuals or groups to take an active part in the process of achieving agreed-upon goals" (Epstein, 1982, p. 2). Transactional outcomes, "in which relationships with followers are based upon an exchange for some resource valued by the follower" (Trofino, 1995, p. 45) were emphasized in these definitions.

More recent definitions of leadership emphasize mutuality, empowerment, and transformational processes (Burns, 1978). Manfredi (1994, p. 51) describes leadership as "an interactive process directed toward mutual goal achievement of leader and follower." Taking issue with the term "follower" as being submissive and inactive, Rost (1994, p. 3) defines leadership as "an influence relationship among leaders and collaborators who intend real changes that reflect their mutual purposes." Gurka (1995) emphasizes change, innovation, and commitment to the growth of self and others. Leaders create a vision that inspires commitment and empower people by sharing authority. They are not satisfied with transactional outcomes; rather, they want to be transformational.

According to Covey (1989, p. 222), the real test of interpersonal leadership is the leader's ability to permit others to validate their own lives, and the ability to "bring most people to a realization that they will win more of what they want by going for what you both want." In transformational leadership, there is "mutual learning, mutual influence, mutual benefits" (Covey, 1989, p. 216). Marquis and Huston (1992, p. 16) synthesized the works of leadership authorities and declare that the transformational leadership process is energized by leaders who identify common values, who are committed, who inspire others with vision, look at effects, and empower others.

In this chapter, *nursing leadership* is defined as a mutual process of interpersonal influence through which a client is assisted to make decisions in establishing and achieving goals toward improved well-being and the professional nurse's practice is validated and professional growth is enhanced. Although leadership can be applied at many different levels of systems complexity—individual, family, groups of clients or professional colleagues, and the larger society—this chapter emphasizes leadership with individual clients and peers.

◎ Current Perspectives on Leadership

The paradigm for leadership has shifted from a transactional one to a transformational one. In this paradigm, the major philosophic tenets are mutuality, empowerment, and transformational change. Effective leadership is based on intervention to meet a client's goals and uses strategies based on the client's motivations. Effective leadership with one's professional peers also is based on the peer group's goals, motivations, and work group culture.

Sherwood (1988) describes five characteristics of a high-performance, high-commitment work culture: delegation; teamwork across boundaries; empowering people; integrating people with technology; and fostering a shared sense of purpose. The result is energy and learning in doing work, as well as improvement in the quality of performance. The focus should be on "enlisting people's heads (intelligence) and their hearts (caring) as integral parts of the work process and not just expect[ing] their hands to be extensions of the technology" (Sherwood, 1988, p. 10). The likelihood of success in leadership is enhanced when the needs of the followers are met at the same time that incentives are provided to motivate them to work toward the leader's goals.

Research findings validate that RNs are more satisfied in their work when they are accorded professional status and autonomy (Johnston, 1991). Brill (1990, p. 220) states that "leadership involves the use of power and is related to position and status on the team," and notes that power is "the ability to act . . . position is the place the team member occupies in the pattern of team life and relates to the function performed . . . [and] status is the rank accorded that position." Indeed, if the health care delivery system serves as an environment in which the professional nurse is expected and supported to be autonomous and responsible, then that system will be one that truly integrates the dictionary definition of the verb "empower"—to invest with power, especially legal power or official authority; that is, to enable (Soukhanov, 1992).

Further, if nurses feel able to act (empowered), they are more likely to share that power with clients by approaching the nursing process as an enabling relationship, in which responsibility and accountability for health are shared with the client. Effective leadership, therefore, is based not only on the client's motivations, but also on the nurse's motivation to enable the client to act responsibly in the pursuit of improved health.

LEADERSHIP AS A PROCESS OF EMPOWERMENT

Perceptions of power and power relationships have changed markedly in the past 20 years. Who will control changes in the future—who will have power—is being redefined (Toffler, 1990). Noting that the rules of the power game are changing and that the nature of power is being revolutionized, Toffler (1990, pp. 7–8) declares that the heyday of physician dominance in health care is over. He notes that physicians no longer can keep "a tight choke-hold on medical knowledge." No longer is the prescription written in a secret code (Latin), no longer are the medical journals and texts restricted to physicians alone, no longer is the information about health and medicine inaccessible to nonprofessional people. Rather, anyone can purchase the state-of-the-art information on drugs, the *Physi-*

cian's Desk Reference (either in book or computerized form); anyone can tune into video versions of material from the *Journal of the American Medical Association;* anyone can find information from the medical journals (such as *The New England Journal of Medicine*) in the newspapers; and anyone with a personal computer and a modem can access data bases such as Index Medicus and obtain scientific papers on almost any topic. Clearly, "as knowledge is redistributed, so, too, is the power based on it" (Toffler, 1990, p. 8).

This shift in power is occurring in all fields. Businessmen now acknowledge that "advances are being made by people who outthink others, not people who buy twice as many machines" (Stewart, 1991, p. 31). Thus, knowledge now provides the key raw material for power. Toffler (1990, p. 18) says that "knowledge has gone from being an adjunct of money power and muscle power, to being their very essence. It is, in fact, the ultimate amplifier."

This power shift provides the nurse with a real opportunity to become a full-fledged professional provider of health care. The nurse becomes a power broker through sharing knowledge and skills with the client. Effective nurse leaders "will ultimately reap the human harvest of their efforts by the simple action of power's reciprocal: empowerment. It puts the duality in motion—power to empowerment, empowerment back to power" (Bennis & Nanus, 1985, p. 80).

Leadership gives energy to the work of nursing. This energy empowers the nurse and the client in the professional process. Thus, empowerment is an outcome of leadership. Bennis (1989, p. 23) says that empowerment is evident in the following four themes (adapted for nursing):

1. People feel significant. All feel that they make a difference and that what they do has meaning and significance. In the nursing process, the nurse and the client are equal in significance; both have meaning and what they do together is mutually signficant.
2. Learning and competence matter. The nurse and the client value learning and mastery. The nurse makes it clear that there is no failure, only mistakes that provide feedback and tell us what to do next.
3. People are part of a community. The nurse, the client, and other health care providers are experienced as a team, a family, a unity. A person does not have to like another to feel a sense of community (striving for a common goal).
4. Work is exciting. The nursing process is stimulating, challenging, and fun. The nurse "pulls" rather than "pushes" a client toward a goal. This pull style of influence energizes the client to "enroll in an exciting vision of the future . . . . It motivates through identification, rather than through rewards and punishments." The nurse articulates and embodies the ideals of health toward which both the nurse and the client strive.

Using Power on the Client's Behalf

Rafael (1996) describes three levels of power as it is exercised in caring. Power in *ordered caring* is associated with:

A patriarchal (male supremacy) ideology
Fostered by separation, strength, and control (esteemed properties of masculinity)
Related to having control over others and nature
Sustains organizational hierarchies
"Vested in certain positions and legitimized as authority over nurses" (p. 8)

Examples include "the increasing use of unlicensed personnel, the American Medical Association proposal for 'registered care technologists,' and the medical lobby opposing nurses as primary health care practitioners" (p. 8).

At the second level, *assimilated caring*, power is gained through "access to male power through assimilation of male characteristics, practices, and values" (Rafael, 1996, p. 12). Assimilated caring is ethically based on "malestream ethics," with its emphasis on application of universal principles such as self-determination, beneficence, and rights-based justice.

Empowered caring, the third level, has the following characteristics:

Both sexes are publicly recognized as at least equal
Credentials are a source of power. (Nurses' credentials must be equally valued and respected as members of other health care disciplines.)
Expertise is closely linked to research and credentials but also develops from practice
Knowledge is distributed so that all may grow (rather than hoarding it to give a few the edge)
"Collegiality that values and respects the expertise and experience of other nurses" (p. 13) and "nurturance of others in recognition that they are integral to one's own existence" (p. 14)
Power is based on respect for and connection with others and nature.
It "involves an awareness of and a commitment to change problematic social and cultural contexts" (p. 14)
It is not invested in a position
Enabling power requires the active and equal participation of the nurse and the client in health care decisions
It is "not consistent with deference to medical or administrative authority" (p. 15)
In a relational way of becoming, both the nurse and the client are transformed during the caring relationship (p. 15)
A relational ethics is contextual (ie, may be guided by principles but is not driven by them)

If professional nurses are expected to fulfill leadership roles, they must analyze their positions about power. These roles as defined in this book mandate that empowerment of clients and others in the delivery system must be our major focus. One cannot be an effective change agent if one wields power over the target of change. Behavioral changes emerging from such a "power" environment are probably rote, not well integrated, and exist over a very short duration. Behavioral changes emerging from an "empowerment" experience are more likely to be realistic, genuine, and well integrated (because the person has fully participated in the process) and may become habitual over an extended period.

The position has been taken that leadership in promoting change in client behavior is best accomplished through the appropriate use of authority and influence, emphasizing the empowerment of self, clients, and other providers. However, nurses also should assume power to exert professional leadership:

1. Power based on knowledge and expertise should be used to affect the organizational climate within which nurses work, using nursing knowledge to promote desirable change. For example, knowledge of rhythm theory and research on the effects of shift changes present a strong rationale for changes in staffing patterns to avoid shift rotation.
2. Power based on legitimate right and authority should be used to affect the quality of the support systems available to the nurse in client care. For example, the staff nurse has a legitimate right to expect that administration will provide sufficient resources and assistance so that nurses' energies and time are not dissipated in nonnursing activities.
3. Nurses can apply referent power (based on identification with the personal qualities of the nurse) to mobilize community resources in support of desired change.

The professional nurse must be an activist in the work setting and in the community, setting an example as a change agent and an advocate for health.

CLIENT ADVOCACY

VIGNETTE

Lisa, a new associate degree graduate, has been caring for a patient who has just been diagnosed with metastatic cancer. The physician has "ordered" the staff not to tell the patient his diagnosis. The patient, however, is asking a number of questions. Lisa wonders how can she advocate for the patient without jeopardizing her job by "rocking the boat."

Meanings of Advocacy

If nurses believe that clients have a right to a nurse–client relationship based on mutuality, shared respect, consideration of information and feelings, and full participation in the problem-solving related to their health and health care needs, then they believe in advocacy. If nurses believe that it is their responsibility to ensure that clients have access to the health care delivery systems appropriate to their needs, then they believe in advocacy. If nurses believe that clients are responsible for their health and that nurses are responsible for mobilizing and facilitating the strengths of clients in achieving the highest level of health possible, then they believe in advocacy. An *advocate* "supports or defends someone or something and recommends or pleads in another's behalf...[and] works to change the power structure so that a situation will be improved" (Douglass, 1988, p. 259).

Nurses cannot be effective advocates unless they believe fully in their own strengths and their peers' or clients' strengths, and hold both themselves and clients responsible for outcomes. Power is shared, and nurses serve as resource persons for clients or peers. Both the nurse and the client have authority and responsibility for advancing the client's health care. Because advocacy requires conviction, it is important for the nurse to overcome personal feelings and beliefs about nurses' "powerlessness" to take the first step in the process of empowerment (Richardson, 1992, p. 38).

EMPHASIS ON MUTUALITY

Evidence is abundant that decisions made for persons by other persons without participation of those affected or those who have the expertise to make the most informed judgments are less likely to be understood or workable. Nurses have both the expertise in health and the ability to help people achieve health. Clients have the expertise in understanding and evaluating their situations; they have control of their lives and their health. It is entirely appropriate that decisions affecting health be made by the client, with full informational support, empathy, and respect from the nurse.

Mutuality means that the nurse and the client together fully describe the client's health situation, agree on the direction and nature of change that the client would like to make, explore alternative ways to achieve the mutually agreed-on goals, and then work together as the client implements the changes. At this stage, the advocate makes sure that technical and informational supports are provided for the client and assists the client in gaining access to the health care services needed.

In almost every identifiable nurse–client situation, it is possible to focus on the client's strengths and to reasonably expect that the client be responsible. For example, in work with bereaved parents following the death of a child, nurses found the potential for positive growth in significant numbers (Miles & Crandall, 1983). The researchers pointed out that focusing on the growth potential in bereaved parents was in no way meant to minimize the pain of grief, rather to help them find meaning in their lives at the time.

How does emphasis on mutuality enter into this nursing situation? It is important because two essential elements of mutuality are respect and sharing. Respecting the client's right to make decisions about working on finding meaning, while emphasizing the client's ability to be responsible for himself or herself, the nurse sets up a relationship based on mutuality. The nurse empathizes with the parents, showing understanding of the pain from loss, respects the strengths of the parents, and gives choices to the family as they mutually establish a goal of reducing the pain of grief and searching for meaning in their lives.

The communication process of empathy is important to understand in the advocate role, because "empathy involves feelings of mutuality with another" (Olsen, 1991, p. 67). Olsen also says that "empathy can exist simply because both parties share humanity" and that "justification of another's humanity would make little sense in the way that justifications of another's actions or feelings do" (Olsen, 1991, p. 70). Thus, empathized humanity is the crux of the nurse–client relationship and the advocate's role.

The most important factor in mutuality is that the nurse and the client are seen as equally able and responsible for the outcomes of the nursing process. Their areas of expertise vary, but their authority and significance in the relationship are equal. Each's potential can be more fully realized in a relationship characterized by mutuality.

EMPHASIS ON FACILITATION

The advocate assumes that every client has strengths, and that the nurse's job is to help the client use those strengths to achieve the highest level of health possible. Several aspects of facilitation have been described.

Snowball (1996) suggests that emphasis on facilitation in the advocacy process requires that the advocate take responsibility to make sure the client has all the necessary information to make informed decisions and to support clients in the decisions they make. King (1984, p. 17) suggests that an effective way for the nurse to facilitate growth in self and others is through values clarification—that is, to help the client think through issues and develop a personal value system that aids decision-making. Hames and Joseph (1980) suggest that facilitation is effected through helping clients understand the tasks before them; ensuring that they experience some success when they are trying to accomplish something; providing an environment that is conducive to learning (one of trust and respect); and offering information and emotional supports.

EMPHASIS ON PROTECTION

Client advocacy has been associated with an assumption that nurses have a responsibility to protect their clients. Commonly, nurses are called on to examine their roles in protecting the client's right to live or die. Bandman and Bandman (1995) report that nurses are commonly caught in an ethical dilemma between physicians and incurably ill or hopelessly disabled persons. The advocate must determine what actions to take in terms of protecting the client from either forced treatments or withholding treatments. Bandman and Bandman (1995) conclude that morality tends to support a client's right to live over letting others decide that the client's life is not worth living; that the welfare of others is not necessarily in conflict with a client's right to die; and that there are cases in which the nurse can legitimately decide to protect a client's wish to end life.

Perhaps the greatest need for the nurse to act as protector is the need to change a condition or situation in the health care delivery system in which either the client is given inadequate care or the environment poses some hazard. Cassidy and Koroll (1994) indicate that in the current environment of cost containment, nurses may need to:

■ Promote access to health care
■ Protect an individual's right to make autonomous or independent life choices
■ Refrain from causing intentional injury
■ Prevent injury from occurring
■ Eliminate potential sources of injury
■ Monitor the quality of client care
■ Intervene in a nonadversarial way when harmful behaviors are observed in any health care worker

However, recently it has been questioned, "by what authority does the nurse assume the obligation of representing the patient's interests or preferences?" (Willard, 1996, p. 65). Also questioned is the "hero model" in which the nurse

> possessing unusual strength and courage, is engaged in a socially visible struggle. This is the nurse under the advocacy model, who both defends patients' rights and seeks to elevate nurses' professional status, in an adversarial struggle against the forces of institutional oppression (Bernal, 1992, p. 21).

Given the personal risks (Snowball, 1996) and the rigorous demands of the advocate role (Willard, 1996), it has been suggested that the client be represented by an independent advocate who is without conscious bias (Kirkpatrick, Hull, Katrabos, & Sherman, 1995).

Challenges and Rewards

For nurses to effectively carry out the role of client advocate, the health care delivery system must be restructured in terms of where the nurse is placed in the total organization. In most delivery systems, advocacy efforts are challenged by the nurse's lack of equality in authority. Equality in responsibility is more likely to be evident among health care disciplines. There is agreement that each discipline is fully responsible and accountable for its own practice. However, as noted throughout this book, authority is more commonly dispersed in a hierarchical manner, in which nursing may occupy a position of disadvantage.

Therefore, nurses attempting to operate as client advocates in a hierarchical system will be more effective if they learn both to negotiate the hierarchy and to develop image-building strategies that promote the significance of their advocacy work. If the nurse perceives the need for equal authority to fulfill the advocate's role as important, he or she must demonstrate both the effectiveness of the advocacy work (such as improved client outcomes and the accomplishment of serving more persons at more affordable cost), and the improvement in satisfaction and retention of nurses.

Emphasis should be placed on the knowledge and skills necessary to assist clients to increase competency in assuming responsibility for their own health. In such a restructured system, the nursing staff would be supported in the following:

1. Development of understanding of clients' responses to various threats to health and development of strategies to respond effectively to these responses
2. Refinement and further development of health promotion and illness prevention abilities, as well as restorative abilities
3. Reevaluation of belief systems about the independent versus dependent role of clients and self
4. Assumption of collaborative responsibility for monitoring the effectiveness of the delivery system, as well as of independent responsibility for evaluating the effectiveness of the nursing interventions in responding to the client's health needs
5. Implementation of interdisciplinary dialogue, with all professional workers sharing equal responsibility and authority for meeting clients' health needs
6. Provision of opportunity for all members of the team to evaluate effectiveness in collaboration, thereby avoiding the establishment of adversary relationships

Work would be viewed in terms of professional responsibilities implicit in the preceding categories. The challenge to professional nursing to restructure the work of the nurse as an advocate includes both gaining acceptance of and placing emphasis on role behaviors for professional nurses. The professional nurse would be expected to do the following:

1. Interact with the client in a manner and quantity that permits:
   a. Exploration of the client's personal responses to health or threats to health
   b. Evaluation of the environmental circumstances in which the client exists
   c. Identification of strengths and limitations
   d. Identification of resources perceived to be needed
   e. Clearly allocate responsibilities of client and nurse, which ensures the client's assumption of responsibility for health and the

nurse's assumption of responsibility for the informational and interactional supports needed

2. Prepare for and implement teaching programs needed by the client
3. Update technical skills as new therapeutic techniques and equipment are made available for health care
4. Discuss beliefs about the client's abilities with professional peers in an effort to evaluate own values about independence and dependence in various states of health
5. Update nursing care plans in an effort to evaluate outcomes of nursing care
6. Participate in nursing research as a consumer and assist in nursing studies conducted in the health care setting
7. Identify all units of the delivery system that need to be involved in the client's care
8. Coordinate efforts of the multiple health care workers involved in the client's care
9. Assess the adequacy of efforts of all workers involved in care, according to the client's stated needs
10. Resolve conflicts that might occur in relation to advocacy efforts for the client by:
    a. Respecting the position of all involved
    b. Gathering data that describes the whole system of client–environment
    c. Promoting expression of conflicts
    d. Participating in the problem-solving process
    e. Allowing the client to make decisions based on data rather than on advice from others
11. Recognize and show appreciation for the contributions of team members to the client's health care
12. Periodically discuss and evaluate the quality of the interactions of health care team members and evaluate own interpersonal effectiveness with the client and team members

Fulfillment of these work role behaviors reflects the professional nurse's commitment to client advocacy as a legitimate role.

To restructure their working conditions, nurses must be advocates both for professional colleagues and for themselves. Chapter 7 suggested that an effective method for gaining control over practice is to develop and use data as a basis for recommending changes. Data, rather than opinion, give strength. Advocacy for anyone is more effective if the advocate is working from a position of strength, armed with data and the belief that what one is trying to accomplish is not only worthwhile for oneself, but also vital to the quality of care the nurse can deliver.

Public support cannot be underestimated. Both a public image of the nurse as competent, and an appreciation of the nurse's advocacy efforts, will build public support. Public support is one of the most powerful forces for change in society. Nursing can use the public's help to restructure the health care delivery system.

As nurses gain the respect of the public they serve, they are more likely to gain the respect of interdisciplinary peers. Such respect is necessary to change the position of nursing in the delivery system, to ensure full participation in decision-making. To fulfill the responsibilities of a client advocate, the nurse must participate in decision-making, achieved through cooperation and coalition-building (Richardson, 1992) and through consensus formation and equality of participation by all involved.

DECISION-MAKING THROUGH CONSENSUS-BUILDING

Shared power and shared responsibility in decision-making are key ingredients of participation in the nursing process. Participatory decision-making is successful to the extent that adequate information is available and the persons involved do not become prematurely concerned with implementing the decision. Conley and Mariano (1991, p. 5) further note that the "selective use or withholding of information influences the possessors' success in persuading the group to select one alternative even though that choice may not be the most effective or appropriate for the identified problem." Such manipulation of information usually represents a conflict over power. Thus, successful participatory decision-making depends on genuine respect between the partners in the relationship and a willingness to share all that is known about the concern on which they are working.

The goal in participatory decision-making is to reach the decision by consensus. In most situations, several options may be effective. Singular solutions are rare in human health concerns. To enable the client to make the wisest choice, the choice that best fits the client's personal situation, the nurse and the client must responsibly and fully explore the client's situation and all of the options available.

For example, in the nursing process between the professional nurse and the client newly diagnosed with early stage breast cancer, consensus is obtained when both the nurse and the client together have sorted and processed all the relevant data, weighed the risks and benefits of various options, understand fully the impact of the various options on functioning, and reach a choice together that is perceived to be the most helpful in the situation (Knobf, 1990). In consensus-building, the commonalities and the connectedness of varying ideas are identified. It is this sense of connectedness that enables both the nurse and the client to feel empowered and to take action.

Connections and feeling connected underlie the process of consensus. If consensus-building is effective in the nursing process, all who participate in the process will feel they played a significant role in the decision(s) made. More importantly, "value results from a total effort, rather than from one isolated step in the process" (Toffler, 1990, p. 83).

Clearly, interdependence characterizes the relationship. The nurse's value is not more important than the client's, nor is the client's value more important than the nurse's. Both have a presence, both have something to say, both inspire each other, and both are respected by the other (Ahern, 1992). Both equally share accountability and responsibility for the quality of the decisions made. The nurse brings expertise in health and health care to the relationship, and the client brings expertise in his or her abilities and the context of his or her health concerns. To reach effective consensus in decision-making, all of these areas of expertise must be fully explored.

Although some studies indicate that both nurses (mostly women) and physicians (mostly men) use command styles rather than participatory styles in attempting to influence decision-making by clients (Taylor, Pickens, & Geden, 1989), some researchers predict that women are more likely to use empowerment and consensus-building as major strategies in helping relationships.

Common themes and meaning between the characteristics of transformational leaders and the attributes of women who are constructed knowers are described in Table 17-1. Barker and Young indicate that constructed knowers

> participate in a network or web that includes caring, moral responsibility, positive self-esteem, and use of both intuition and logic. Both transformational leaders and women seek to establish an environment that generates empowerment in self and/or others (1994, p. 20).

As a change agent, the professional nurse works with the client to identify when and what change is needed, and helps to facilitate desired change to promote better health.

TABLE 17-1

Transformational Leadership and Feminine Attributes

Transformational Leaders	Constructed Female Attributes
Relationships: engaged	Relationships: network/web
Individual consideration	Caring
Leader as moral agent: values and needs	Moral responsibility
Mutual dependence/trust	Reciprocity and cooperation
Communication	Integration of voices
Builder of self-esteem	Positive self-esteem
Listens to intuition, balances with analysis	Use of intuition and logic
Empowerment	Empowerment

From Barker, A. M., & Young, C. E. (1994). Transformational leadership: The feminist connection in postmodern organizations. *Holistic Nursing Practice, 9,* 20. Used with permission of the publisher.

CHANGE AGENCY

Psychological Stages in Coping With Change

"Resources and energy from within individuals are necessary to help accomplish [organizational] change" (Perlman & Takacs, 1990, p. 33). Change has an emotional meaning for people and is often associated with feelings of loss or pain (Davis, 1991). Based on the Kübler-Ross model of death and dying, Perlman and Takacs (1990) propose a 10-stage model to explain the psychological problems associated with change (Table 17-2).

1. Equilibrium: Because people are vested in the *status quo*, they are comfortable and contented.
2. Denial: Because change "produces a sense of uneasiness, a lack of direction, a sense of unfinishedness, insecurity, and a lack of closure" (Perlman & Takacs 1990, p. 33), energy is now channeled into active resistance of the change.
3. Anger: Others are blamed, which is stressful.
4. Bargaining: People attempt to negotiate away the change and restore the old *status quo*.
5. Chaos: Diffused energy, feelings of powerlessness, and a sense of disorientation spread and intensify.
6. Depression: Fear of loss causes reactive depression, while preparatory depression facilitates eventual acceptance.
7. Resignation: The need for the change is accepted although people are not happy about it.
8. Openness: People are ready to learn about the change.
9. Readiness: People experience emotional letting-go.
10. Reemergence: People reinvest in the organization.

In another model, Carnall (1990, pp. 141–146) proposes five steps in coping with change:

Stage 1: denial of the validity of new ideas
Stage 2: defense (experiencing depression and frustration)
Stage 3: discarding (acknowledging change as inevitable or necessary)
Stage 4: adaptation (feeling anger)
Stage 5: internalization

The Perlman and Takacs model and the Carnall models are compared in Table 17-3.

Change Roles

ROLES OF THE CHANGE AGENT

Based on a comparative analysis of the literature, Wooten and White (1989) have identified five basic change roles: (1) educator/trainer, (2) model, (3) researcher/theoretician, (4) technical expert, and (5) resource linker. The role of educator/trainer "is the focal point for the change

TABLE 17-2

Growing With Change: The Emotional Voyage of the Change Process

	Charted Summary	
Phase	Characteristics/Symptoms	Interventions
1. Equilibrium	High energy level. State of emotional and intellectual balance. Sense of inner peace with personal and professional goals in sync.	Make employees aware of changes in the environment which will have impact on the status quo.
2. Denial	Energy is drained by the defense mechanism of rationalizing a denial of the reality of the change. Employees experience negative changes in physical health, emotional balance, logical thinking patterns, and normal behavior patterns.	Employ active listening skills, (eg, be empathetic, nonjudgmental, use reflective listening techniques). Nurturing behavior, avoiding isolation, and offering stress management workshops also will help.
3. Anger	Energy is used to ward off and actively resist the change by blaming others. Frustration, anger, rage, envy and resentment become visible.	Recognize the symptoms, legitimize employees' feelings and verbal expressions of anger, rage, envy and resentment. Active listening, assertiveness, and problem-solving skills needed by managers. Employees need to probe within for the source of their anger.
4. Bargaining	Energy is used in an attempt to eliminate the change. Talk is about "if only." Others try to solve the problem. "Bargains" are unrealistic and designed to compromise the change out of existence.	Search for real needs/problems and bring them into the open. Explore ways of achieving desired changes through conflict management skills and win–win negotiation skills.
5. Chaos	Diffused energy, feeling of powerlessness, insecurity, sense of disorientation. Loss of identity and direction. No sense of grounding or meaning. Breakdown of value system and belief. Defense mechanisms begin to lose usefulness and meaning.	Quiet time for reflection. Listening skills. Inner search for both employee and organization identity and meaning. Approval for being in state of flux.
6. Depression	No energy left to produce results. Former defense mechanisms no longer operable. Self-pity, remembering past, expressions of sorrow, feeling nothingness and emptiness.	Provide necessary information in a timely fashion. Allow sorrow and pain to be expressed openly. Long-term patience, take one step at a time as employees learn to let go.
7. Resignation	Energy expended in passively accepting change. Lack of enthusiasm.	Expect employees to be accountable for reactions to behavior. Allow them to move at their own pace.
8. Openness	Availability to renewed energy. Willingness to expend energy on what has been assigned to individual.	Patiently explain again, in detail, the desired change.
9. Readiness	Willingness to expend energy in exploring new events. Reunification of intellect and emotions begins.	Assume a directive management style: assign tasks, monitor tasks and results so as to provide direction and guidelines.
10. Re-emergence	Rechanneled energy produces feelings of empowerment and employees become more proactive. Rebirth of growth and commitment. Employee initiates projects and ideas. Career questions answered.	Mutual answering of questions. Redefinition of career, mission and culture. Mutual understanding of role and identity. Employees will take action based on own decisions.

From Perlman, D., & Takacs, G. J. (1990, April). The ten stages of change. *Nursing Management, 21,* 34. Used with permission of the publisher.

TABLE 17-3	
Comparison of Stages in Coping With Change	
Perlman and Takacs	**Carnall**
Equilibrium	Denial
Denial	
Anger	Defense
Bargaining	
Chaos	
Depression	Discarding
Resignation	
Openness	Adaptation
Readiness	
Reemergence	Internalization

process" (Wooten & White, 1989, p. 655). The change agent must model appropriate behaviors in an atmosphere of trust and openness, accept responsibility for getting data in an appropriate manner, provide skills and expertise, and link needed resources in ways that make the intervention effective. The selection and timing of particular roles depend on the specific needs of the situation.

ROLES OF THE CLIENT SYSTEM
Wooten and White (1989) also describe four basic roles of the client system: (1) resource provider, (2) supporter/advocate, (3) information supplier, and (4) participant. The client system provides effort, time, and money resources; advocates the change; provides information involving self and others; and participates in the change process. It is crucial that the change agent and the client collaborate to promote effective change.

MUTUAL ROLES
Wooten and White (1989, p. 657) indicate that "mutual role enactment is at the heart of the change process." The mutual roles include (1) problem-solver, (2) diagnostician, (3) learner, and (4) monitor. Instead of investing the change agent alone with the responsibility for the entire change process, this model focuses on joint responsibility and action.

Problem-solving involves identifying a problem, generating alternatives, and testing assumptions. Diagnosis necessitates sensitivity to issues in the relationship. Learning includes knowledge, skills, or new attitudes, and monitoring involves "remain[ing] aware of alternatives, ascertain[ing] the consequences of action, gaug[ing] the effectiveness of the change effort and relationship at each stage of the intervention" (Wooten & White, 1989, p. 657). Each role can be adopted independently, as well as at the same time as other roles.

Categories of Change Strategies
EMPIRICAL–RATIONAL STRATEGIES

The empirical–rational category assumes that persons will act in a way that is rational and in their own self-interest. These strategies are aimed at educating a person about the available options, assuming that the individual will change behavior because he or she knows that the new behavior will be desirable.

For example, in-service education may include a demonstration of the latest techniques available for a particular task, with the expectation that nurses will then apply that knowledge to improve their care of clients. Because persons do not always act rationally, these strategies are frequently not successful in facilitating a lasting change when used alone (Haffer 1986).

NORMATIVE–REEDUCATIVE STRATEGIES

The normative–reeducative category assumes that sociocultural norms are fundamental to a person's behavior. In addition to rationality and intelligence, change must involve modification of attitudes, values, skills, and significant relationships. This is the basis for the belief that the change process must be based on mutuality and collaboration between the client and the change agent. This allows for the problem-solving and personal growth believed necessary to promote effective change. According to Haffer (1986, p. 20), "if beliefs, attitudes, and values are the target of the needed change, then these strategies should be used."

POWER–COERCIVE STRATEGIES

The third category, power–coercive strategies, is based on the use of power. It is believed that despite the need for knowledge and for modification of attitudes and values, change will occur only when it is supported by power. This rationale is the basis for much political action, and it may imply the use of legitimate channels of authority or violent, nonsanctioned methods (Chin, 1976). This strategy effects change more quickly than other strategies, but the change that results usually is not lasting (Haffer, 1986).

FACILITATIVE STRATEGIES

Facilitative strategies are used to make clients aware of the availability of help in sufficient detail and clarity so that they know exactly what is available and where and how assistance may be obtained. Facilitative strategies are appropriate when there is openness to change, but they are relatively ineffective when resistance is expected. Examples of this type of strategy are:

1. Simplifying data, providing feedback, and providing other necessary tools to help the client to recognize a problem
2. Providing multiple potential solutions to the problem
3. Involving the client and others in the decision-making process

These strategies produce greater commitment to change, but the agent must be sure that there are sufficient resources, commitment, and capability to maintain the change after the agent has withdrawn from the process.

REEDUCATIVE STRATEGIES

Reeducative strategies are based on empirical–rational theory. Relatively unbiased presentation of fact is assumed to provide a rational justification for action. This type of strategy is necessary when effective use of an advocated change requires skills and knowledge that the client does not possess. It is also desirable when resistance is prevalent and based on inaccurate information and when the change involved is a radical departure from past practices and there is a great deal of uncertainty about the ability to successfully perform the new practices. However, in themselves, reeducative strategies are inadequate to bring about change unless there is a strongly felt need and a strong motivation to satisfy that need.

Reeducative strategies work slowly and thus are feasible only when time is not a pressing factor. Examples of reeducative strategies are creating awareness that a problem exists by indicating how much better off the client could be, connecting symptoms with causes to aid in problem identification, and demonstrating alternative possible solutions to an identified problem. Reeducative strategies heighten awareness of a problem and possible solutions, but they do not heighten the need or motivation to change. This requires persuasive strategies.

PERSUASIVE STRATEGIES

Persuasive strategies attempt to bring about change partly through bias in the manner in which a message is structured and presented. Reasoning, urging, and inducement through incentives are examples of this type of strategy.

Persuasive strategies are more effective for those who are less open to change, and they can be used to increase both attitudinal and behavioral commitment. Knowledge about the client can help the change agent be more persuasive, especially in combating resistance to change. A persuasive strategy is indicated when the proposed change is risky, not amenable to limited or small-scale trial, is technically complex, has no clear relative advantage, and must be implemented in a short time. These strategies are especially useful in situations where the change agent has limited resources with which to initiate and sustain a change.

POWER STRATEGIES

Power strategies imply the use of coercion. They typically result in compliance, which indicates a low level of commitment to the change but leads to adoption of the induced behavior because the person expects to gain specific rewards and avoid punishment by conforming. Power strategies may be necessary if the client or target group has limited resources and is generally unwilling to allocate available resources to the continued implementation of a change. However, forced compliance requires surveillance to maintain the change. This is not an appropriate approach if the goal is to produce a self-sustaining change.

◎ The Nurse as Leader

Adapted from Bennis and Nanus's (1989) description of organizational leadership, leadership is what gives nursing its vision and its abilities to transform clients' health. This transformation occurs through the leader's translation of vision into reality with clients. These leadership transformations are the heartbeat of professional nursing. In this transformational relationship, the nurse leader is the coordinator of communication.

According to Bernhard and Walsh (1990, p. 65):

> the interactions between the nurse leader and an individual client is a specific type of relationship often called a therapeutic relationship . . . . The interaction between the nurse leader and another member of the health care organization is also a specific type of relationship, ideally a collaborative relationship.

Essential in both types of relationships is the ability to establish open communication based on mutual trust.

In a *transformational relationship*, characterized by the sharing of power rather than the wielding of power by the nurse over the client, both participants influence each other. Yukl (1981) describes different forms of influence that have been adapted to the nurse–client relationship:

1. Legitimate request: responding to legitimate power; that is, the client complies with the nurse's request because he recognizes her right to make such a request. The client's compliance represents internalized values of obedience, cooperation, courtesy, respect for tradition, and loyalty to the organization.
2. Instrumental compliance: responding to reward power; that is, the client complies because the nurse has made an explicit or implicit promise to ensure some tangible outcome that the client desires.
3. Coercion: responding to the threat of aversive outcomes such as economic loss, embarrassment, or expulsion. Because the influence is motivated by fear, it is most effective when it is credible.
4. Rational persuasion: responding to a logical argument. The client is convinced that the nurse's suggested behavior is the best way to satisfy needs or attain objectives.
5. Rational faith: acting out of faith in the nurse's expertise and credibility. Such a response is based on expert power.
6. Inspirational appeal: responding to expressions of values and ideals without any tangible reward. The client acts from obedience to authority figures, reverence for tradition, self-sacrifice, and so forth.

7. Situational engineering: responding to manipulation of relevant aspects of the physical and social situation. The nurse must have control, and the client must accept the situation.

8. Personal identification: based on referent power. The client imitates the behavior of an admired nurse.

9. Decision identification: the influence derived from involvement in decision-making.

In transformational leadership, rational persuasion and decision identification are the most valid forms of influence because the they reflect empowerment through information and the sharing of power in relationships characterized by mutuality and respect. The nurse assumes leadership by initiating, facilitating, and successfully terminating professional influence in the process. Following is a discussion of the competencies a nurse needs to be a transformational leader.

COMPETENCIES NEEDED TO BE A LEADER

Gurka (1995, p. 170), synthesizing research findings, has identified three qualities of the transformational leader:

- Individual consideration—exhibited by promoting others' growth, recognizing and supporting others' needs and feelings, and giving positive feedback and recognition
- Charisma—exhibited by inspiring and motivating, demonstrating enthusiasm, and communicating in a positive manner
- Intellectual stimulation—exhibited by creating a questioning environment, acting as a mentor, and challenging others to grow and learn

Gurka (1995, p. 170) also identifies three qualities of the transformational leader that have been proposed experientially:

- Vulnerability—exhibited by communicating authentically and openly, expressing emotions as well as ideas, and sharing self with others
- Knowledge, concern, and courage—exhibited by seeking knowledge through study and experience, showing concern and caring for others, and being willing to take risks
- Feminine attributes—exhibited by maintaining accessibility, paying attention to process as well as outcomes, and practicing balance in lifestyle

Based on transformational leadership concepts (Bennis & Nanus, 1985), the following actions reflecting competency in practice are proposed. The competent professional nurse:

1. Exhibits an intense concern for the client's health and couples that intensity with a commitment to help

2. Communicates that the client is capable of participating meaningfully, that what the client can do is meaningful, and that the relationship builds on both of their strengths.
3. Pays close attention to the client's ideas and insights while sharing the nurse's own ideas and insights, leading to a sense of unity in the work together.
4. Enthusiastically relates a compelling image of health and the client's ability to be responsible for achieving improved health behaviors.
5. Explores shared meanings and interpretations of the client's health realities to facilitate coordinated actions.
6. Uses various teaching–learning strategies to shape meanings that lead to alignment of goals and enabling behaviors for improved health.
7. Independently thinks ahead of time about what is to be done, what ought to be done, and why it ought to be done to communicate positive meanings in the relationship (searches out and builds own knowledge base).
8. Establishes trust with the client by making self known to be genuine and predictable (eg, keeps promises, makes positions known, and keeps at those positions).
9. Recognizes own strengths and compensates for weaknesses.
10. Keeps working on and developing own professional skills.
11. Carefully discerns the fit between own skills and knowledge and what the particular client requires in the nursing process.
12. Accepts clients for what they are, on their terms, rather than judging them.
13. Approaches relationships and problems on the basis of the present rather than on the past.
14. Treats colleagues in the health care delivery system with the same courteous attention afforded strangers and casual acquaintances (eg, hearing what is said and giving feedback to indicate attentiveness).
15. Focuses clients as well as self on strengths and ability to embrace positive goals and encourages clients to put their energies into that task, not to look behind and dredge up excuses for past health-related events or behaviors.
16. Empowers clients and other professional colleagues to translate intention into reality and sustain it (ie, to take actions and then keep "working at it").

These continuous actions become parts of the nurse's character called habits. Because habits are powerful forces in determining health, professional nurses focus extensively on health habits. Leadership habits of the nurse also determine the effectiveness of the nurse in practice. The next section presents a brief discussion of the seven habits of leadership as envisioned by Covey (1989). When developed by a professional nurse, these habits should enhance the ability to be a transformational leader.

HABITS OF THE EFFECTIVE LEADER

Defined as the intersection of knowledge, skill, and desire (Covey, 1989, p. 47), a habit has great power in a person's life. Covey (1989, p. 47) describes knowledge as the theoretical paradigm, the "what to do" and the "why"; skills as the "how to do"; and desire as the motivation, the "want to do." He warns that even if a person knows something (eg, that we need to listen) and has developed the necessary skills (eg, to listen intently), this is not enough to form an effective habit. Unless the person wants to listen, listening will not become a habit.

Effective habits are the internalized principles and patterns of behavior that reflect the three interrelated factors of knowledge, skills, and desire. All the habits that Covey (1989) designates for effective leadership are based on the theoretical premise of sequential growth moving people from dependence to independence and finally to interdependence, the phase in which true mutuality can occur.

The seven habits identified by Covey (1989) are listed below and briefly described in terms of the professional nurse's relationship with clients.

1. Be proactive. Nurses need to set a goal and work to achieve it. They commit themselves to the client's perceptions and serve as a model for health, not a critic of those with expressed concerns. They accept their own ability to be "response-able" in dealing with clients' whole human responses to their health concerns. They believe that "it's not what happens to us, but our response to what happens to us that hurts us" (Covey, 1989, p. 73).

2. Begin with the end in mind. The nurse should identify what is really important and try to be and to do what really matters the most every day. The nurse also must differentiate management from leadership: management, representing the bottom line, focuses on how the nurse can best accomplish certain things with the client, and leadership, representing the top line, focuses on what the nurse wants to accomplish. "Management is efficiency in climbing the ladder of success; leadership determines whether the ladder is leaning against the right wall" (Covey, 1989, p. 101).

3. Put first things first. The formula for the nurse who wants to stay focused on the important business of nursing and give less energy to the unimportant is to prioritize, organize, and, finally, perform. The challenge for the nurse is to manage time in such a way that most of the time is used for urgent important activities, such as crises, pressing problems, and deadline-driven projects, as well as the not urgent but important projects, such as health promotion/illness prevention, relationship building, recognizing new opportunities, planning, and recreation (Covey, 1989, pp. 149–151).

4. Think win–win or no deal. Interdependency is the most mature goal for any relationship; thus, in professional relationships, interdependency would emphasize mutual benefits. Activities would reflect a commitment to both parties' growth, development, and satisfaction. For example, a client benefits from being empowered by the professional nurse providing informational support, and the nurse benefits by having the interventions validated and the sense of presence with the client valued. When such mutuality is experienced, neither person in the relationship loses or feels powerless (Covey, 1989, pp. 213–234).

5. Seek first to understand, then to be understood. Empathy is the habit reflected in this principle. The ability to focus on the client's reality as he experiences is vital to positive communication. Empathy is discussed in detail in Chapter 15. Credibility problems, such as the client's feeling that "you just don't understand," are prevented to the extent that the nurse empathizes with the client (Covey, 1989, pp. 236–260).

6. Value differences and bring all perspectives together. Respect is the characteristic that enables the nurse to develop this habit. Respect is discussed further in Chapter 15. To the extent that the nurse facilitates respect for differing perspectives, the client is likely to feel more free to seek the best possible alternative. If the nurse also experiences respect for his or her perspectives, synergistic relationships are enhanced. Using the principle of synergy, the nurse and client multiply their individual talents and abilities, and the outcome of their efforts is greater than the sum of the parts (Covey, 1989, pp. 277–284).

7. Have a balanced, systematic program for self-renewal. Consistency in having a regularly planned and balanced program for self-renewal prevents weakening of the body, mechanization of the mind, exposure of raw emotions, and desensitization of the spirit. Clearly, nurses' leadership ability is enhanced if they consistently participate in activities that renew four aspects of the self: physical, mental, emotional–social, and moral being. Renewal energizes capabilities that are necessary for productive helping relationships in nursing (Covey, 1989, pp. 288–304).

Additionally, Prestwood and Schumann (1997, p. 68) suggest that the personal growth and state of mind needed for leadership require an understanding of the following principles:

1. Know who you are—what you know and do not know about yourself, resistance and tolerance for change, fears, preferences, and skills and abilities

2. Let go of what you have hold of—discover chains that bind you to the past

3. Learn your purpose—based on values, unfolding through a lifelong process of learning

4. Live in the question—understand relationships, be open to the potential of the unknown, avoid the quick fix
5. Learn the art of "barn raising"—need to work with and through others, shared purpose
6. Give "it" away—ennoble, enable, empower, and encourage yourself and others
7. Let the magic happen—let go of the demands of the ego

Habits represent the integrated principles of the professional nurse. The following section presents an overview of the leadership behaviors that are actualized in professional nursing.

NURSING LEADERSHIP BEHAVIORS

Leadership as a Change Agent Using the Nursing Process

Promoting change is an important component of nursing care, with principles and strategies to promote change integrated into all phases of the nursing process. Because "paradoxes and ambivalent feelings are a normal component of the change process" (Davis, 1991), it is important to build in the client's strengths, promote the client's ability to be self-empowering, and perceive change as a challenge and an opportunity for growth.

ASSESSMENT

The assessment phase of the nursing process involves identifying client characteristics, including openness and motivation for change. The client's culture and social group are important sources of data about possible biases. Influences of the client's family, significant others, and the environment should also be considered. These data are then shared for validation with the client and key persons in the situation. The client must share the nurse's perception that a problem exists and that change is desirable, or the change process will not be successful.

The variables that should be assessed are related to the client, the nurse–client relationship, and the environmental situation. Some factors that must be considered include the:

1. Client's status and potential for health
2. Client's health goals
3. Client's strengths and weaknesses in achieving health goals
4. Client's needs
5. Client's available resources (including significant others)
6. Nurse's goals and their congruence with the client's goals
7. Nurse's knowledge and skill relative to the client's goals
8. Openness and adequacy of communication among the client, nurse, and significant others
9. Environmental influences that have an impact on the situation

If clients do not recognize the existence of a need, nurses should identify the perceived problem and the needed change. Clients will be influenced by their perception about their ability to use a particular change, about the degree of commitment that will be required, and about the degree of control they will have over the change process. These factors may all selectively influence their perception and retention of the information shared with them. Nurses are unlikely to be successful if they try to impose their opinion on clients. Rather, the major goals in this phase should be to create or stimulate the client's perception of a problem.

People usually have some resistance to change. Habits are behaviors that have become comfortable; thus, the anticipation of change creates discomfort. People are more likely to seek or be open to change if they feel deprived by a felt unmet need and if they perceive control over the change process. Thus, the nurse should try to actively encourage the client to be concerned about resolving the problem.

The change process is often time-consuming and difficult, and it requires commitment from the nurse and client. Personal resources are important aspects for consideration. The nurse must have the appropriate knowledge and skills to follow through until the change is successfully implemented. The nurse also must have a relationship with the client based on trust and respect and must be aware also of the personal motivation for wanting to promote a particular change. Is the nurse's motivation genuine concern for the client's well-being, or is the nurse influenced by desire for recognition, power, or possibly change simply for the sake of change? Building on client strengths can facilitate the change process.

The nurse–client relationship is critical to the success of the process. Trust must be established. The nurse should assess the degree of congruence between the nurse's and the client's values. If there are basic differences, it may not be possible for the nurse to be an effective change agent for that particular client.

The principle of mutuality must be an integral part of the relationship. As data are collected, the nurse should validate the accuracy of perceptions with the client. The client and nurse must have the same perception of a problem, and clients must understand that it is their responsibility to decide whether or not to implement possible solutions. Client should know what the nurse expects and they should be able to share their expectations of the nurse. The client must be an informed and equal participant from the beginning of the change process (Wilson, 1988).

Relating, a critical element in communication, is used to initiate and maintain an appropriate flow of information. Deciding, an application of knowledge and judgment, is used to analyze and organize data as they are collected; this moves the process into the planning phase.

PLANNING

The essence of the planning phase is to negotiate jointly determined goals with the client and to develop appropriate strategies to accomplish the goals. These purposes require judgment and decision-making ability (deciding); ability to influence the client toward goals that promote well-being (influencing); ability to facilitate the planning process through the therapeutic relationship (facilitating); and communication with professional colleagues and client support systems (relating).

One of the greatest potential problems in the planning phase is the lack of clearly defined goals. This can lead to ambiguity, uncertainty, and anxiety. The nurse and the client must be clear about the objectives for change that has been identified, and they should be sure that the client and other key persons are informed of, understand, and accept the goals. This involvement will facilitate commitment to support the change process.

A strategy comprising steps to be taken, by whom, and on what timetable must be established. This plan should set specific goals, with deadlines that establish the time by which the objectives should be achieved. It also may be desirable to design a trial period to test the proposed plans. At the end of the trial period, the goals, methods, and timetable can be reassessed and modified, if necessary.

An important component of the planning phase is identifying potential support systems for the client, to facilitate the proposed change. Time is an important resource that is often overlooked. The amount of time available to implement and support the change has a major influence on strategies that should be used. Setting a trial period for the change can be an effective technique to reduce resistance. Key influential persons are a resource that should be cultivated to develop allies, although the informal structure (nonhierarchical relationships) can be effective as well.

Personal characteristics of the change agent are essential to the development of relationships that inspire confidence, avoid defensiveness, and create support for the change process. Such qualities include respect for others, the ability to empathize, and genuineness in interactions. The specific roles assumed by the change agent are influenced by the nurse's special abilities and personality.

The phases of the change process to this point have been concerned with decision-making about whether or not a particular change is needed, desired, and feasible. At this point, the decision-making shifts to considering how to implement the change.

INTERVENTION

The intervention (implementation) phase includes instituting the change strategies and then maintaining the change once it has begun. The change agent must maintain a balance between leading the change process and developing the capabilities of the client and significant others to promote continuation of the process. Nurturance, constructive criticism, positive feedback, and rewards for progress may be helpful strategies at this time.

The change agent may function in various ways, depending on the particular situation. In some cases, the nurse may function as an expert role model by demonstrating how a particular skill should be performed; in others, the agent may function as a teacher, group leader, caretaker, or catalyst. Frequently, the nurse change agent acts as a facilitator by promoting effective communication and helping move the process toward its goals.

It is important that the nurse, the client, and others involved in the change process have the same expectations of each other's roles. If, for example, the client expects the nurse to do a procedure for him, and if the nurse perceives her role as that of a teacher and facilitator, it is obvious that there will be conflict and misunderstandings that could jeopardize the success of the project. The nurse needs to validate perceptions with the client frequently to ensure that communication remains open.

It is helpful to guard against the desire to implement too much change too quickly. Each aspect of change must be assimilated and accepted before the new equilibrium allows the system to consider additional changes. If a large change appears necessary, it may be desirable to break this change into smaller steps for implementation. The simplest solutions should be used whenever possible. The change agent should always have contingency plans ready in case the original plan hits unanticipated snags.

Recall of strategies to avoid or reduce resistance is important at this phase. Communication is critical so that everyone knows his or her role. Self-esteem, autonomy, and sense of security must be promoted. Conflict should be avoided while an open atmosphere is maintained. It is probably realistic to assume that optimal rather than minimal time will be needed to promote change in a manner that does not increase resistance.

Once the change has been implemented, it must be maintained. This is an especially delicate phase. It takes time before the new procedure or process feels comfortable, and some persons may wish to return to the old ways of doing things. Expectations may be unrealistic, and it may appear that the desired outcomes are not being realized, when in fact they have not had sufficient time to be demonstrated. The change agent may act to support the change and to reenergize the client's commitment to continue the change.

The client must be the one who actually maintains the change. The change agent must slowly withdraw from the situation, allowing the client to take over all aspects of the change. At this point, it will become clear whether the client and key others have been involved fully in the process and whether they have the power and authority to maintain the change. Unless the client is committed to it, the change will not succeed.

The change agent should keep the client informed about when the relationship will be terminated and whether there will be any future relationship between the nurse and the client. Joint evaluation of the process and its outcomes is desirable before the relationship is terminated. Through joint assessment of the relationship's significance, the nurse and client can focus on the strengths gained rather then on a sense of loss at its termination. It may also be helpful to develop a written summary of the change project to help ensure its survival and to serve as a source of information for future reference.

EVALUATION

Evaluation should be done during all phases of the nursing process. The possibility of the plan not working must be anticipated, and there should be a way to reverse the process or implement alternative plans if needed. The plan must be open to revision during all phases, and the change agent should be aware in advance of what modifications she is willing and able to make.

Evaluation involves a judgment about whether or not the change process has been successful. This decision requires assessing the effectiveness of the change process in relation to the objectives for change. Effectiveness is a subjective dimension that concerns attitudes toward the change process. Degree of adoption of the change is more objective; it relates to whether the change has made a measurable impact and has been continued.

Yura, Ozimek, and Walsh (1981, pp. 188–198) suggest a number of criteria for evaluation of nursing leadership. Some pertinent questions are:

1. Does the leader demonstrate a mastery of the nursing process?
2. Does the leader demonstrate sensitivity to the impact of self on others, leading to effective use of self?
3. Does the leader demonstrate mastery in the use and determination of verbal and nonverbal communication?
4. Can the leader initiate, maintain, and terminate effective relationships?
5. Can the leader effectively modify his or her own behavior and that of others?
6. Can the leader delegate action to be accomplished by selected knowledgeable persons?
7. Is the leader able to develop resources as needed to facilitate action?
8. Does the leader demonstrate accountability and morality in application of the leadership process?

If the change has been adopted and internalized, the change agent is ready to terminate the relationship and withdraw from the scene. The agent should ensure that the client and key others have the ability to maintain the change. The nurse should also determine, in collaboration with the client, whether she will have any future contact with the client.

APPLICATION TO GROUPS OR LARGER SYSTEMS

The nursing process has focused on the role of the nurse in promoting change in the health of an individual client. The nursing process is just as applicable when the change involves groups or larger systems. There are more variables to assess and a larger number of interrelationships for which to plan, but the principles and process remain the same.

◎ Conclusion

Effective nursing leadership is critically needed at all system levels. Through expert and ethical use of leadership behaviors in conjunction with nursing and change processes, clients are empowered and thus enabled to achieve their goals for improved health, and nurses are enriched in their practice and thus enabled to advance in their own career development.

THOUGHT QUESTIONS

1 Do nurses have power and authority in your practice setting? How can you enhance your power on behalf of clients?

2 Do you feel that you can advocate for clients? Should you assume the role of client advocate?

3 Do you have leadership qualities? How can you develop your ability to be a leader?

4 What is your opinion of Steven's view of leadership in the vignette at the beginning of the chapter?

REFERENCES

Ahern, J. (1992, Spring). Your presence is requested. *Revolution: The Journal of Nurse Empowerment, 2,* 80–82.

Bandman, E. L., & Bandman, B. (1995). *Nursing ethics through the life span* (3rd ed.). East Norwalk, CT: Appleton & Lange.

Barker, A. M., & Young, C. E. (1994). Transformational leadership: The feminist connection in postmodern organizations. *Holistic Nursing Practice, 9,* 16–25.

Bass, B. M. (1991). *Stogdill's handbook of leadership.* New York: The Free Press.

Bennis, W. (1989). *Why leaders can't lead: The unconscious conspiracy continues.* San Francisco,: Jossey-Bass.

Bennis, W., & Nanus, B. (1985). *Leaders: The strategies for taking charge.* New York: Harper & Row.

Bernal, E. W. (1992). The nurse as patient advocate. *Hastings Center Report, 22,* 18–23.

Bernhard, L. A., & Walsh, M. (1990). *Leadership: The key to the professionalization of nursing* (2nd ed.). St. Louis: Mosby.

Brill, N. I. *Working with people: The helping process* (4th ed.). New York: Longman.

Burns, J. M. (1978). *Leadership.* New York: Harper Colophon Books.

Carnall, C. A. (1990). *Managing change in organizations.* New York: Prentice-Hall.

Cassidy, V. R., & Koroll, C. J. (1994). Ethical aspects of transformational leadership. *Holistic Nursing Practice 9,* 41–47.

Chin, R. (1976). The utility of systems models and developmental models for practitioners. In W. G. Bennis, K. D. Benne, & R. Chin (Eds.). *The planning of change* (3rd ed., pp. 90–122). New York: Holt, Rinehart, and Winston.

Conley, A., & Mariano, C. (1991, June). Participatory decision-making: Issues and guidelines. *Journal of the New York State Nurses Association, 22,* 4–8.

Covey, S. R. (1989). *The 7 habits of highly effective people.* New York: Simon & Schuster.

Davis, P. S. (1991). The meaning of change to individuals within a college of nurse education. *Journal of Advanced Nursing, 16,* 108–115.

Douglass, L. M. (1988). *The effective nurse leader manager* (3rd ed.). St. Louis: Mosby.

Epstein, C. (1982). *The nurse leader: Philosophy and practice.* Reston, VA: Reston Publishing.

Gurka, A. M. (1995). Transformational leadership: Qualities and strategies for the CNS. *Clinical Nurse Specialist 9,* 169–174.

Haffer, A. (1986, April). Facilitating change: Choosing the appropriate strategy. *Journal of Nursing Administration, 16,* 18–22.

Hames, C. C., & Joseph, D. H. (1980). *Basic concepts of helping—A wholistic approach.* New York: Appleton-Century-Crofts.

Johnston, C. L. (1991, August). Sources of work satisfaction/dissatisfaction for hospital registered nurses. *Western Journal of Nursing Research, 13,* 503–513.

King, E. C. (1984). *Affective education in nursing.* Rockville, MD: Aspen Systems.

Kirkpatrick, M. K., Hull, A., Katrabos, S., & Sherman, C. (1995). Patient representative: More than an advocate. *Nursing Management, 26,* 92–94.

Knobf, M. T. (1990, November). Early-stage breast cancer: The options. *American Journal of Nursing, 90,* 28–30.

Manfredi, C. M. (1994). Leadership preparation: An examination of master's degree programs in nursing. *Holistic Nursing Practice, 9,* 48–57.

Marquis, B. L., & Huston, C. J. (1992). *Leadership roles and management functions in nursing.* Philadelphia: Lippincott.

Miles, M. S., & Crandall, E. K. (1983). The search for meaning and its potential for affecting growth in bereaved parents. *Health Values: Achieving High Level Wellness, 7,* 19–23.

Olsen, D. P. (1991). Empathy as an ethical and philosophical basis for nursing. *Advances in Nursing Science, 14,* 62–75.

Perlman, D., & Takacs, G. J. (1990, April). The 10 stages of change. *Nursing Management, 21,* 33–38.

Prestwood, D. C. L., & Schumann, P. A. (1987). Seven new principles of leadership. *The Futurist, 31,* 68.

Rafael, A. R. (1996). Power and caring: A dialectic in nursing. *Advances in Nursing Science, 19,* 3–17.

Richardson, P. (1992, Spring). Hospital practices that erode nursing power by promoting job dissatisfaction. *Revolution: The Journal of Nurse Empowerment, 2,* 34–39.

Rost, J. C. (1994). Leadership: A new conception. *Holistic Nursing Practice, 9,* 1–8.

Sherwood, J. J. (1988, Winter). Creating work cultures with competitive advantage. *Organ Dynamics, 16,* 5–27.

Snowball, J. (1996). Asking nurses about advocating for patients: 'Reactive' and 'proactive' accounts. *Journal of Advanced Nursing, 24,* 67–75.

Soukhanov, A. H. (Ed.) (1992). *The American heritage dictionary of the English language* (3rd ed.). Boston: Houghton Mifflin.

Stewart, T. A. (1991, January, 14). Now capital means brains, not just bucks. *Fortune, 123,* 31–32.

Taylor, S. G., Pickens, J. M., & Geden, E. A. (1989, January/February). Interactional styles of nurse practitioners and physicians regarding patient decision making. *Nursing Research, 38,* 50–55.

Toffler, A. (1990). *Powershift: Knowledge, wealth, and violence at the edge of the 21st century.* New York: Bantam Books.

Trofino, J. (1995). Transformational leadership in health care. *Nursing Management, 26,* 42–47.

Willard, C. (1996). The nurse's role as patient advocate: Obligation or imposition? *Journal of Advanced Nursing, 24,* 60–66.

Wilson, C. K. (1988). The impact of utilization review programs on consumer expectations, decision-making, and access to health care. *Nursing Administration Quarterly, 12,* 51–56.

Wooten, K. C., & White, L. P. (1989). Toward a theory of change role efficacy. *Human Relations, 42,* 651–669.

Yukl, G. A. (1981). *Leadership in organizations.* Englewood Cliffs, NJ: Prentice-Hall.

Yura, H., Ozimek, D., & Walsh, M. B. (1981). *Nursing leadership: Theory and process.* New York: Appleton-Century-Crofts.

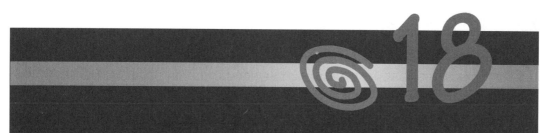

Management of Client Care

LEARNING OUTCOMES

By the end of this chapter, the student will be able to:

1 Discuss how to implement the client care management skills of critical thinking, time management, communication, conflict management, collaboration, coordination, consultation, coaching, mentoring, facilitating, and delegation.

2 Differentiate between quality assurance, quality improvement, and total quality management.

3 Identify ways to enhance the quality of client care.

In today's health care delivery system, management language has become very current. For example, systematic efforts to integrate and coordinate the financing and delivery of health care in a way that controls cost and maximizes quality is called *managed care* (Grimaldi, 1996). Coordination and integration of health services for clients with complex or extraordinarily costly medical problems is called *case management* (Grimaldi, 1996). *Care management* is a specific model for identifying variances from critical pathways for an entire client population in a given area (Hurt, 1995).

VIGNETTE: JUDY

Judy has been working on a pediatric unit for 6 months since graduating from an associate degree nursing program. She says, "I like patient care. I don't want to be a manager because I would have to move away from the bedside."

This chapter will discuss the professional nursing role of management of the care of individual or family clients. Management "relates to the activities needed to plan, organize, motivate, and control the human and material resources" needed to achieve patient care outcomes (Bleich, 1995, p. 4).

In the past, management was not viewed as a staff nurse role, but was associated with tasks done by the head nurse or other middle manager to accomplish institutional objectives. More recently, the term *patient care manager* has been used to describe a process of planning, organizing, and directing of human and physical resources to coordinate, integrate, and monitor patient care (Parkman, 1996). Management of client care is a vital part of every professional nurse's role in any practice setting.

Client Care Management Skills

According to Parkman (1996, pp. 126–127), "three attributes—professional standards, strong patient care values, and critical thinking—are the underlying role aspects necessary to forge an understanding of the professional nurse role in patient care management." Four general managerial skills that enable the nurse to manage most effectively (Douglass, 1992; Parkman, 1996) are:

- Technical skills—what things are done, and the ability to use technology
- Human skills—how things are done and the ability to work with others in goal achievement
- Conceptual skills—why things are done, and linking the work of nursing with the work of others to achieve patient goals

■ Diagnostic skills—ability to specify why something occurred, including analysis and examination of particular circumstances or conditions

Within these four categories, a number of specific skills are integrated for effective management of client care. Some of these specific skills are:

■ Critical thinking
■ Time management
■ Communication
■ Conflict management
■ Collaboration
■ Coordination
■ Consultation
■ Coaching, mentoring, and facilitating
■ Delegation

Each of these skills will be discussed in the following sections.

INTRAPERSONAL SKILLS

Critical Thinking

Jones (1996, p. 3) describes critical thinking as "a skill developed in looking for alternative solutions to problems and adopting a questioning approach." Problem-solving and decision-making are processes used in critical thinking. "Problem solving, which includes a decision-making step, is focused on trying to solve an immediate problem . . . . Decision making is a purposeful and goal-directed effort using a systematic process to choose among options" (Welch, 1995, p. 110).

Before attempting to solve a problem, certain key questions should be asked (Welch, 1995, p. 111):

1. Is it important?
2. Do I want to do something about it?
3. Am I qualified to handle it?
4. Do I have the authority to do anything?
5. Do I have the knowledge, interest, time, and resources to deal with it?
6. Can I delegate it to someone else?

If the answer to questions one through five is "no," a conscious decision can be made to ignore the problem, refer or delegate it to others, or consult or collaborate with others.

A number of processes for problem-solving and decision-making have been identified. One process, which might be labeled the *routine process*, consists of five steps (Jones & Beck, 1996; Marriner-Tomey, 1996; Sullivan & Decker, 1992):

1. Identification of the problem—includes gathering all pertinent facts and establishing goals for the decision

2. Seeking alternatives—includes determining the most desirable alternative
3. Selection of an alternative
4. Implementing the decision—includes setting a timeline and assigning tasks to others
5. Evaluation of the solution—was the solution effective in solving the issue or problem?

A second process, which might be labeled the *creative process*, focuses on creating unique solutions as opposed to generating choices of solutions. The creative process also consists of seven steps (Jones, 1996; Marriner-Tomey, 1992):

1. Identifying a felt need—what is the problem?
2. Preparation—generating numerous creative and innovative potential solutions
3. Incubation—taking time to review the information that has been collected
4. Illumination—the discovery of a solution
5. Verification—the solution refined and advantages and disadvantages of the chosen alternative assessed
6. Implementation of the chosen solution
7. Evaluation of the solution

A third approach to problem-solving and decision-making, which might be labeled the *intuitive process*, is based on a continuum of competence (Benner, 1984). Novice and advanced beginner nurses use a rational, step-by-step analytical approach like the routine process outlined earlier. However, by the proficient and expert levels of practice the nurse demonstrates intuition in perceiving the client's situation as a whole. Aspects of intuitive judgment include (Benner & Tanner, 1987; Jones, 1996):

■ Pattern recognition—perceptual ability to recognize configurations and relationships among variables in a situation
■ Similarity recognition—ability to recognize similarities and differences between previous and current situations
■ Common sense understanding—deep grasp of the culture and language of an illness experience from direct observation of patients
■ Skilled know how—ability to juggle many concurrent considerations in a situation
■ Sense of salience—ability to recognize which events are most important
■ Deliberate rationality—selective attention to salient events

The *cognitive nursing process* is a problem-solving process that is similar to the routine process outlined above. In step one, assessment data are collected. In step two, diagnosis, the problem is defined. In step three, planning, strategies to solve the problem are selected. Bleich (1995, p. 11) suggests that the following activities are part of planning once a client care goal has been established:

1. Deciding on a course of action
2. Determining the chronology of events that must occur to meet the goal(s)
3. Determining the talent and skills needed to accomplish the goal(s) and assigning these tasks to individuals who can most effectively meet the needs
4. Assessing the time requirements to accomplish the goal(s) and coordinating tasks around deadlines
5. Considering the driving and restraining forces that will affect goal attainment

The process is concluded with the implementation and evaluation steps.

Another primarily intrapersonal skill is time management.

Time Management

Busyness and time urgency are common complaints among nurses. One recent study found that nurses perform 93 different activities in a day. In comparison, pharmacists are involved in an average of only 26 different activities in a typical workday (*American Journal of Nursing*, 1992). Another study found that only 35% of nurses' time was spent in direct client care (including care planning, assessment, teaching, and technical activities) (Brider, 1992). Tappen (1995, p. 128) states that although "categories change from study to study, [but] the amount of time spent on direct care is usually less than half of the workday." It is clear that nurses need help with ways to use their clinical time effectively.

Several strategies that may be helpful have been proposed (Cummings, 1996; Tappen, 1995):

1. Setting your own personal and career goals that will provide guidelines for deciding how to spend time
2. Organizing your work using "to do" lists, schedules, blocks of time, and a filing system for paperwork
3. Setting limits by saying "no" to nonpriority demands on your time, eliminating unnecessary work, keeping your goals reasonable, and delegating work when appropriate
4. Streamlining work by keeping a time log, reducing interruptions, avoiding recurrent crises, finding the most efficient way to perform a task, automating repetitive tasks when possible, and breaking down large projects into small pieces
5. Matching tasks with your energy level by accomplishing routine tasks when energy is low

The determination of goals is the first and most important step. Once goals are known, priorities can be set. Wise (1995, p. 208) suggests that "although there are many routine tasks of any work, the tasks that have priority should be those related to the goals and priorities." You should try to address the most important goals and not get sidetracked on what may seem easier, but has a lower priority. Two obstacles to be avoided if possible are putting off to another time (procrastinating), or never finishing anything because it is not quite good enough (perfectionism).

It is especially important for professional nurses to learn how to balance life goals, including mental, physical, and social/emotional goals and activities (Cummings, 1996). The most important thing may be to relax and avoid stress and worry.

INTERPERSONAL SKILLS

Communication

Communication in nurse–client helping relationships was discussed in depth in Chapter 15. In addition, the nurse communicates with physicians, other professionals, assistive staff, and family members. In all of these relationships, how the message is communicated influences the communication. Empathy, respect, and genuineness are essential principles of communication in all relationships.

Management of assistive personnel is a vital element in current professional nursing practice. Strategies for communication with unlicensed assistive personnel (UAP) such as personal care assistants or certified nursing assistants (CNAs) include (Walton & Waszkiewicz, 1997; Wywialowski, 1995):

1. Support members of the work group by communicating that they are valued
2. Try to maintain an open mind and willingness to listen to others' viewpoints
3. Try to maintain a positive perspective and focus on solving problems rather than finding fault
4. Treat team members as "dignified people . . . without biases for their organizational position or credentialing statuses" (Wywialowski, 1995, p. 327)
5. Actions communicate expectations more consistently than words
6. Nonprofessional workers "may have greater need for concrete, context specific information" (Walton & Waszkiewicz, 1997, p. 25)
7. Clearly define tasks and expectations
8. Give clear instructions
9. Identify task priorities, rationale, and time frame for completion of the task
10. Be clear about the rationale for completing tasks on time
11. Provide an opportunity for questions and clarifying instructions
12. Ask for help instead of telling (Walton & Waszkiewicz, 1997)

13. Listen to suggestions

14. Recognize differences in educational and cultural backgrounds

It has been suggested (Warfel, 1995) that there has been a breakdown in nurse–physician communication. Not surprisingly, suggestions for communication with physicians are somewhat different from those given above for communication with UAP. Some suggested strategies (Cummings, 1996, p. 191) include:

1. Consider yourself and the physician partners on the health care team

2. Focus on the task or issue, not personal differences

3. Maintain improvement of patient care as the goal for the interaction

4. Establish clear roles for the physician, staff, and yourself

5. Communicate assertively

6. Make direct suggestions rather than subtle hints. Avoiding conflict and preserving the "omniscient physician notion" is "a game"

There are times in most relationships when differences lead to conflict. The management of conflict might be considered a special communication application.

Conflict Management

There is a potential for conflict whenever people communicate. Individuals have unique ways of perceiving situations and understanding information. When perceptions and understandings of situations or information differ, conflict occurs (Roe, 1996). According to McElhaney (1996), managers spend an average of 20% of their time dealing with conflict. The goals of conflict management include being able to work together more effectively and generating new ideas and new solutions to difficult problems (Roe, 1996).

Keenan and Hurst (1995) describe four stages of conflict, with movement possible in either direction between stages: frustration, conceptualization, action, and outcomes.

Frustration occurs when people perceive that their goals may be blocked. Frustration may escalate into anger or deep resignation. "When frustration occurs, it is a cue to stop and clarify the nature of major differences" (Keenan & Hurst, 1995, p. 342). Anger may occur as the result of a perceived threat. "Although anger is a common response to conflict, it can become a barrier to conflict management because it is difficult to problem solve rationally while feeling intense emotions" (Roe, 1995, p. 155). Roe (1995) recommends a rational problem assessment and intervention process to control emotion and manage conflict effectively.

Everyone involved has a *conceptualization* and interpretation of what the conflict is and why it is occurring. People may differ on four aspects of a conflict (Keenan & Hurst, 1995):

Facts
Goals
Methods to achieve goals
Values or standards used to select goals, priorities, and methods

Most often these interpretations are different and involve the person's own perspective. However, regardless of its accuracy or clarity, the conceptualization forms the basis for everyone's reaction to the frustration (Keenan & Hurst, 1995). At this stage, it is most important to accurately define the conflict.

Action, in the form of intentions, strategies, plans, or behavior results from the conceptualization (Keenan & Hurst, 1995). Approaches to handling conflict include (Keenan & Hurst, 1995; McElhaney, 1996):

Avoiding—simply not addressing the conflict, a lose–lose situation
Accommodating—meets goals of the other person, a lose–win situation (may be appropriate when the issue is more important to someone else, the person is more powerful, or when the person is wrong [p. 49])
Competing—pursuing own goals at the expense of another, a win–lose situation (may be appropriate when a quick or unpopular decision has to be made)
Collaborating—finds mutual agreeable solutions, a win–win situation
Compromising—combines assertiveness and cooperation, a lose–lose situation (may be effective when persons are of equal power and an expedient answer is needed)

A match between the nature of the conflict and the action is most likely to result in resolution with desirable results.

Strategies for the professional nurse to facilitate conflict resolution between other persons may include (Cummings, 1996, p. 195):

■ Protect each person's self-respect.
■ Focus on issues, not personalities.
■ Do not blame participants for the problem.
■ Encourage open and complete discussion of the issues.
■ Allow equal time for all parties to participate.
■ Encourage expression of both positive and negative feelings.
■ Encourage active listening and understanding among all parties.
■ Summarize key themes in the discussion.
■ Assist in the development of alternative solutions.
■ At a later point in time:
    ■ Follow up on progress in resolution of the conflict.
    ■ Give positive feedback related to problem-solving styles.

Outcomes are consequences that result from the action. Productivity and efficiency may increase, decrease, or stay the same. Relationships may be strengthened, weakened, or ended. Four questions that can be used to assess the degree of conflict resolution are (Johnson & Johnson, 1994; Keenan & Hurst, 1995):

1. Are the relationships stronger and are people better able to interact?
2. Do the members like and trust each other more?
3. Are all the members satisfied with the results of the conflict?
4. Have group members become more able to resolve future conflicts with one another?

Depending on the nature of the conflict, urgency for resolution, and the balance of power, collaboration is the desired approach to conflict management. As Keenan & Hurst (1995, p. 351) state, "collaborating . . . is the position of the wise owl."

Collaboration
Collaboration is viewed as "the opposite of both avoiding and competing" (Keenan & Hurst, 1995, p. 351). In contrast to the mutual concessions of compromise, in collaboration no one is asked to give up anything. The goal is to have both parties win. The problem-solving process continues until each individual is satisfied with the resolution. This process is growth producing, but it takes a considerable amount of time (Roe, 1995).

The following defining characteristics of collaboration have been identified (Henneman, Lee, & Cohen, 1995, p. 105):

- Joint venture
- Cooperative endeavor
- Willing participation
- Shared planning and decision-making
- Team approach
- Contribution of expertise
- Shared responsibility
- Nonhierarchical relationships
- Shared power (based on knowledge and expertise rather than role or title)

Collaboration is an important intervention when the individuals (like team members) must work together over a long period of time and therefore have an investment in solutions that satisfy all important concerns and goals to be achieved. For trivial issues, collaboration and consensus-seeking are not needed. Examples of strategies for collaborative process include:

- Mutual respect is essential
- Use positive confrontation to verbalize facts, assumptions, and feelings
- Listening skills permit each party to "be heard"
- Seek open and creative solutions

- Replace "who has more power" with "what does the client need" and "where does each of us fit into the plan" (Keenan & Hurst 1995, p. 351)
- Be clear about the desired goal, using objective criteria
- Send consistent signals
- Ensure that agreements are clearly stated at the end of the negotiation

Communication among individuals and groups is the basis for most other manager skills, such as coordination, with either clients and their families or with colleagues.

Coordination

Coordination is the ability to achieve unity of effort or teamwork across individuals, departments, and organizations. It is an integrative or synchronizing function that links all the services needed by the client and ensures that all services and caregivers provide their part at the right time and place for each client. Effectiveness in this "integrator role is partially dependent on the creation of communication linkages between the providers who will render those services" (Alfred, Arford, & Michel, 1995, p. 22). Coordination among multiple providers with diverse skills, experience, and information can:

Foster information exchange
Minimize uncertainty
Encourage unity of effort
Promote efficiency of client care services

The nurse coordinates people while coordinating client care. Alfred and coworkers (1995) identify three programming mechanisms and three feedback mechanisms for coordination, as described in Table 18-1. "Programming mechanisms specify in advance the activities to be performed, the education required, or the outcomes expected relative to the work. Feedback mechanisms specify the manner in which information is exchanged between individuals" (p. 23).

"Nurses will have increased accountability for coordinating care with an increasing number of specialists across institutional boundaries and in a way that minimizes hospital length of stay while attaining predetermined quality outcomes" (Alfred et al., 1995, p. 27). Some structural strategies that maximize coordination across boundaries include (Alfred et al., 1995):

- "Direct line" communication channels to administrators
- Protocols, standards of care, or critical pathways for routine services
- Triage, admission, and discharge protocols
- Daily team care planning care conferences

TABLE 18-1

Mechanisms for Coordination

Mechanism	Definition	Example(s)
Programming Mechanisms		
Standardization of work	Specifies in advance activities to be performed	Rules, policies, schedules, procedures, protocols, textbooks
Standardization of skills	Specifies in advance the type of training or education required to perform the job	Certification, educational degree requirements, inservice education, orientation
Standardization of outputs	Specifies in advance the outcome of the work	Nursing standards or critical pathways
Feedback Mechanisms		
Direct supervision	Oral or written exchange of information between two people in a hierarchical relationship	A staff nurse instructing and/or monitoring the work of a patient care assistant
Mutual adjustment	Oral or written exchange of information between two people not in a hierarchical relationship	Face to face discussion/communication that may take place between a case manager, physician, or social worker and nurse, when making discharge plans, etc.
Group coordination	Exchange of information between three or more people through an integrating device found in the formal work structure	Staff meetings, rounds, shift report, patient care conferences, liaison positions, or project teams

Alfred, C. A., Arford, P. H., & Michel, Y. (1995). Coordination as a critical element of managed care. *Journal of Nursing Administration, 25,* 23.

- Opportunities for face-to-face discussions between hospital and community providers for complex client care situations
- Hospital–community integrator positions
- Cross-training of various staff categories
- Linking providers via integrated information systems
- Incentives and rewards that recognize team-related performance and outcomes

Another communication-based management skill is consultation.

Consultation

Consultation is an interactive communication process that involves the sharing of advice or information by someone with specialized expertise. The staff nurse recognizes that help is needed to resolve a client care problem. Once a consultant has been identified, the steps of the formal consultation process are (Parkman, 1996):

- Assessment of the problem
- Preparation of a consultation report
- Implementation of the recommendations
- Follow-up

According to Parkman (1995, p. 148):

> the staff nurse does not give up the problem during consultation, but retains responsibility in assisting with assessing the problem, choosing the best interventions, and ensuring that the interventions are indeed carried out. The staff nurse also discusses issues with the consultant during follow-up and evaluation of the interventions and the process.

The staff nurse role in the consultation process is (Parkman, 1995) to:

- Identify the problem
- Request consultation
- Assess the problem
- Choose interventions from those recommended
- Carry out interventions
- Conduct follow-up and evaluation with the consultant

A formal consultation process is not necessary for all client care problems. The client or the client's family might provide informal expertise. Staff may also consult with each other. Peer consultation is an excellent way for experienced nurses to help newer colleagues to learn and to address similar situations in the future. Experienced nurses can use the skills of coaching, mentoring, and facilitating to help newer colleagues.

Coaching, Mentoring, and Facilitating
Coaching is an instructional skill by which the professional nurse teaches or trains clients and their families to help them to improve their performance and capabilities. Rodriguez (1995, p. 314) points out that "coaches are distinguished by their absence on the playing field. They let others do the job. Yet they are visible on the sidelines and readily accessible when problems occur." According to Parkman, 1996, p. 151), while coaching the client and family, the nurse is responsible for:

- Explaining why the skill being taught or coached is important to the client
- Answering any questions regarding the skill
- Explaining how to do the skill or procedure
- Demonstrating how to do the skill or procedure
- Giving the client and family an opportunity to practice the skill or procedure until it can be performed safely
- Giving constructive feedback, both positive and negative

Coaching of colleagues can be effective in supporting professional development, giving recognition, and facilitating improvement in clinical performance. In short-term coaching for developmental opportunities, the coach "guides the interactive problem-solving process and uses constructive feedback to develop or improve effective behavior, facilitate problem solving, and enhance individual effectiveness" (Cummings, 1996, p. 199).

In constrast, long-term coaching to correct performance deficiencies of team colleagues is usually focused on a specific behavior and is planned rather than spontaneous. Peer consultation may help the novice manager to prepare for this type of coaching situation. Specific strategies include (Cummings, 1996):

- Identify the desired outcome before the session
- Clearly articulate performance standards
- Give colleague accurate feedback about current performance and opportunities for improvement
- Create a developmental plan with the colleague
- Monitor progress after a plan has been agreed to and has been implemented
- Give both positive and corrective feedback
- Give recognition as performance outcomes warrant
- Incorporate coaching within disciplinary action if mutually agreed on performance objectives are not attained

Coaching is considered to be high in the directive behaviors of structuring, controlling or supervising, and also high in the supportive behaviors of praise, listening, and facilitating (Ulrich, 1995). Coaching may be used with clients or with colleagues. In contrast, *mentoring* is associated with professional development. Mentoring, which is based on mutual positive regard, involves role modeling and supporting, guiding, and counseling a less experienced colleague. Some of the functions of a mentor include (Gray, 1995):

- Facilitate the career of the mentee
- Provide psychosocial support
- Volunteer or nominate the mentee for additional responsibilities
- Teach "unwritten rules about how things are done"
- Provide information about how to improve performance (coaching)
- Help mentee to learn technical and management skills
- Role model as a career example
- Counsel to allow the mentee to explore personal concerns

The mentor facilitates the growth and development of the mentee. *Facilitation* is a skill that makes it easier for people to mobilize their own resources. Facilitation focuses on a person's human needs enabling them to grow and develop. Some guidelines for using facilitation as a managerial technique with clients or colleagues include (Davidhizar, 1994):

- Practice active listening in contrast to giving advice, instruction, or actually "taking over"
- Communicate genuine interest and concern
- Provide the person with adequate information
- Provide the person with ideas through suggestion
- Use the person's words in formulating the plan of action

- Use techniques that maximize feelings of self-respect
- Focus on the person's ability to help self
- Do not minimize the value of time
- Praise competent performance

McCloskey, Bulechek, Moorhead, and Daly (1996) differentiate between the "provider of client care" role, which they label *direct care*, and the "manager of the care environment" role, which they label *indirect care*. They state that studies show that "hospital nurses spend approximately one-third of their time in direct patient care, one-half in indirect and unit management [combined], and about 14% to 17% in personal time" (McCloskey et al., 1996, p. 23). A direct care intervention is performed in interaction with the client. An indirect care intervention is performed away from the client, but on the client's behalf. McCloskey and colleagues (1996) found that the most frequent indirect interventions used by nurses were documentation in a clinical record, and delegation of responsibility for specific client care tasks.

VIGNETTE: MICHELLE

Michelle is an experienced staff nurse in the emergency room. She says, "Lately I am so angry I have trouble making myself come to work. The hospital is laying off nurses and hiring UAPs. They expect me to supervise these workers, but my license is at risk. I used to love nursing, but managed care has taken all the fun out of it."

Delegation
Delegation is defined as "transferring to a competent individual authority to perform a selected nursing task in a selected situation" (Hansten & Washburn, 1994, p. 1). Delegation depends on a balance of responsibility, accountability, and authority. Responsibility and authority must be delegated equally—the RN sets the limits and allows the caregiver to decide how to achieve the goals (Boyle, 1995). According to Hansten and Washburn (1994, pp. 2–8), the activities of delegation are to:

- Know your world
- Know your organization
- Know your practice
- Know yourself
- Know your delegate
- Know what needs to be done
- Prioritize, and match the job to the delegate
- Know how to communicate
- Know how to resolve conflict
- Know how to give feedback
- Evaluate and problem solve

KNOWING YOUR WORLD AND ORGANIZATION

In today's managed care environment, the role of the professional nurse in the hospital is to guide patients through the shortest possible stay, ensuring maximal benefit from needed care (Boyle, 1995). An organization supports delegation downward from manager to staff, laterally from peer to peer, and upward from staff to manager to ensure the best possible use of various skill levels. A staff nurse delegates to get work accomplished in a timely manner. Given the increasing hospital use of UAP, delegation between nursing staff and assistants on the unit "is the most significant aspect of delegation for the professional staff nurse" (Parkman, 1996, p. 153).

KNOWING YOUR PRACTICE

Many nurses are afraid that their license to practice nursing will be jeopardized by delegating to UAP. Therefore, it is important for nurses to understand the nurse practice act in their state as it affects delegation. All states have adopted language that either explicitly or implicitly include delegation within the definition of nursing.

The National Council of State Boards of Nursing (NCSBN, 1987, p. 227) has issued the following definition of delegation, "nurses entrusting the performance of selected nursing tasks to competent unlicensed persons in selected situations. The nurse retains the accountability for the total nursing care of the individuals." Some of the key elements of this definition are:

1. When you delegate a task to an unlicensed assistant, you remain accountable for the client's total care. This means that you are answerable for your decision to delegate the task.
2. The assistant is responsible for performance of the task for which he or she has been trained.
3. Nurses must know the competencies of the delegate. Boards of nursing usually have developed rules on determining competence, level of supervision necessary, and which acts may be delegated.
4. If you delegate a task to someone whom you know is not competent, you will be in violation of the standard of practice in any state (Hansten & Washburn, 1994).
5. Supervision includes the initial direction given to the assistant and periodic checking and follow-up. The nurse who delegates a task is responsible for supervision whether the nurse is physically present or not (eg, home health, community, long-term care settings).
6. Your professional license is only "on the line" if you delegate inappropriately. You are not expected to assume responsibility for the personal performance of all individuals on the health care team (Hansten & Washburn, 1994).
7. The employer may suggest, but cannot decide, which nursing acts can safely be delegated and to whom. "Employee policies cannot override the law and rules of nursing and will not protect the nurse who is following policy but acting outside of the practice

act" (Hansten & Washburn, 1994, p. 61). It is in the best interests of the nurse to resolve any differences of expectation with the employer.

8. Specific limitations to interventions that may not be delegated to UAP (eg, medications, suctioning, surgical asepsis) are determined by each state.
9. Delegation to a licensed practical nurse (LPN) must meet the same rules. States differ in whether or not the LPN is allowed to delegate to a UAP.

KNOWING YOURSELF

The thought of delegating to other health care workers causes many nurses to have negative feelings (Hansten & Washburn, 1994, p. 97), including:

Fear
Anger
Loss of trust in management
Loss of control
Concern about quality
Burnout
Stress
Feeling overwhelmed
Lack of enjoyment in work
Feeling betrayed
Feeling abandoned
Decreased job satisfaction

Many of these feelings are related to the nurse's individual response to work life changes and the method by which the change took place. Given that the addition of new unlicensed workers is often accompanied by lay-offs of nurses, the rage and pain can be debilitating and destructive. Some other possible barriers to effective clinical delegation are (Boyle, 1995; Hansten & Washburn, 1994, pp. 108–114):

Risk aversion
Being able to trust others
Letting go of some technical tasks or amenities
Fear of loss of control
Overcoming old habits
Needing to cross tasks off a list
"If I don't do what I'm used to doing, what's left for me to do?"
Thinking "I can do it better myself"
Needing help with organization of work
The supernurse syndrome—trying to "do it all"
Wanting to be liked
The supermartyr syndrome—needing to be needed and indispensable
Uncertain about rules or regulations
"It takes too much time"

Denial

Am I still a real nurse when I delegate?—shifting from clinical expert to manager

No role models

Hansten & Washburn (1994, p. 116) also indicate some of the potential benefits of delegation that have been cited by nurses:

More personal time (eg, breaks, lunch)

Personal growth

Empowerment and growth of the UAP

Making better use of brain power and assessment skills

More time for professional nursing interventions such as

    Educating patients

    Emotional support

    Coordination of care

    Planning

    Communication with other professionals and family

    Discharge planning

Less stressed out with "doing it all"

More sense of team and support of each other

Collegiality

Someone to help gather data, answer lights

Better job satisfaction

KNOWING YOUR DELEGATE

Before nurses can delegate specific tasks, they must know the strengths and weaknesses of the person to whom they are delegating. Strategies for determining the competency of the delegate include:

1. Know the official job description expectations for each worker category
2. Review the competency checklist that new workers complete
3. Know the unofficial expectations for each worker category
4. Ask the person about strengths, but validate these perceptions through observation
5. Ask for feedback about what the person feels uncomfortable doing, or what he or she needs to learn more about
6. Listen to others, but use your own judgment
7. Assess the worker's motivation and preferences
8. Understand cultural diversity and perceptual ethnocentrism (Walton & Waszkiewicz, 1997)
9. Clarify questions and perceptions
10. "Communicate, communicate, communicate" (Hansten & Washburn, 1994, p. 179)

KNOWING WHAT NEEDS TO BE DONE, PRIORITIZING, AND MATCHING THE JOB TO THE DELEGATE

Hansten & Washburn (1994) suggest several strategies for getting the job done:

1. Assess the situation. Get a global idea of the outcomes you would like to achieve during the shift.
2. Take a few minutes at the beginning of each shift to plan. Determine optimal goals, what is reasonable, and priorities.
3. Analyze the knowledge, skills, and personal traits needed for each job. Focus on the outcome desired rather than the task. In making assignments, consider:
    a. Complexity of client care—how involved is the care required?
    b. Dynamics—how often is the client's condition changing?
    c. Complexity of assessment
    d. Technology involved
    e. Degree of supervision needed
    f. Availability of supervision
    g. Infection control and safety precautions
4. Match the job and the delegate.
5. Evaluate effectiveness and efficiency. Were the desired outcomes achieved?

KNOWING HOW TO COMMUNICATE

A major element of effective communication related to delegation is effective assignment giving. Hansten & Washburn (1994) suggest consideration of who, what, when, where, how, and why:

- Who—involves to whom the job should be delegated and who is the client or receiver of the task
- What—be clear, specific, and take the time to explain the task thoroughly. What exactly do you want done? You may be able to show (teach) the delegate rather than tell.
- When—what is the time frame for completion? Under what circumstances should the delegate notify you?
- Where—anatomically (eg, clean the graft incision on the calf with Betadine) or geographically (eg, ambulate Mrs. Jones from her room to the nurses' station and back)
- How—be specific (eg, take a rectal temperature)
- Why—what is the reason that a task has to be carried out in a particular way?

KNOWING HOW TO RESOLVE CONFLICT

Hansten & Washburn (1994) suggest the following sources of conflict regarding delegation:

- Ambiguous jurisdiction—not knowing who should be doing what, and how roles and duties overlap

- Conflict of interest—personal values influence care methods and priorities
- Communication barriers
- Dependence of one party on another
- Disagreement related to work interaction (without communication to resolve the disagreements)
- Unresolved prior conflicts

GIVING FEEDBACK

A method for giving feedback has been proposed by Hansten and Washburn (1994, p. 241):

1. Get the delegate's input before proceeding
2. Give credit for the delegate's efforts
3. Share your perception of what you have observed, read, assessed
4. Explore the situation more fully with the delegate: discuss gaps in perceptions, causes of the problem
5. Get the delegate's solution to the problem
6. Agree on an action plan
7. Set a time to check on progress

When giving a feedback message to a delegate, it is helpful to remember the following criteria:

1. Be specific rather than general
2. Direct the message toward behavior that can be changed
3. Consider the needs of the receiver and the giver of the message
4. Feedback should be appropriately timed
5. Ideally, feedback is solicited rather than imposed
6. Clear communication and understanding is ensured by asking the receiver to rephrase the message
7. Share positive feedback but keep negative feedback private
8. Never reprimand in public

Both ongoing and periodic evaluation are essential to assess how the delegation process is proceeding. And then, "recognize your unique contribution to this world, and recognize all the people that help make it happen. And celebrate the success of the team!" (Hansten & Washburn, 1994, p. 281).

This chapter has been based on the belief that management of client care is an integral part of nursing, and therefore, is essential to quality care.

◎ Management of Quality in Client Care

The Joint Commission on Accreditation of Healthcare Organizations develops standards for *quality assurance* for hospitals. According to Miller (1995, p. 203), "the term quality assurance frequently indicates a focus on clinical aspects of care rather than on the full series of interrelated governance, managerial support, and clinical processes that affect patient outcomes."

In contrast, *quality improvement* (QI) is defined as "the ongoing study and improvement of the processes of providing health care services to meet the needs of patients and others" (Miller, 1995, p. 203). QI focuses on whole systems, not just the performance of individual practitioners (Tappen, 1995). *Total quality management* (TQM) is an application of QI, in which "through continual examination of and focus on patient outcomes, the goal is to deliver the highest quality product or service" (Miller, 1995, pp. 203–204). Regardless of which program is used, the goal is to improve the results of client care and services.

Biggs (1996) identifies the following principles for implementing QI: organizational commitment; process improvement; use of a scientific approach; and employee involvement and empowerment. Three different aspects of health care can be evaluated in a QI or TQM program (Tappen, 1995, pp. 464–466):

- Structure (setting and resources)
  - Facilities (comfort, convenience of layout, accessibility of support services, safety)
  - Equipment (adequate supplies, state-of-the-art equipment, staff ability to use it)
  - Staff (credentials, experience, absenteeism, turnover rate, staff–client ratios)
  - Finances (salaries, adequacy, and sources)
- Process (actual activities carried out by health care providers)
- Outcomes (results of activities)

The long-term goals of QI are to

achieve optimal patient outcomes in terms of both improved well-being (to the extent possible given the patient's condition) and patient satisfaction with care within a well-functioning system while keeping costs to a minimum . . . . The more immediate purposes of any quality improvement activity are to improve the efficiency and the effectiveness of the services rendered (Tappen, 1995, p. 462).

Quality in health care is defined as "meeting or exceeding the customer's needs and fulfilling his or her expectations" (Biggs, 1996, p. 305).

◎ Conclusion

The survival of a health care organization depends on the ability to improve care and service while reducing costs. The professional nurse plays a pivotal role, through management of client care and participation in QI activities.

THOUGHT QUESTIONS

1 What are the differences between the routine process, the creative process, the intuitive process, and the cognitive process for problem-solving and decision-making?

2 Is time management compatible with professional and personal balance in life?

3 How do processes differ when communicating with UAP versus physicians?

4 How might you modify conflict management approaches based on different situational factors?

5 How similar are your feelings to those of Michelle (in the delegation vignette)? What can you do to resolve any negative feelings and improve work satisfaction?

REFERENCES

Alfred, C. A., Arford, P. H., & Michel, Y. (1995). Coordination as a critical element of managed care. *Journal of Nursing Administration, 25,* 21–28.

American Journal of Nursing. (1992). RNs do 93 different jobs says hospital study. *American Journal of Nursing, 92,* 9.

Benner, P. (1984). *From novice to expert: Excellence and power in clinical nursing practice.* Menlo Park, CA: Addison-Wesley.

Benner, P., & Tanner, C. (1987, January). Clinical judgment. How expert nurses use intuition. *American Journal of Nursing, 87,* 23–31.

Biggs, J. (1996). Quality improvement. In C. E. Loveridge & S. H. Cummings (Eds.). *Nursing management in the new paradigm* (pp. 300–334). Gaithersburg, MD: Aspen.

Bleich, M. R. (1995). Managing and leading. In P. S. Y. Wise (Ed.). *Leading and managing in nursing* (pp. 3–21). St. Louis: Mosby-Year Book.

Boyle, C. C. (1995). Delegation—The path to professional practice. In K. W. Vestal (Ed.). *Nursing management: Concepts and issues* (2nd ed., pp. 87–100). Philadelphia: Lippincott.

Brider, P. (1992). The move to patient-focused care. *American Journal of Nursing, 92,* 27–33.

Cummings, S. H. (1996). Role of the professional nurse: Organizational management. In C. E. Loveridge & S. H. Cummings (Eds.). *Nursing management in the new paradigm* (pp. 176–220). Gaithersburg, MD: Aspen.

Davidhizar, R. E. (1994). Using facilitation as a managerial technique. *Journal of Nurse Management, 2,* 193–196.

Douglass, L. M. (1992). The effective nurse: Leader and manager. St. Louis: Mosby-Year Book.

Gray, J. J. (1995). Role transition. In P. S. Y. Wise (Ed.). *Leading and managing in nursing* (pp. 460–477). St. Louis: Mosby-Year Book.

Grimaldi, P. L. (1996). A glossary of managed care terms. *Nursing Management Supplement, 4,* 5–7.

Hansten, R. I., & Washburn, M. J. (1994). *Clinical delegation skills: A handbook for nurses.* Gaithersburg, MD: Aspen.

Henneman, E. A., Lee, J. L., & Cohen, J. I. (1995). Collaboration: A concept analysis. *Journal of Advanced Nursing, 21,* 103–109.

Hurt, L. W. (1995). Care management: Providing a connecting link. *Nursing Management, 26,* 27–33.

Johnson, D. W., & Johnson. F. P. (1994). *Joining together: Group theory and group skills* (5th ed.). Englewood Cliffs, NJ: Prentice-Hall.

Jones, R. A. P. (1996). Processes and models. In R. A. P. Jones & S. E. Beck (Eds.). *Decision making in nursing* (pp. 3–24). Albany, NY: Delmar.

Jones, R. A. P., & Beck, S. E. (Eds.) (1996). *Decision making in nursing.* Albany, NY: Delmar.

Keenan, M. J., & Hurst, J. B. (1995). Conflict: The cutting edge of change. In P. S. Y. Wise (Ed.). *Leading and managing in nursing* (pp. 338–361). St. Louis: Mosby-Year Book.

Marriner-Tomey, A. (1996). Guide to nursing management and leadership. St. Louis: Mosby-Year Book.

McCloskey, J. C., Bulechek, G. M., Moorhead, S., & Daly, J. (1996). Nurses' use and delegation of indirect care interventions. *Nursing Economics, 14,* 22–33.

McElhaney, R. (1996). Conflict management in nursing administration. *Nursing Management, 27,* 49–50.

Miller, R. (1995). Quality management. In K. W. Vestal (Ed.). *Nursing management: Concepts and issues* (2nd ed., pp. 195–213). Philadelphia: Lippincott.

National Council of State Boards of Nursing. (1987). *Statement of the nursing activities of unlicensed persons. Book of reports* (pp. 221–229). Ninth Annual Convention, August 25–29, 1987.

Parkman, C. A. (1996). Role of the professional nurse: Patient care manager. In C. E. Loveridge & S. H. Cummings (Eds.). *Nursing management in the new paradigm* (pp. 123–175). Gaithersburg, MD: Aspen.

Rodriguez, L. Selecting, developing, empowering, and coaching staff. In P. S. Y. Wise (Ed.). *Leading and managing in nursing* (pp. 300–317). St. Louis: Mosby-Year Book.

Roe, S. (1995). Managing your work setting: Positive work relationships, conflict management, and negotiations. In K. W. Vestal (Ed.). *Nursing management: Concepts and issues* (2nd ed., pp. 147–162). Philadelphia: Lippincott.

Sullivan, E. J., & Decker, P. J. (1992). Effective management in nursing. Redwood City, CA: Addison-Wesley.

Tappen, R. M. (1995). *Nursing leadership and management: Concepts and practice* (3rd ed.). Philadelphia: Davis.

Ulrich, B. T. (1995). Leadership and management. In K. W. Vestal (Ed.). *Nursing management: Concepts and issues* (2nd ed., pp. 67–85). Philadelphia: Lippincott.

Walton, J. C., & Waszkiewicz, M. (1997). Managing unlicensed assistive personnel: Tips for improving quality outcomes. *MEDSURG Nursing, 6,* 24–28.

Warfel, W. M. (1995). Communication in complex organizations. In K. W. Vestal (Ed.). *Nursing management: Concepts and issues* (2nd ed., pp. 49–66). Philadelphia: Lippincott.

Welch, R. A. (1995). Problem solving and decision making. In P. S. Y. Wise (Ed.). *Leading and managing in nursing* (pp. 108–128). St. Louis: Mosby-Year Book.

Wise, P. S. Y. (1995). *Leading and managing in nursing.* St. Louis: Mosby-Year Book.

Wywialowski, E. (1995). Communicating and collaborating. In P. S. Y. Wise (Ed.). *Leading and managing in nursing* (pp. 318–335). St. Louis: Mosby-Year Book.

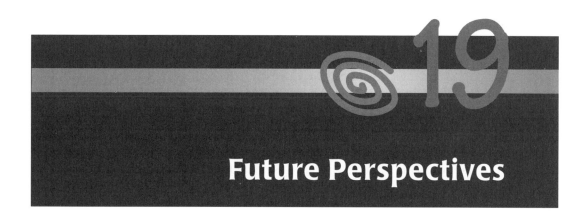

Future Perspectives

LEARNING OUTCOMES

By the end of this chapter, the student will be able to:

1 Identify forces that will affect the direction of change in health and health care delivery between now and the year 2005.

2 Understand the implications of change for nursing practice, education, and scholarship.

Chapter author: Carol R. Sando, R.N., D.NSc.

> Some men see things as they are and say "why?"
> I dream things that never were and say "why not?"
> (John F. Kennedy, as quoted by Robert Kennedy in Schlesinger, 1978)

During the past 15 to 20 years, dramatic societal and professional changes have influenced nursing practice, education, and scholarship. Some of the forces influencing changes have been detailed throughout the preceding chapters. This chapter discusses selected trends to provide a perspective on the implications for the nursing profession at the beginning of the 21st century.

Future Scenarios

Scenarios are forecasts, "a model of an expected or a supposed sequence of events" (Soukhanov, 1992, p. 1612). They raise awareness of the wide range of possible implications of external forces, sensitize people to potential threats and opportunities, and allow examination of alternative options for action. Projecting existing trends, Bezold (1996, pp. 35–39) developed four scenarios that describe radically different potential pictures of the health care delivery system at the start of the 21st century: the business as usual, hard times, buyer's market, and healthy healing communities scenarios.

BUSINESS-AS-USUAL SCENARIO

The business-as-usual scenario assumes continued technological ingenuity, sophisticated communication, and high levels of consumption. Although the majority of Americans are better off, the percentage of poor continues to rise. Health care reform has been left to the states, which in turn leave it to the marketplace. Advances in biomedical knowledge and technology make it possible to forecast, prevent, and manage illnesses earlier and more successfully. High-tech interventions such as performance-enhancing bionic implants and organoids (a new organ or organ part grown outside the body and then implanted) are widely available to those who can pay for them. Hospitals become smaller and their numbers decline, reducing the number of hospital beds by two-thirds in two decades. Health care delivery becomes more efficient, so health care's percentage of the gross national product (GNP) stabilizes at 15%.

In this scenario, which is an extension of the current environment, nursing education could be highly individualized (but also depersonalized) through the use of computers, with little traditional face-to-face instruction. Fewer nurses would be employed primarily in institutional settings, caring for acutely ill and long-term clients. Salaries would be higher, but lack of work satisfaction and low prestige would perpetuate recruitment problems, leading to intensified labor shortages.

HARD TIMES SCENARIO

This scenario assumes that times are tough for the economy as a whole and for health care. Although health care costs have been stabilized at 15% of the GNP, only 80% of the population has health care coverage. As unemployment increases, pressure is placed on the federal government to create universal access to a frugal basic package of care. Health care innovation slows dramatically, as do heroic measures to prolong life. A two-tier health care system emerges for the health haves and have-nots.

Nursing care of acutely ill clients would be important in this scenario, but nurses would be poorly paid and have little prestige. Consequently, the majority of nurses would be from lower socioeconomic groups and from foreign countries. Clients who could pay would be cared for in the home by private-duty nurses. Technology would be limited to reliable established treatments; thus, education would be shorter, more standardized, and more focused on technical interventions and measures designed to increase client comfort.

BUYER'S MARKET SCENARIO

In this scenario, responsibility for health and health care expenditures have been returned to the consumer. Insurance coverage includes a tax to help pay for the cost of care given to the poor. Health care providers are now certified by the state on the basis of knowledge and competence. People have greater freedom from health care providers and have better tools for changing their lifestyles and preventing or managing illnesses. Various types of providers and treatments are often sought by consumers for illness prevention.

This scenario offers real potential for nursing to achieve greater power and influence than it now has. By accessing consumers directly, nurses would have a major role in promoting health. Education would emphasize ways of teaching consumers how to promote individual, family, and community health.

HEALTHY HEALING COMMUNITIES SCENARIO

This scenario involves a focus on "healing the body, mind, and spirit of individuals and communities" (Bezold, 1996, p. 38). Neighbors look out for each other, and people work together to eliminate problems such as drugs, teenage pregnancy, and the effects of poverty. However, as information makes workers more productive—or replaces workers altogether—unemployment grows to 25%. Health care organizations help to make communities environmentally and financially sustainable, with the help of unpaid volunteers. Older persons have rewarding ways to contribute to the community, reducing disability and the time in long-term institutions. Advanced technologies have led to a comfortable life for most people, and bionics, robotics, smarter homes, and more caring neighborhoods allow disabled elderly to remain in their homes. Consumers are involved in decision-making regarding their health. The emphasis is on wellness and development of full human potential, with rejection of anonymity, artificiality, manipulation, and unnecessary size or complexity.

Nurses would be full partners with consumers in this scenario, helping people with self-care and providing information to support fully informed decision-making. Older persons would be valued and would be cared for at home. Various information sources to support health would be available at home through computer networks. Nurses would be highly educated professionals, whose contribution would be valued for its effectiveness.

IMPLICATIONS FOR NURSING

Through advocacy of the principles in its Agenda for Health Care Reform (American Nurses Association [ANA], 1991), nursing has the opportunity to help to shape its future. "Nursing offers just what the American health consumer hopes for" (Porter-O'Grady, 1994, p. 38). If nurses communicate effectively as a cohesive group with consumers, legislators, and other policymakers to influence decisions affecting health care delivery, the result will be enhanced opportunities for authority, regardless of which scenario dominates the delivery system. Otherwise, the agendas of others will take precedence, and professional nursing and nurses will be at risk.

Hadley (1996, p. 6) describes five challenges that nursing faces:

- Demonstrating that nurses provide cost-effective, high-quality care that can be measured
- Adopting uniform licensure and educational requirements for the profession and establishing simpler, fewer titles
- Overcoming the mentality of an oppressed minority
- Accepting job insecurity
- Sustaining a commitment to lifelong professional learning

◎ Changes in Health Care and Health Care Delivery

Demonstrable shifts are occurring in the causes of mortality from infectious diseases and chronic diseases and diseases associated with life stress. For example, acquired immunodeficiency syndrome (AIDS) and related illnesses are a major cause of death. Influenza and pneumonia are still the sixth highest cause of death in children aged 1 to 14 years, but the leading cause of death in childhood—unintentional injuries—is preventable. Homicide and suicide are major causes of death in adolescents and young adults (aged 15–24). Coronary heart disease, cancer "and the other top causes of death between the ages of 25 and 65—unintentional injuries, stroke, and chronic liver disease and cirrhosis—have all been associated with risk factors related to lifestyle" (U.S. Department of Health and Human Services, 1990, p. 19). Infant deaths are closely related to maternal smoking, alcohol, drug use, and poor nutrition.

Every indication is that these trends will continue, if not accelerate, concomitant with an ever-increasing life span and the rapid pace and increasingly technological emphasis of modern life. These kinds of health problems are especially suited to nursing expertise in care. There has also been a demonstrable increase in people's interest in assuming responsibility for self-care and in activities such as diet, exercise, and stress reduction that are critical to health promotion. This trend offers great potential for nursing to assume leadership in helping people experience well-being and prevent illness.

In the past, hospitalization was often prescribed because nursing care was needed. Until fairly recently, common reasons for hospitalization included diagnostic laboratory testing, routine care, or rehabilitation, in addition to treatment of illness. Increasingly, however, the high cost and highly specialized medical technology associated with hospitalization have led to the use of hospitals primarily for diagnosis and attempted cure of serious acute illnesses and acute treatment of chronic disease.

Minor illness and illness prevention are increasingly provided through separately contracted ambulatory care in clinics, doctors' offices, and people's homes. There is an opportunity for nursing to exert a much-needed influence in long-term institutions, nursing homes, and home settings.

Central to the current organization of the health care delivery system is the concept that the client contracts with the physician for care, while nursing is supplied by the hospital as part of a package of services. The system is still structured for the facilitation of medical cure or stabilization. In the future, the system could move toward either increased centralization or increased decentralization of services. The decentralized model, comprising a number of laterally linked components separate from the hospital, could facilitate entrepreneurial nursing delivery systems, for example, independent nursing practices and partnerships between nurses and various other health care professionals.

Some systems are building point-of-service networks to broaden consumer choice and embracing 'disintegration' (Goldsmith & Goran, 1996). With direct third-party reimbursement from private or federal insurers, nurses could contract directly with clients for the provision of nursing services. Through contractual agreements, nurses could provide essential professional services as autonomous providers rather than as employees.

However, given the power, influence, and control of the medical–hospital industry, it is unlikely that the health care delivery system will be completely restructured in the near future. Some hospitals have moved toward centralization of services in care centers that include ambulatory services as well as inpatient care. This model accentuates the current status of most nurses as employees and further consolidates the financial control of "health care" by hospitals and physicians. The challenge for nursing would be to gain autonomy within the system. For this, nurses would need equality with other health professionals, which can be accomplished only through comparable educational qualifications and an equivalent allocation of authority.

The movement toward prospective payment is bound to become the standard for third-party reimbursement by private and public agencies, for physicians and other professionals, and for hospitals and other care institutions. Nursing must actively promote the cost benefits and care outcomes of educated, highly skilled professionals in the system, or the trend toward replacement of RNs by less highly salaried, less qualified, and unlicensed workers will be accelerated.

It is critical that the nursing profession emphasize the cost effectiveness of competent care and assume initiative in documenting the unique contribution of nursing to the restoration of well-being and prevention of illness in clients. Nursing's "ability to articulate specific and refined costs of nursing activity and compare them to achieved outcomes will have a direct relationship to the ability of nurses to render measurable, achievable, and cost-effective care" (Porter-O'Grady, 1986, p. 205). One positive aspect of prospective payment is the potential of clear labeling of the distinct contribution made by nursing to restoration of well-being, which promotes the valuing of nursing services by the public.

Porter-O'Grady (1986) has suggested that nursing will shift away from dependent, illness-fixed, delegated, and narrowly defined roles that include institutionally defined and prescribed care and safety responsibilities in direct-care, physician-dominated, interruptive functions. New roles will be interdependent and health based, with flexible applications. The nurses' accountability for health prescription will be determined by the client or the community, supported by new teletechnology such as home health monitors and personalized computer cards (Millett & Kopp, 1996). Functions will be multidisciplinary, aimed toward prevention or correction, and defined by standards (Fig. 19-1).

These shifts in roles, responsibilities, and functions are possible if nurse leaders (1) are aware of changes in the delivery system; (2) interpret and share changes with peers; and (3) provide support, information, and direction for desirable action. However, of major concern is the fact that "many RNs lack the education to work autonomously outside the hospital and institutional settings" (Hadley, 1996, p. 9).

◎ Changes in Nursing Education

The knowledge base and technology used in providing nursing care will continue to increase, as will nurses' need for skill and ability in:

- Intensely acute aspects of care
- Diagnostics and decision-making
- Client teaching

```
┌─────────────────────────────────────────────────────────────────┐
│                                                                   │
│                 Nursing Professional Transition                   │
│                                                                   │
│            Current                        Next Century            │
│                                                                   │
│         Role                           Role                       │
│            Dependent                      Interdependent          │
│            Illness fixed                  Health based            │
│            Delegated                      Assumed (a priori)      │
│            Narrowly defined               Flexible application    │
│                                                                   │
│                                                                   │
│         Responsibility                 Accountability             │
│            Care and safety                Health prescription     │
│            Institutionally defined        Community defined       │
│            Prescribed                     Self–client determined  │
│                                                                   │
│                                                                   │
│         Function                       Function                   │
│            Direct care                    Policy, legislation,    │
│                                              direct care          │
│            Physician dominated            Team interactive        │
│                                              (multidisciplinary)  │
│            Interruptive                    Preventive, maintenance,│
│                                              and corrective       │
│            Policy based                   Standards defined       │
│                                                                   │
│                          Future Direction                         │
│                                                                   │
└─────────────────────────────────────────────────────────────────┘
```

FIGURE 19-1. Role transition into the 21st century. From Porter-O'Grady, T. (1986). *Creative nursing administration: Participative management into the 21st century* (p. 204). With permission of Aspen Publishers.

- Coordination of and delegation to less-skilled workers
- Collaboration with clients and health care professionals to improve the quality of health

In the future, more than ever, nurses will need a broad-based education, assertiveness skills, technical competence, and the ability to deal with rapid change.

Since the 1960s, there has been an intensive national effort to promote the baccalaureate degree as the entry level for professional nursing. In that time, although there has been an increase in the number of nurses prepared at the baccalaureate level, there has also been a dramatic increase in the percentage of nurses prepared at the associate degree level. More than 70% of nurses are still being prepared at the technical level of nursing. Further, previously educated nurses account for more than a third of baccalaureate enrollments.

Entry to nursing could conceivably occur at one of four levels: the associate degree, the baccalaureate degree, the master's degree, or the doctoral degree. Thus, there are at least four different patterns of education for nursing that might predominate in the future.

The current pattern—entry at the associate level, with professional education at the baccalaureate degree level—might be perpetuated. Nursing is a profession that has been closely associated with upward mobility, especially for women. Most associate degree programs are located in community colleges and, thus, are financially and geographically accessible. Demand can readily be met by an increased supply of licensed workers in a short time.

Before their baccalaureate studies, many RN students perceive nursing education at the baccalaureate level as additional and partially redundant rather than as different and enriching. Little incentive for professional education is provided by the delivery system, which lacks differential salary structures or clearly articulated differences in job expectations. Licensure as an RN after associate degree education has reinforced this model.

Some propose that education for entry to professional nursing be moved to the master's level rather than the baccalaureate level. This level of education would prepare the student for a combination of specialized and generalized practice appropriate for the developing delivery system. All students would need prior general education and possibly a bachelor's degree for entry into nursing, which would strengthen the liberal arts and science base for practice, prepare an educated person, encourage recruitment of students from other fields, and raise the status and authority of the profession. This model for nursing education would probably include the associate degree or baccalaureate degree for nursing assistants and the master's degree for licensed professional nurses.

There are currently three doctoral programs leading to a Doctor of Nursing (ND) as the first professional degree. Aydelotte (1992, p. 470) summarizes the possible problems of this type of program as follows:

- Goals of the program are not understood
- The differences between the ND and other doctoral programs in nursing, such as the PhD or DNSc, are not perceived
- Employers expect the ND graduate, as an entry level practitioner, to perform in traditional nursing roles
- The "nursing and health communities" are hesitant "to accept general professional nursing knowledge as meriting a practice doctorate"

The purpose of the ND degree program is to prepare a generalist in professional nursing. The student enters the program as a nonnursing college graduate. Following the program, the ND graduate would continue into a master's degree program as preparation for specialized practice and into a PhD or DNSc program as preparation for research and advanced role specialization.

Arguments for a nursing doctorate as the degree for entry into professional nursing practice include the following (Aydelotte, 1992, pp. 447–478):

1. The content for professional nursing practice and socialization for the role merit doctoral preparation
2. An entry nursing doctorate would clearly differentiate between technical and professional programs and roles

3. Educational preparation for nursing would be on an educational level with other health professionals (eg, medicine, pharmacy, clinical psychology). Credentials are important to status and influence
4. Reorganization of health care systems will require mature, articulate professionals "who command attention because of their knowledge base and skill"

However, considering the continued resistance to any upgrading of the current educational preparation for licensure, it is unlikely that either the entry master's or the entry doctorate model will achieve widespread acceptance in the foreseeable future.

A fourth possibility is that the baccalaureate degree will finally become the entry level credential for professional practice and be recognized as such with the appropriate licensure, as is the case currently in South Dakota. Most major nursing organizations, including the ANA and the National League for Nursing (NLN), have now endorsed this goal. An increasing number of nurses are seeking baccalaureate education and the credentials to practice at the professional level.

The nursing profession needs to better articulate and publicize (both internally and to the general public) the contributions of professionally educated practitioners to health promotion and restoration and illness prevention. This book has identified the knowledge base and values that characterize the professional nurse, in the hope that this will be the first step toward acceptance of scholarship and demonstration of professional competence in practice. If the baccalaureate or a higher degree does become the entry level for professional practice, the associate degree will probably become the accepted credential for nursing assistants.

Regardless of which model is accepted, all educational programs must continue to modify their curricula to include changes in the theoretical and technical data base for nursing. For example, computer technology is making an enormous impact on discovery, communication, and storage of information. Yet relatively few nurses are computer literate, and not all schools include computer courses in their curricula. Further, little attention has yet been paid to the moral implications of a computerized society that engenders feelings of isolation associated with nonpersonal communication and invasion of privacy.

In recent years, there has been criticism of the basic model for nursing education. With its emphasis on behavioral objectives, "education is directed toward the preparation for a 'job' rather than for life as a professional" (Aydelotte, 1990, p. 469). Critics encourage:

1. Emphasis on intellectual skills rather than on mechanistic and technical abilities
2. A learning environment that incorporates caring, compassion, and values
3. Attention to pattern recognition and the role of intuition in addition to "rules"

4. Active involvement in learning rather than passive transmission of knowledge
5. More attention to professional socialization and ethics
6. Content relevant to emerging needs and the redesign of the delivery system
7. Concern with process, not just with content

All nurses need to be familiar with such areas as "health care economics, management of human resources, community needs assessment, peer governance, health care agencies, systems management, cost control, cost-effectiveness, strategies, and cost accounting" (Porter-O'Grady, 1986, p. 216), as well as with policy information and areas of developing knowledge. The continuing development and testing of the theory will lead to knowledge that must be integrated into educational curricula.

Nursing Scholarship

Rapid development in nursing theory and research over the past 20 to 25 years points to a promising outlook for the future. Most needed is the explication of theory that is predictive of nursing outcomes. Increasingly, models and theories for nursing care are being validated by research and used in practice as bases for care. If this trend continues, then the promise for the future of professional nursing as described in this book will have become a reality.

Conclusion

The end of the 20th century and the beginning of the 21st century will be characterized by tremendous changes in health and the health care delivery system. These changes will provide threats and opportunities for nurses to finally be recognized as informed professional partners in the provision of care to meet society's evolving health needs.

THOUGHT QUESTIONS

1 How do you think the health care delivery system will look 10 years from now? How might projected changes in health care delivery affect nursing care?

2 What do you expect to be the educational entry level for professional nursing in the future? What are the implications for the nursing profession?

3 What do you consider to be the most important areas for knowledge development in nursing? What is the current state of the art in those areas?

REFERENCES

American Nurses Association. (1991, June). Nursing's agenda for health reform. Kansas City: Author.

Aydelotte, M. K. (1992). Nursing education: Shaping the future. In L. Aiken & C. Fagin (Eds.). *Charting nursing's future: Agenda for the 1990s* (pp. 462–484). Philadelphia: Lippincott.

Bezold, C. (1996). Your health in 2010: Four scenarios. *The Futurist, 30,* 35–39.

Goldsmith, J. C., & Goran, M. J. (1996). Managed care mythology: Supply side dreams die hard. *Healthcare Forum Journal, 39,* 42–47.

Hadley, E. H. (1996). Nursing in the political and economic marketplace: Challenges for the 21st century. *Nursing Outlook 44,* 6–10.

Millett, S., & Kopp, W. (1996). The top 10 innovative products for 2006: Technology with a human touch. *The Futurist, 30,* 16–20.

Porter-O'Grady, T. (1986). *Creative nursing administration: Participative management into the 21st century.* Rockville, MD: Aspen.

Porter-O'Grady, T. (1994). Building partnerships in health care: Creating whole systems change. *Nursing and Health Care, 15,* 34—38.

Schlesinger, A. M. (1978). *Robert Kennedy and his times.* New York: Houghton Mifflin.

Soukhanov, A. H. (Ed.). (1992). *The American heritage dictionary of the English language* (3rd ed.). Boston: Houghton Mifflin.

U.S. Department of Health and Human Services. (1990). *Healthy People 2000.* (Public Health Service Publicaiton No. 91-50213). Washington, DC: U.S. Government Printing Office.

Index

Page numbers followed by f *indicate figures. Those followed by* t *indicate tables.*